Nutrient Availability:
Chemical and Biological Aspects

Special Publication No. 72

Nutrient Availability:
Chemical and Biological Aspects

Edited by
D. A. T. Southgate, I. T. Johnson, and G. R. Fenwick
AFRC Institute of Food Research, Norwich

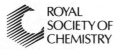

ROYAL
SOCIETY OF
CHEMISTRY

Federation of European Chemical Society Event 128

The Proceedings of Bioavailability 88: Chemical and Biological Aspects of Nutrient Availability organised by The Food Chemistry Group of the Royal Society of Chemistry, The Working Party on Food Chemistry of the Federation of European Chemical Societies, and The Federation of European Nutrition Societies, held 21–24 August 1988 in Norwich, England.

British Library Cataloguing in Publication Data

Bioavailability 88–Chemical and Biological Aspects of Nutrient Availability
  Nutrient availability.
  1. Man. Nutrition. Biochemical aspects
  I. Title   II. Series
  612'.3

  ISBN 0–85186–856–8

Published by the Royal Society of Chemistry, Thomas Graham House, Cambridge, CB4 4WF

Printed in Great Britain by Henry Ling Ltd., at the Dorset Press, Dorchester, Dorset

Preface

Bioavailability '88 was the title of a multi-disciplinary conference
organised by the AFRC Institute of Food Research and held at the
University of East Anglia in Norwich, England, from August 21-24 1988.
Until relatively recently it has been a common assumption that the
nutritional value of foods and diets was more or less synonymous with
their nutritional composition as determined by chemical analysis.
The limitations of this simple picture first became obvious in
relation to trace element nutrition, but recently many lines of
research have emphasised the need to understand and quantify the
intestinal absorption and subsequent metabolism of all the major
nutrient classes.   The purpose of the conference was to emphasise
the value of nutrient bioavailability as a unifying concept, and to
draw together the many threads from chemistry, physics and the
biological sciences which are essential to its proper understanding.

Bioavailability '88 was held under the auspices of the Food Chemistry
Group of the RSC, the Working Party on Food Chemistry of the
Federation of European Chemical Societies, and the Federation of
European Nutrition Societies.   Despite this strong European base,
the conference was truly international in spirit, and succeeded in
bringing together nearly 300 scientists from almost fifty countries.
This volume contains the proceedings of the programme, which
consisted of invited plenary lectures, short oral presentations and
posters, and workshop meetings with written reports which were made
available to the whole conference for discussion at the closing
session.   No distinction between posters and oral contributions
has been made in preparing this volume.   The short papers from both
types of presentation are arranged in chapters which in most cases
are introduced by the appropriate plenary lecture.   The final
chapter consists of edited versions of the workshop reports;   it is
hoped that these give an accurate "snapshot" of the current state
of this particular art.

The editors are very grateful to all those who contributed to the
success of Bioavailability '88, and particularly to the sponsors,
who are listed separately.   Many members of the Institute's staff
and their relatives and friends deserve special thanks for giving
up their spare time to assist with the conference in ways too
numerous to mention.   Finally we would like to thank all the authors
who have made this volume possible, especially the great majority who
conscientiously observed the editors' requests for short and accurate
typescripts.

I T Johnson
G R Fenwick
D A T Southgate

March 1989

The following are thanked for their generous
sponsorship of Bioavailability 88: -

Beecham Products

British Sugar plc

Finnigan MAT Ltd

General Foods Ltd

Gist-Brocades N.V.

Jacobs Suchard

Kellogg Company of Great Britain, Ltd

Metal Box plc

McCain Foods (GB) Ltd

Nestle S.A.

Rowntree Mackintosh Confectionery Ltd

J. Sainsbury plc

Unilever Research (Research and Engineering Division)
Appeals Committee

The Royal Society of Chemistry

The Royal Society of Chemistry - Food Chemistry Group

Foreword

Professor P. Richmond, Chairman, Food Chemistry Group,
Royal Society of Chemistry.

Lifestyles everywhere have been shaped over many
hundreds of years by advances in food preparation.
Underdeveloped nations continue to have problems of
supply; affluent nations have quite different problems
that arise from economic prosperity. Science and
Technology continue to offer new benefits that, adopted
wisely, can further improve human well-being throughout
the world.

But, how do we "adopt wisely"? What constitutes an
adequate diet? Nutritional science and physiology lie
at the heart of these questions and over the years
there has been much progress in our understanding.
However, it is clear that there is much more to do.

For example, current prescriptions for RDAs are gross
assessments; but populations, groups, and individuals
are all known to differ in their requirements for the
many components that make a sensible diet. In recent
years, there has been a revolution in our ability to
make quantitative physical measurements of food
components taken up by the body, using methods such as
NMR and mass-spectrometry. This conference, organised
by the Federation of European Chemical Societies,
Working Party on Food Chemistry (FECS event No. 128),
Federation of European Nutrition Societies, Royal
Society of Chemistry and the Society's Food Chemistry
Group and first mooted in 1986 by Professor Czedik and
Professor Hautvast, was designed to bring together for
the first time physical and nutritional scientists, to
stimulate discussion and increase professional
interaction between these diverse groups. The fact that
280 scientists from 44 countries chose to attend

Bioavailability '88 testifies to the interest and
activity in the subject.

It is appropriate here, to acknowledge the hard work of
the Scientific Committee, the help from the Organising
Committee and the many unsung heroes from the Institute
of Food Research, Norwich Laboratory, who made the
meeting at the University of East Anglia run so
smoothly.

The intense discussion at the meeting suggests that the
next few years will see yet more pertinent advances in
our understanding which will be to the benefit of
mankind everywhere. Another meeting, in the not so
distant future, seems certain to be even more
successful.

Contents

Part 4   The Importance of Speciation

**Part 5   The Bioavailability of the Trace Minerals
Iron and Zinc**

xiii

Part 6   The Bioavailability of Other Minerals and Toxic Metals

Part 8 The Workshop Reports

The Concept and Significance of Nutrient Bioavailability

NUTRITIONAL SIGNIFICANCE OF BIOAVAILABILITY

A. E. Bender,

2, Willow Vale, Fetcham, Leatherhead, Surrey KT22 9TE

1   INTRODUCTION

Probably the most important and at the same time the most difficult task of the nutritionist is to assess the nutritional status of an individual.   We know when people are severely malnourished because they exhibit characteristic signs but in the western world we do not meet such cases.   We know what the average individual should ingest to ensure an adequate intake but RDA's apply to population groups and have extremely limited relevance to individuals.   Since RDA is 20% greater than average needs presumably the individual ingesting less than 60% of RDA is at nutritional risk.

We want to know whether an individual is obtaining less than his optimal requirements.   Our usual criteria for assessing nutritional status are clinical examination and biochemical measures, supported by dietary intake – which should be verified by a change (improvement) on giving the indicated supplement.   Any improvement that we might expect to observe is difficult to measure and probably impossible to distinguish from a placebo effect.   Such a battery of tests is very rarely undertaken and we rely heavily on dietary intake – which is known to be subject to a host of inaccuracies.

Food consumption can most accurately be assessed from a 7–day weighed intake repeated four times during the seasons.   However we then proceed to sacrifice accuracy by resorting to food composition tables to calculate nutrient intake and rarely carry out direct analyses of the foods.

Errors in estimating the macronutrients in this way are estimated at about 10%.   A comparison of 300 calculated and analysed values showed that for 50% of the foods reported, energy and protein agreed within 10%;   for fats only 25% of the values agreed within 10%[1].   Errors for micronutrients are so large that we would often be more realistic to ignore micronutrient "intakes".

3

2   ANALYTICAL PROBLEMS

Even if we had the facilities to analyse the food consumed we have
many problems.   Perhaps the most surprising to the non-specialist
is that we do not have satisfactory methods for more than four of
the thirteen vitamins.   A review of methods that can be recommended
because they have been used successfully in the hands of experienced
experts reported that such validated methods are available only for
beta-carotene, thiamin and vitamins A, C and E.   Only tentative
methods are available for riboflavin, pyridoxine and vitamin D –
these have been tested with only a few food items or are not
sufficiently sensitive to cover the whole range.   For folic acid
and niacin only references are given "since it was felt that the
time was not yet ripe to include detailed descriptions of a method"[2].
For the remaining four vitamins, B12, K, biotin and pantothenate,
neither methods nor references are given.

The next problem is the existence of vitamers – the authors
include eight vitamers of vitamin A commonly found in foods, five
of thiamin and nine of vitamin E.   The analyst is faced with the
possibilities (1) of using a method that will measure all the
vitamers, irrespective of their relative biological potency;   (2) of
measuring the vitamer that is quantitatively or biologically most
important;   (3) of converting, where possible, the vitamers into one
form before the determination.

It is not practical, except in a research project, to determine
each vitamer and even then there is the problem of the different
potencies which might not always be known.

Chemical versus Biological Determination of Vitamins.

We use two types of methods, chemical/physical which depend on
the properties of a specific chemical grouping or a biological assay
of total vitamin potency.   Chemical/physical methods have the
advantages of high reproducibility and speed and low cost, and some
are sufficiently specific to be carried out on crude extracts.
However, they measure only the specific chemical grouping and are
subject to interference which can give erroneously high or low
results.

The true measure of vitamin activity is the biological assay of
the characteristic function.   This, of course, was the means whereby
the vitamins were originally recognised and then measured by
comparison with the standard.   Unfortunately bioassays are not only
lengthy but subject to enormous biological variation.

Biological methods had to be used to validate the rapid chemical/
physical methods.   Microbiological assay also measures total vitamin
potency but only for the particular micro-organism, and also has to
be validated by animal bioassay.   All this ignores any differences
between test animals and man but it is the best that we can do.
Presumably if a "new" food were developed and thought likely to

replace a traditional food to a significant extent, the nutrients would have to be assayed biologically both on test animals and on man, then the usual chemical/physical methods validated before we could routinely apply them to the new food.

So far we have discussed what might be described as the routine problems of the analyst in the laboratory, and the method of choice, correction factors and acceptance of limitations depend on the purpose of the analysis – to analyse foodstuffs, to determine nutrient intake in nutrition surveys, to follow changes on storage, processing and cooking, to select new strains of plants and better methods of animal husbandry, or for legal purposes. For nutritional purposes we add the problems of bioavailability.

Obviously it is not enough to know how much of a nutrient is present in the food, or even its total biological potential but we need to know how much of that potential can be realised when the food is eaten.

3   BIOAVAILABILITY

Definition

Bioavailability has been defined as the proportion of the nutrient[3] that is digested, absorbed and metabolised through normal pathways.

It is not clear why both terms, digestion and absorption are included. If the nutrient is present in an absorbable form it does not need digesting; materials that are hydrolysed in the intestine are not necessarily absorbed.

As regards the term metabolised there are substances that are absorbed but cannot be metabolised and are subsequently excreted so the definition should include absorbable and metabolisable. If an individual is unable to metabolise the nutrient for genetic reasons or because of a disorder or interference by drugs this is an individual physiological effect and not a property of the food. Consequently I would suggest that the definition should read "the proportion of a nutrient capable of being absorbed and available for use or storage"; more briefly "the proportion of a nutrient that can be utilised".

Parallels with Drugs

Some parallels may be drawn with drugs. The bioavailability of a drug is defined as the amount of the substance that reaches the circulation intact and the rate at which this occurs. The rate depends on particle size, the chemical form of the drug and the absorption (if taken orally). The extent of bioavailability depends

on the absorption and the extent of metabolism before it reaches the
target organs.   The latter can be affected by malnutrition, gastrointestinal disease and the presence of inhibiting substances including
dietary fibre.   In addition first pass metabolism in, for example,
the intestinal mucosa or liver can take place before the drug enters
the systemic circulation and may result in compounds of enhanced or
decreased activity.

In addition there are limitations imposed by plasma protein
binding, blood flow to organs, passage through membrane barriers and
absorption into adipose tissue which affects the rate and amount
distributed through the body.

To what extent do these limitations apply to nutrients?   We
tend to assume that our physiology is optimal for available nutrients,
meaning that we can make maximum use of nutrients so long as they
reach the bloodstream but is this necessarily so?   Drugs are foreign
substances that are tailor-made to have their maximal effect but can
the nutrients all survive the physiological hazards?   A surprise
discovery early in the life of vitamin A was that higher results were
obtained in bioassay if vitamin E were included with the vitamin A;
it served as an antioxidant but it was surprising that a vitamin could
suffer oxidation inside the body (if the intestine is so considered)
after it had been consumed.   It is difficult enough to ascertain the
stability of nutrients before they are consumed let alone afterwards.

In theory at least we require a constant flow of nutrients to
the tissues but, quite apart from "night starvation" we know that
adequate or even optimal health can be maintained with an erratic
flow of nutrients, e.g. one adequate meal per day.   In this way
nutrition appears to differ from drug pharmacology.

Many nutrients are transported in the bloodstream in a bound form
and we know, for example, that retinol deficiency can arise despite
a plentiful supply of retinol (or carotene) when protein deficiency
limits the production of retinol-binding protein or the carotene-
converting enzyme, carotenoid dioxygenase.   Are there any problems
associated with the release of nutrients bound in the plasma?   Can
nutrients be "lost" in the adipose tissue?   Can losses take place
through oxidation, reduction, hydrolysis before the nutrients perform
their function?   Can this explain the enormous variations found in
bioassays?

Proteins

So far it might appear that problems of measuring bioavailability
apply particularly to the vitamins but the problem with proteins has
been appreciated for many years although the term protein quality is
generally used rather than bioavailability.

The quality of a protein depends largely on its amino acids and their availability to the tissues. Chemical analysis is preceded by acid hydrolysis which liberates amino acids that may not be liberated during intestinal digestion, and from complexes that are not usable in the body. Chemical analysis may also yield erroneous results if some amino acids liberated early in the hydrolysis are damaged subsequently. For these reasons enormous efforts have been devoted over the last eighty years to methods of measuring protein quality, and particularly to abbreviated methods to provide an index of quality; methods depending on enzymic liberation of amino acids in vitro are still being developed.

The conversion of amino acids to D-forms on heating will considerably alter bioavailability since, while these can be deleterious, they are sometimes beneficial[4].

There is another problem regarding availability of protein because the body is unable to store amino acids for more than a very limited period (apart from the amino acid pool) and has a limited capacity for protein synthesis. So if the definition of bioavailability includes utilisation this means that above a certain intake of protein there is an absolute limit to its "bioavailability" since the amino acids in excess of immediate use are wasted by oxidation to provide energy. In other words the "bioavailability" of proteins would be greater when ingested as three small meals than as one large equivalent meal.

Starch

Starch might appear to be straightforward but many factors influence its digestibility, namely particle size, nature of the starch (amylose and amylopectin content, degree of gelatinisation, processing) interaction with fats and proteins, dietary fibre, phytate, anti-nutrients (lectins, tannins, saponins and enzyme inhibitors) - supported by physiological evidence[5].

Mineral salts

Minerals present severe and well-recognised problems since the amount absorbed depends not only on the chemical form of the mineral in the food but on other ingredients in that food and of the rest of the diet and also on physiological factors.

Furthermore it appears that the body can adapt to the inhibitory effects of dietary fibre and phytate on mineral availability and perhaps to the inhibitory effects of other factors as well.

Further complications arise from the observation that fibre affects various minerals such as calcium, magnesium, phosphate, zinc and iron differently so making it difficult, if at all possible, to ascertain the effects on the ingredients of a mixed meal.

The problems of minerals are multiplied by their own interactions. For example, the absorption of copper is depressed by a large excess of zinc, iron and calcium. A summary of data[6] shows that as zinc intake is increased from 5 to 20 mg per day the requirement for copper is increased by 75%. However, it is difficult to draw conclusions or make generalisations at present since reports are inconsistent.

More Problems

Some further examples from vitamin A exemplify the complexity of the problems. The bioavailability of carotene has long presented a problem and different conversion factors have been used to determine retinol equivalent. More recently it has been shown (in rats and chicks) that the conversion factor diminishes as the intake of beta-carotene increases[7]. It is suggested that the FAO/WHO figure of 6 μg beta-carotene for 1 μg retinol should apply only to intakes between 1500 and 400 μg, and that it should be lower for intakes below 1500 μg and higher for intakes greater than 4000 μg.

These authors point out that the types of trials carried out in earlier years to determine conversion rates made use of vitamin A-deficient subjects which is no longer possible for ethical reasons so that we are now dependent on extrapolation from animal experiments.

Another problem thrown up by retinol availability is the lower efficiency of conversion of carotene to retinol in women, which leads to lower blood levels of retinol.

Conclusions

The problems listed are so numerous as to appear almost insurmountable. Rao, for example,[9] lists the factors that influence fluoride availability as: - (1) nature of the food and beverage, (2) concentration and chemical form, (3) the presence of other elements and constituents, e.g. Al, Ca, Mg and chloride which reduce uptake and P and sulphate which increase uptake, (4) previous and concurrent exposure to F from other sources and (5) physiological state of the individual (including age, acid-base balance status and urine pH). On the other hand the very fact that these factors are now known makes it possible to derive some principles. Indeed the author refers to a suggested nomogram[10] "that permits estimation of the permissible intake of food depending on the desired or planned F supply".

Research on the absorption of iron from which the pool concept was developed led to the recognition that increased iron absorption can be achieved not only by increasing the amount of iron in the diet but by altering the proportions of various inhibitory and enhancing factors. So it is likely that principles will come to light that will enable us to apply similar solutions to our problems.

It will, of course, complicate matters if these substances have a different effect on other nutrients.

REFERENCES

1. Whiting, M.C. and Leverton, R.M. (1960) Amer. J. Publ. Hlth. 50. 815–832.
2. Brubacher, G.B., Muller-Mulot, W. and Southgate, D.A.T. (1985) Methods for the Determination of Vitamins in Food. Elsevier. Applied Science Publishers.
3. Fairweather-Tait, S.J. (1987) Nutr. Res. 7. 319–325.
4. Man, E.H. and Bada, J.L. (1987) Ann. Rev. Nutr. 7. 209–225.
5. Jenkins, D.J.A., Jenkins, A.L., Wolever, T.M.S., Thompson, L.H. and Venkat Rao, A. (1986) Nutr. Rev. 44. 44.
6. Stanstead, H.H. (1982) Amer. J. Clin. Nutr. 35. 809–814.
7. Brubacher, G.B. and Weiser, H. (1985). Internat. J. Vit. Nutr. Res. 55. 5–15.
8. Mauron, J. (1977) in Physical, Chemical and Biological changes in Food caused by Thermal Processing. Ed. Hoyem, F and Kvale,O. p.330.
9. Rao, G.S. (1984) Ann. Rev. Nutr. 4. 115–136.
10. Siebert, G. and Trautner, K. (1983) Caries Res. 17. 171.

CONCEPTUAL ISSUES CONCERNING THE ASSESSMENT OF NUTRIENT BIOAVAILABILITY.

D.A.T. Southgate

AFRC Institute of Food Research
Norwich Laboratory
Colney Lane
Norwich NR4 7UA

Recognition that the ingested nutrients in the diet could not be completely used occurred early in the emergence of the nutritional sciences. For example Atwater[1] used the concept of availability in connection with the energy value of the diet and later in their classical review of the carbohydrates in foods, McCance and Lawrence[2] developed the concept of "available carbohydrate" for those carbohydrates that when digested and absorbed provided the body with carbohydrate.

Since then there has been an increasing volume of evidence, that with very few exceptions[3], only a proportion of the total ingested nutrients in a diet or food is capable of being used - or 'available' and the term 'availability' has come into use for the proportion of the intake that is available. Particular interest has focussed on the availability of inorganic constituents, especially the trace elements but availability concerns all aspects of quantitative nutritional study.

The prefix 'Bio' denotes that a biological attribute is being discussed and not availability in the market place or food supply. In this paper I will use availability as being synonymous with 'bioavailability', and I will argue that because availability is of such importance to quantitative nutrition we need to define it in a formal way. Starting from a formal definition of the term I propose to explore the implications of the definition for the experimental study of availability.

In order for a nutrient to be capable of being used - or available it must either be present in the diet in a form that can be transported across the mucosa, or the

10

ingested forms must be capable of being transformed into transportable forms (digestion in a strict sense) and the nutrient must be absorbed in a form that can be utilised in normal metabolism[4]. Absorption is not synonymous with availability because some well absorbed constituents, for example, xylose and some iron chelates, are well absorbed and do not contribute to metabolism or nutritional status.

This definition has two important corollaries. First, availability is not a property of the diet or food per se but the response of the individual to the diet or food[5].

Second, observed availability, therefore represents an integration of the various components of the processes whereby an ingested nutrient becomes available - the determinants of availability. It is therefore possible to formalise an intuitive equation that defines availability in terms of these determinants; the proportion that can be converted to absorbable species (D), the integrated ratio of enhancers to inhibition (Σ E/I), the proportion transported (T) and the proportion of the transported nutrient utilised (U).

Thus Availability = fD.Σ E/I .T.U.
At the present time it is not possible to define this function; for a few nutrients many of the terms are unity eg Na and for many nutrients the proportions utilised are identical with the proportions transported. In addition for some nutrients the proportion transported is a function of the nutritional status of the individual consuming the diet - introducing another term into the equation.

This analysis has further implications for the experimental study of availability. Speciation in the food or diet is important only as a determinant of whether an ingested nutrient is capable of being converted into an absorbable species. The crucial stage where speciation is important is in the intestinal contents and at the mucosal surface. In vitro studies of simulated digestion provide a method for the study of the term, D - although with real foods the interactions between the nutrient and enhancers and inhibitors can rarely be separated. Such studies depend on a knowledge of, or an intuitive judgement about, the nature of the absorbed species. They are limited by the lack of a transporting system removing absorbable species and altering the equilibria set-up in in vitro studies.

Studies with physiological preparations incorporate the transport component and permit the evaluation of direct interactions between diet and the transport system which is very important where competition for transport sites occurs.

In the formal analysis, however, an *in vivo* biological assessment provides the only true measure of availability, but the range of measurements and techniques available and widely used often only measure approximations of availability.

The formal definition indicates that availability can be measured by changes in functional status, which provides an unequivocal indicator of utilisation. For this approach to be successful good indicators of functional status are required and where these are available the rate of change of functional status with intake is a function of availability.

This is a primary reason why the study of availability is a key to quantitative nutritional studies. Because, if one accepts that the nutritional sciences are concerned with evaluating the response of the organism to food and nutrients[6] - the function that related to response to intake has availability as a determinant of the slope of the relationship.

REFERENCES

1.   W.O. Atwater, On the digestibility and availability of food materials. Conn (Storrs) Exp Sta 14 Ann Report. 1901. pp179-
2.   R.A. McCance and R.D. Lawrence. The Carbohydrate Content of Foods. MRC Spec Rep Ser No 135 HMSO Lond 1929.
3.   A.A. Paul and D.A.T. Southgate. McCance and Widdowsons The Composition of Foods 4th Edition HMSO London 1978 p33.
4.   D.A.T. Southgate. Guidelines for the preparation of national tables of food composition. Karger Basel 1974.
5.   S. Southon; S.J. Fairweather-Tait and T. Hazell. Proc. Nutr Soc 1988, 47 27-
6.   H. Himsworth, Bibl. Nutritia et Dieta 1969, 13 1.

IMPORTANCE OF NUTRIENT AVAILABILITY IN RELATION TO TRENDS OF FOOD PRODUCTION AND CONSUMPTION

H.R. Mueller

Nestec Ltd.
Research Department
1800 Vevey / Switzerland

The main objective for studying the bioavailability of nutrients must be the prevention of nutritional inadequacies. This can be of particular importance with regard to modern life style and new eating habits. Today, nutritional problems often arise from overconsumption and nutritional imbalances rather than from any specific deficiency. In addition, the current tendency for low energy consumption and other dietary restrictions may well lead to new nutrient deficiency symptoms.

Nutritional adequacy has been defined by the Recommended Dietary Allowances and nutrition goals or guidelines are promoted to guide consumers towards healthy diets and sound eating habits. In man, however, one finds a good deal of nutritional individuality and, human behaviour is not readily standardized. Therefore, an estimation of available nutrients must take into account the practical terms of dietary intakes, the losses or interactions of nutrients during food preparation and industrial processing and the critical limits of essential nutrients according to the present consumption patterns in our modern industrial society.

1 THE CHANGING PATTERN OF FOOD CONSUMPTION

The amounts of nutrients available from a particular pattern of food depends on three crucial factors: the choice of foods available in the market, the food consumed by the individual person and the bioavailability of the nutrients.

13

In analysing patterns of food consumption and nutritional status in the populations of industrialised countries over the last century, two distinct phases can be detected: an earlier period when consumption patterns were mainly determined by socio-economic factors such as employment, income and food prices, followed by a shorter phase after World War II, characterised by higher living standards, abundant food supply and a prevalence of chronic degenerative diseases. With growing affluence, many changes in production, distribution and consumption occurred, with direct consequences on the quantity, variety and quality of foods eaten. The introduction of modern technology into agricultural production in particular has led to an ever increasing input of cereals in order to meet the higher level of consumption of animal products desired by the modern consumer. The scene has also changed with regard to health. Obesity, once primarily a disorder of the higher social classes, became increasingly a general phenomenon and is now more often associated with the poorer classes. At the beginning of this century, nutritional problems were mainly linked to general undernutrition and to specific vitamin and mineral deficiency states like rickets in the UK and goitre in the Alps, but today they are of a quite different nature and not as obvious. This is not only because more food is available, but also because we have a better understanding how to prevent nutrient deficiency diseases, following the discoveries of vitamins, essential amino acids and trace elements. During the same period, consumption of industrially manufactured foods in the diet has greatly increased, especially in urban areas. The overall changes in food consumption during phase 1 included a reduction of staple foods like bread, potatoes and legumes, and their replacement by more energy dense foods of animal origin, but also increases in the consumption of fruit, vegetables, sugar and alcohol.

Although dietary differences are likely to persist due to cultural, psychological and other factors, phase 2 has seen most european countries adopting more and more similar patterns in the use of the main food groups: a lower intake of cereals and starchy foods and an increase of meat, egg and milk products as shown in figure 1 (1).

Since food habits are closely related to traditional and behavioural parameters, it is particularly interesting to see how much health policies, nutritional recommendations and dietary guidelines contribute to the changes in food consumption. Recent reports on this

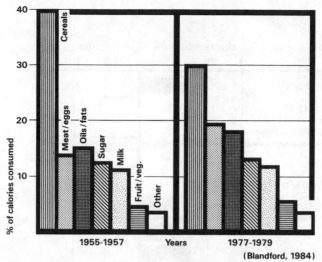

<u>**Figure 1**</u>　　Changes in Dietary Structure in the OECD Area

subject seem to confirm some positive effects, or at
least, a growing awareness about diet and health concerns
starting to have an impact on the consumers' consumption
habits (2). Figure 2 summarizes some of the new findings
from several highly industrialized countries of Europe and
the USA since 1975 (3,4,5,6). Although people of these
countries have attained a total fat consumption as high as
40-43% of dietary energy, they show still a trend to
slight increases in consumption of meat and meat products.
There is, however, a clear tendency towards leaner meat
and poultry. Full cream milk is losing market share, but
the decrease is more than compensated by low fat milks,
yoghurts and cheeses. The most pronounced changes appear
with vegetables and fruit, especially with impressive increases in consumption of frozen vegetables and fruit
juices. Bread consumption is still declining, but there is
more interest to find a more "nutritious" bread, e.g.
brown bread or speciality breads, and to adopt "muesli"-
type products. The trend to consume more vegetables,
fruits and brown bread adds more fibre to the diet. Even
if some of the changes are only marginal, for the longer
term they will probably lead to a reduction in total fat
consumption, thus following the proposed nutritional
guidelines. The reappraisal of vegetables, fruits and
whole grain products could also mean that highly refined
foods of animal origin have attained saturation and that a
swing back to consuming more plant food materials may soon
begin.

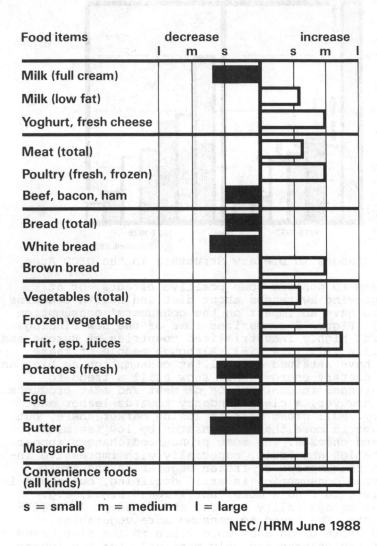

Figure 2 New Trends in Food Consumption: Volume Increases and Decreases of Main Food Groups (after 1975)

An important factor in the development of these trends is the wider availability of more variety of foods in fresh, refrigerated and frozen forms. Such products are highly attractive and of natural appearance and taste, as well as convenient in use (e.g. prepared dishes, yoghurts, fresh cheeses, frozen vegetables). Prepacked goods offer many practical advantages such as single portion packs and easy and rapid preparation in the household. They also offer additional nutritional qualities, due to careful selection of raw materials, rapid professional handling during harvesting, processing and distribution. The cold chain combined with suitable packaging ensures good keeping quality without the addition of preserving agents. Recent surveys confirm that, for the consumer the price of a given foodstuff is less determinant than high quality and convenience in use.

2 THE PEOPLE AT RISK

In the developed countries, there are abundant quantities of food available so that everybody can be fed correctly. In spite of this apparent abundance nutritional surveys continue to report the existence of groups with borderline nutrient intakes. Today this is no longer a question of the methods used for such investigations, but rather of understanding the motives for the particular nutritional behaviour of such people. The human body in good health adapts readily to temporarily lower or higher food intake and can compensate for short-term negative nutrient inter-actions. However, people who have adopted the habit of an unbalanced diet run the risk of nutrient deficiency diseases. They may be found especially in the following groups:

- individuals with unusual food habits, dieters and people who are consuming unbalanced diets.

- elderly people, who eat less frequently and in smaller quantities or are taking medications which lead to negative interactions.

- people in need of a higher intake, such as during pregnancy, lactation or in a period of rapid growth as in infancy or adolescence

- heavy alcohol consumers and heavy users of drugs.

Lack of understanding of basic nutrient requirements often explains the malnutrition seen in many people with

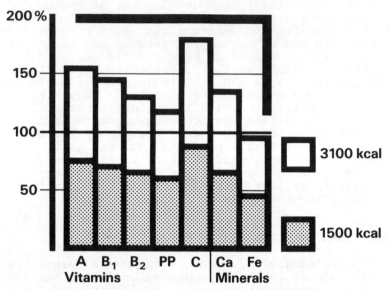

(G. Brubacher, 1987)

<u>Figure 3</u>   % Nutrient Coverage of Average Food Supply (CH)

unusual consumption habits. Another culprit is reduced
physical activity, leading to lower energy needs and
limited total food intakes. Unfortunately, food is more
often chosen for reasons of taste and convenience than for
nutritional quality and nutrient density. Diet plans aimed
at reducing the energy value or at lowering the animal fat
intake often cut out basic food items like full cream
milk, eggs and meat. Even if such measures are quite in
accordance with proposed dietary guidelines, they underestimate the limited margin of error in reduced nutrient
intakes. A too drastic change in the consumption of
important nutrient sources, like those listed in Table 1,
could easily result in a diet falling below the critical
requirements of certain essential nutrients.

3 THE CRITICAL NUTRIENTS

One can define critical nutrient limits as the minimum
amounts necessary to satisfy the body's requirements over
a reasonable time period. If for some particular reason,
individuals do not consume enough foods known to be
necessary sources of specific nutrients, they may develop
typical, although often marginal deficiencies. The
following example may illustrate the point: The estimated

Table 1   Critical Nutrients and Antinutritional Effects

Food consumption: +/-	Nutrients concerned:
- milk	calcium, vitamins A, B12, B2
- potatoes	potassium, vitamin C
- meat (red)	iron, vitamins B12, B1
- egg	protein, vitamin D
- fats	vitamins A and E
+ fibres	minerals (incl. trace elements)
	Interactions of antinutrients
+ vegetables, fruits, legumes	phytate, goitrogens, oxalates, polyphenolics, etc.

average food supply at the level of 3100 kcal/person/day reported in the 2nd Swiss Nutrition Report (7) covers the requirements of critical nutrients by 100 to 180% (Fig.3). Cutting the consumption of the same food range to 1500 kcal per day would result in a coverage of 47 to 88% of the selected nutrient requirements (8).

Slimmers and dieters not only restrict their energy intakes, but they also ban from the food list some basic foods like milk, potatoes, pork, bread and other items. They thus eliminate essential nutrient sources and aggravate the already insufficient supply of critical nutrients. The main areas of concern are listed in Table 1 where also possible gaps of nutrients are indicated. A typical example to mention is the shortage of thiamin by a voluntary suppression or reduction of pork, bread and potatoes, the three main contributors of thiamin in an average diet (covering normally about 70% of the needs). An even more critical area of concern is the loss of bone mass in the elderly which is sometimes due to low calcium intakes. For calcium as well as for a few other critical nutrients, e.g. vitamins A, B12, B2, milk and milk products represent the most important dietary pool. Anemia and low iron status can have a rather complicated aetiology. However, the reduction or omission of red meat one of the major sources of iron (heme iron) without a reasonable compensation by other means could be of critical importance for people belonging to the risk groups like pregnant and lactating women. Vegetarians are of particular interest in this regard. They have high intakes of fibres and vitamin C, their body weight and

blood cholesterol are lower than in non-vegetarians. Being
rather health-conscious people,vegetarians normally choose
a greater variety of vegetables to cover their needs.
Those using regularly milk or milk products and eggs can
achieve a well balanced diet (9). However, this is not the
case for vegans who fall short on vitamin B12, calcium and
iron without an adequate supplement.

The new "health" movements have created the habit to
consume nutrients from supplements and not from food. Such
practices must be carefully examined. Water-soluble vitamins as well as fat-soluble vitamins can be toxic in high
doses. Abuse of vitamins (A, B6 and D or nicotinic acid)
has recently been described in several scientific reports
(10,11).

The above examples show that under- or over-supply of
critical nutrients may occur more often than we might
expect. The numerous factors interfering with the physiological and the behavioural aspects complicate the identification of the real problems in food selection and, particularly, the determination of critical nutrient limits.
Obviously, in many of the food restricted diets, the bioavailability of particular nutrients remains to be studied.

    4 NUTRIENT INTERACTIONS, HIGH FIBRE DIETS AND MINERAL
      RETENTION

Sensitive components of foods like proteins, vitamins and
trace elements are prone to many possible interactions,
either in the food itself, or in our body. Such interactions have a major influence on the final bioavailability, absorption and utilisation of nutrients, some being
beneficial while others harmful. The great number of
interactions between macro- and micronutrients, and
naturally occurring antinutrients, such as enzyme
inhibitors, vitamin antagonists, goitrogens, saponins,
polyphenolics, oxalates, etc. has offered good oppor-
tunities for interesting research, so that today we are
able to identify many of the favourable and unfavourable
food combinations. The standard example of such an interaction is that of iron where concomitantly absorbed
dietary components can as well as physiological conditions
enhance or inhibit its absorption (Table 2). Another
important positive interaction is that between vitamin D
and calcium. Vitamin D is required for calcium absorption.
Milk, the most widely used calcium source, is therefore
fortified with vitamin D, and vitamin D is often included
in calcium supplements.

<u>Table 2</u> Iron Availability

A. Dietary factors enhancing (+) inhibiting (-)

Ascorbic acid	+	Tannins	-
Citric acid	+	Phosphates	-
Meat, fish	+	Bran, phytate	-
Alcohol	+	Egg yolk (cooked)	-

B. Relative bioavailability of iron sources (12)

Ferrous sulphate	100	Ferric saccharate	97
Ferrous fumarate	101	Ferric pyrophosphate	58
Ferrous succinate	119	Electrolytic iron	44

Fibre-containing foods and various types of fibres can have inhibitory effects on the absorption and retention of minerals such as zinc, calcium and manganese. It has also been demonstrated that phytates inhibit the absorption of non-heme iron. The dietary use of brans rich in phytate could have a detrimental effect on the iron-status of people at risk e.g. pregnant woman, elderly people. Of particular importance is iron absorption in cereal-based weaning foods, where iron pyrophosphate commonly used for fortification has poor bioavailability. Organoleptic and technological limitations preclude the use of iron sulfate, the best absorbed chemical form of iron. Now it has been demonstrated that the bioavailability of iron in such a dietary environment can be markedly improved by the use of iron fumarate or iron succinate (12). Some of the frequently consumed dietary components like whole grain bread, brown rice, wheat germ, <u>etc</u>. are characterized by relatively high contents of fibre and phytate. But they are also good sources of minerals and therefore one can assume that the small changes in absorption are partially offset by the higher mineral contents of such foodstuffs. In addition to this, Hallberg (13) has shown that ascorbic acid added to a meal (50 to 100 mg) strongly counteracted the inhibitory effect of phytates on iron bioavailability. The same could be demonstrated by adding meat (82 g as a hamburger) to the high phytate containing wheat rolls. Thus the latest results suggest that it is possible to increase the amount of fibre in our diet by consuming more cereals, vege-tables, fruits and flour with higher extraction rates

without interfering too much with iron balance. Numerous
interactions among minerals could well be more important.
High levels of calcium can depress magnesium, iron and
zinc utilization under certain conditions. The high
calcium consumption of 1000 to 1500 mg/day suggested to
woman by an official health recommendation in the USA must
be critically reviewed because the regular use of calcium
supplements may well interfere with the availability of
other nutrients. Well studied interactions concern the
competition between iron, copper and zinc with reference
to their bioavailability (14). Many of the mentioned
interactions remain to be further elucidated, especially
with regard to reduced food intakes (slimming) and for
particular requirement situations.

5 CHANGES OF NUTRIENT AVAILABILITY THROUGH FOOD PREPARATION AND PROCESSING

Keuning and Beek (15) estimate that in industrialized
countries 80% of the food basket is made up of processed
foods. With such an important contribution it is essential
to know if the foods available offer an adequate supply of
nutrients, especially in relation to present consumption
trends. The first objective of processing is the prevention
of food spoilage, and heat is the most frequently used
method to achieve this. Different time/temperature conditions are applied for various technological reasons and
to ensure the wholesomeness of the product. In the same
applications, heat can have other desirable effects, such
as:

. favourable alterations of product characteristics,
  texture and flavour changes or increased palatability

. destruction of undesirable food compounds such as peroxidase, thiaminase, ascorbic acid oxidase, trypsin inhibitor, avidin, etc. and

. improvement in nutrient availability e.g. increasing
  digestibility of proteins or gelatinising starches.

Finally, some of the undesirable effects of heat
treatment cannot be overlooked. They include changes in
the availability of proteins and amino acids, especially
lysine and threonine, and in lipids, carbohydrates,
vitamins and minerals.

Nutrient losses occurring during food preparation and
processing have always been a matter of concern. They are

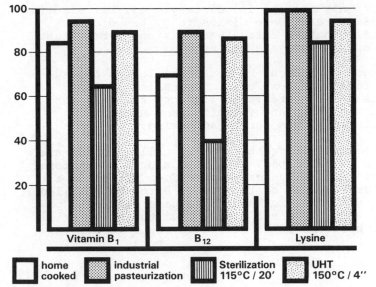

<u>Figure 4</u> Milk Processing: Residual Nutrient Content
          According to Heat Treatment

the result of various operations like washing, peeling,
boiling, milling and drying, some occurring in the household preparations as well as in industrial production. For
the food industry the question of minimising nutrient
losses has been an important challenge for a long time,
and progress has been achieved in many areas:

. by more careful selection of food raw materials.

. by better monitoring and improved methods and equipment
  for processing of foodstuffs from the place of harvest
  to the moment of use by the consumer. The flash heat
  treatments used for milk sterilisation (uperisation)
  compared to the classic in-can sterilisation (Fig. 4)
  are a typical example. Similarly, combining several processing treatments e.g. blanching and freezing, pasteur-
  isation and drying, with suitable packaging, heat damage
  can be reduced to a minimum. The refrigeration chain and
  new techniques like aseptic filling and packaging under
  inert gases have also led to new nutritionally improved
  food products. The gentler methods of processing used in
  order to improve the flavour, colour and texture offer
  in addition good protection to nutritive values.

. by the creation of an extended range of formulated

foods, not only for special dietary uses, but also in
the fields of ready-made dishes (e.g. based on
nutritional concepts like "Lean Cuisine"), breakfast
cereals, nutritional snacks, etc.

. through food enrichment by restoring losses and additional fortification: e.g. milk enriched with
vitamins A and D, cereals for infants and children
fortified with iron and vitamin C and vitamin
restoration in flours for bread making.

. With the demand for fresher foods, chilled foods are
certain to be developed. This brings both nutritional
advantages and new dangers. Space does not allow a
detailed development of this topic here, but chilled
foods are difficult to handle and have short and potentially variable shelf lives. Thus there are still
important problems to be solved in the future.

6 CONCLUSIONS

Food consumption patterns have changed more in the last
30 years than over the whole of the previous century. The
food market offers today a large, extended range of
different kinds and qualities of foods. This means that
problems related to nutrient availability are more often
located in areas of particular eating habits, voluntary
restrictions of food intakes and behavioural changes than
in inadequate foods. Although the growing importance of
processed foods in our diet will call for further efforts
to minimize nutrient losses through processing, the
achievements with new preservation techniques, better
handling and formulations have brought a marked
improvement in the availability of critical nutrients.

However, one has to admit that the abundancy of food
in the market place does not facilitate the consumer's
choice. Therefore, an important priority is improving the
consumer's knowledge of individual requirements and the
extent to which individual portions of different foods
satisfy daily needs. A second aim is to encourage better
selection of food sources for given nutrients. It is in
general preferable to eat a wide variety of foodstuffs
including restored or supplemented foods, than to have
recourse to pure supplements. Well presented nutrition
information and nutritive value declarations on food
labels can help to avoid particular shortcomings.

REFERENCES

1. D. Blandford, European Review of Agriculture
    Economics, 1984, 11, 43
2. J. Frank and V. Wheelock, British Food Journal, 1988,
    90, 22
3. "Nationwide Food Consumption Survey", CSFII, US
    Department of Agriculture, Hyattsville Md, 1986,
    Report No. 85-3
4. "Household Food Consumption and Expenditure",
    Ministry of Agriculture, Fisheries and Food, London,
    1986
5. "Ernährungsbericht", Deutsche Gesellschaft für
    Ernährung, Frankfurt, 1984
6. "Diet Nutrition and Health", British Medical
    Association, London, 1986
7. H. Aebi, A. Blumenthal, M. Bohren-Hoerni,
    G. Brubacher, U. Frey, H.R. Müller, G. Ritzel,
    M. Stransky, "Zweiter Schweizerischer Ernährungs-
    bericht", Hans Huber, Bern, 1984
8. G. Brubacher, Schriftenreihe Schweiz. Vereinigung für
    Ernährung, 1987, 59, 43
9. H. Rottka, Schriftenreihe Schweiz. Vereinigung für
    Ernährung, 1987, 59, 55
10. L. Aldaheff, C.T. Gualtieri and M. Lipton, Nutr.
    Rev., 1984, 42, 33
11. C.D.H. Evans and J.H. Lucey, Br. Med. J., 1986, 292,
    509
12. R.F. Hurrell, D.E. Furniss, J. Burri, P. Whittaker,
    S.R. Lynch, J.D. Cook, Am. J. Clin. Nutr., 1988 (in
    press)
13. L. Hallberg, in Symposium "Dietary Fibre with
    Clinical Aspects", Tricum AB, Sweden, 1986
14. N.W. Solomons, in "Nutrient Interactions",
    C.E. Bodwell, J.W. Erdman, Jr (Eds), Marcel Dekker,
    Inc., New York, 1988
15. R. Keuning and W.J. Beek, "Proceedings of the Fourth
    European Nutrition Conference 1983", E.M.E. van den
    Berg, W. Bosman, B.G. Breedveld (Eds), The Hague,
    Voorlichtingsbureau voor de Voeding, 1985, 51

IMPORTANCE OF NUTRIENT AVAILABILITY TO FOOD PRODUCTION AND CONSUMPTION

Golam Mowlah and Abdul Malek

Institute of Nutrition and Food Science
University of Dhaka[2] Bangladesh

1 INTRODUCTION

Information on food intake patterns of different countries
should provide us with keys in formulating national nutritional guidelines. Undoubtedly sound food and related
information will be helpful in reducing the nutritional
problems. In this paper attempt has been made (a) to
elaborate the nutrition aspects existing in the developed
world; (b) to make awareness through stating the food
production, availability, nutrient intake pattern of a
developing country; and (c) to state some expert opinions
and suggestions for international co-operation and activities in this field.

2 NUTRITIONAL CONSCIOUSNESS IN THE WESTERN WORLD

United States, E.E.C. countries, Japan and other developed
countries have always surplus food productions.   The
developed countries are concerned about establishing a safe
level of nutrient intake to prevent diseases associated
with ageing, cancer and cardiovascular diseases. Undoubtedly, for overcoming and reducing the diseases of the affluent society, the U.S. dietary goals (1977) could be effective.

3 FOOD PRODUCTION AND NUTRIENT INTAKE PATTERN

The developing countries like Bangladesh have many nutritional problems due to food deficiencies, in addition to
the ones more or less similar to those which exist in the
developed parts of the world.   In food deficiencies, food
production and supply is an important factor of nutrition
and health. The existing situation in terms of production

is shown in Table 1.

Table 1   Major food production in Bangladesh
           (production X 100000, tons)[2]

	1982/83	1983/84	1984/85	1985/86
Rice	139.91	145.07	146.20	150.37
Wheat	10.78	12.11	14.64	10.42
Sugar	18.14	15.14	8.79	8.29
Potato	11.31	11.48	13.00	12.98
Sweet potato	7.02	7.12	8.00	8.24
Pulses	2.10	1.96	2.15	2.00
Oil seeds	2.49	2.63	2.90	3.00
Vegetables	10.01	10.23	10.65	9.00
Fruits	1.38	1.38	1.70	1.85

According to Table 1, although there is a trend of increasing production, the national food balance sheet of 1986-87
indicated an import need of 1850 X 1000 tons of grain food.

Most of the developed countries have a clear picture
of dietary and nutrient intake for different age and socio-
economic groups. In these cases it is easier because of
the existence of co-operative and institutional food service
systems and maintenance of family food charts and food consumption table. In developing countries, the task is not
so easy due to sociocultural and socioeconomic factors.
However, to know and evaluate the nutritional status of
a country is a necessity. In Bangladesh, we have some
nutrient intake data generated through different studies.[5]

Although governmental and non-governmental organizations are studying the data for various purposes, controversy often exists about the usefulness of such information,
due to methodology and sampling technique, way of analysis
and interpretation. However, it gives some information
about the food intake pattern and any drastic deviation
due to existing situations, environments and natural calam-
ities. To locate the status of the individual country and
to formulate the nutritional guideline, it is necessary to
know the food intake of some countries. Table 2 may be
useful in this respect.

Table 2   Annual per capita intake of macronutrients
           in some countries of the world

	Netherland[3] (1975)	Switzerland[4] (1972/73)	Bangladesh[5] (1975/76)
Energy (Kcal)	2925	3224	2094
Protein (gm)	88	88	58.5
Fat (gm)	129	136	12.2
Carbohydrate (gm)	353	371	439

4   GLOBAL NUTRITIONAL ASPECTS AND VIEWPOINTS

There are opinions that 'the protein gap is a myth and what
really exists is a food gap and an energy gap'[6]. Protein
deficiency is known primarily as a result of low calorie
intake and people can have sufficient protein by eating
enough of a cereal/pulse diet to meet their energy
demands.[7,8]

The remark of Hautvast on the year 2000 as being the
year in which the nutrition revolution will have shown its
real face,[3] and its expected success, is very encouraging.
Hollingsworth[9] quoted that the nutritional gaps between
the 'haves' and the 'have-nots' continue to widen, and the
nutrition and food problems in the developing countries is
becoming vulnerable. Now, if every scientist is a member
of the global scientific community, there is urgent need
for endeavour of international co-operation and research
to have food for all.

REFERENCES

1. US Senate, Select Committee on Nutrition & Human Needs, Dietary
   Goals for the United States', US Government Printing Office,
   Washington, DC. 1977.
2. Bangladesh Agricultural Production Statistics. Bangladesh,1985/86
3. J.Hautvast,Problems in Nutrition Research Today,Academic Press,
   New York, 1981.
4. F. Gutzwiller,Problems in Nutrition Research Today, Academic
   Press, New York, 1981.
5. Nutrition Survey of Bangladesh, Inst. of Nutrition & Food Science,
   University of Dhaka, Bangladesh, 1962/64,1975/76,1981/82
6. J.C.Waterlow & P.R.Payne, Nature, 1975, 258, 113.
7. C.Clark & J.B.Turner,Man Food & Nutrition,CRC Press, London 1973.
8, P.V, Sukhatme, Indian J.Agric.Econ.,1972, 28, 1.
9. D.F.Hollingsworth, Problems in Nutrition Research Today,
   Academic Press, New York, 1981.

Physical and Chemical Techniques for the Measurement of Bioavailability

USE OF ICP-MS TO ASSESS THE BIOAVAILABILITY OF TRACE ELEMENTS IN THE HUMAN DIET

B.G. Dalgarno, R.M. Brown and C.J. Pickford

Chemical Analysis Group
Environmental and Medical Sciences Division
Harwell Laboratory
Oxfordshire
OX11 ORA

1 INTRODUCTION

A new mass spectrometric technique[1,2] is being applied to the measurement of trace element isotope ratios in biological samples such as blood and urine. Methods involving the use of stable isotopes as tracers have been developed, which allow an assessment of the bioavailability of trace elements in the human diet. Strontium is a minor dietary constituent with similar chemistry to that of calcium and therefore human uptake, retention and excretion experiments performed using strontium allow a comparison to be made of the metabolism of these two elements.

A human volunteer uptake experiment has been conducted in order to demonstrate that ICP mass spectrometry is a suitable technique for monitoring the uptake and excretion of trace elements such as strontium.

2 EXPERIMENTAL

Two volunteers each consumed 1 mg ^{86}Sr as a solution (5 ml) of strontium carbonate dissolved in dilute hydrochloric acid and mixed with cold milk (150 ml). One milligram corresponds to the normal daily dietary intake. Blood and urine samples were then taken at discrete time intervals following ingestion. By adopting a pre-concentration method, the total strontium concentration in blood and urine samples was raised to ca. 150 ng ml^{-1}. This would improve measurement precision in addition to removing the bulk of the matrix elements. ICP mass spectrometry is susceptible to matrix effects caused by high concentrations of matrix elements, particularly univalent cations. This extraction method also has the advantage of separating strontium from rubidium.

   The ICP–MS uses a high–temperature plasma as an efficient
atmospheric pressure ionization source for a quadrupole mass
spectrometer. Samples are introduced to the plasma as aqueous solutions in the form of an aerosol. Five consecutive measurements
(peak area) were made of the strontium isotope ratio in each sample.

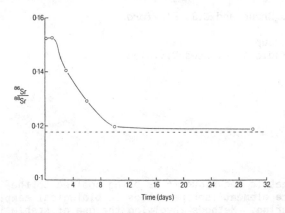

**Fig. 1   Graph of $^{86}Sr/^{88}Sr$ ratio _versus_ time following ingestion
(blood analysis)**

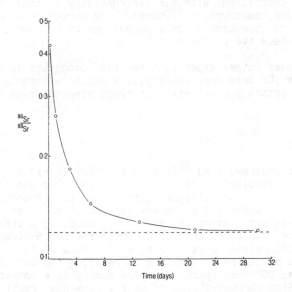

**Fig. 2   Graph of $^{86}Sr/^{88}Sr$ ratio _versus_ time following ingestion
(urine analysis)**

3 RESULTS

The isotope ratio data for the blood and urine samples from one of the volunteers have been plotted as ratio _versus_ time curves as shown in Figures 1 and 2. The horizontal line shows the natural $^{86}Sr:^{88}Sr$ ratio. Measurement precisions (1σ) of $\pm0.20\%$ and 0.98% (average values) were achieved for the urine and blood analyses respectively, with 15 min data acquisition times. The relative difference in these figures (factor of 5) is due to the greater mass of strontium measured, in turn caused by the greater volume of urine sample available.

4 CONCLUSIONS

The ICP-MS technique can measure isotope ratios ($^{86}Sr:^{88}Sr$) in blood and urine samples with high precision following simple separation and preconcentration of strontium. Measurement precision appears to be limited by counting statistics, which indicates that substantial improvement will only result from an increased ion count, achieved either through improved instrumental sensitivity, increasing the sample size, or by longer acquisition times. The approach is an extremely viable one for stable isotope uptake studies. Unlike thermal ionization mass spectrometry, the ion source is external to the spectrometer, and consequently isotope ratios may be determined economically as a relatively high through-put of samples is possible. Furthermore, the high measurement precision achieved made it possible to discriminate between the measured and natural ratios in samples well down the biological decay curve, thereby allowing levels of tracer in blood or urine to be followed for times comparable with those achieved by other techniques such as radiotracer methods. In urine, the ratio did not return to normal until several weeks after ingestion.

ACKNOWLEDGEMENTS

The authors are grateful for the advice and encouragement given by Dr J.S. Hislop (Harwell). This work is funded by the Department of Health and Social Security (Hannibal House, Elephant and Castle, London SE1 6TE), but the views expressed in this publication are those of the authors and do not necessarily represent those of the DHSS.

REFERENCES

1. A.L. Gray and A.R. Date, Analyst, 1983, _108_, 1033.
2. J.A. Olivares and R.S. Houk, Anal. Chem., 1986, _58_, 20.

THE USE OF ICP-MS TO ESTIMATE ABSORPTION OF IRON DURING NORMAL HUMAN PREGNANCY

Whittaker PG, Lind T, *Williams J and *Gray A,

University Department of Obstetrics and Gynaecology,
Princess Mary Maternity Hospital
Newcastle upon Tyne
*ICP-MS Unit
Chemistry Department
Surrey University
Guildford

The increasing availability of stable isotope compounds and mass spectrometers is opening the way to investigate safely many aspects of human pregnancy and the problems that can occur. Determination of the extent to which oral iron absorption increases throughout normal pregnancy will help to resolve the problem of whether normal pregnant women need routine iron supplements. This is important as the absorption of other elements, such as magnesium and zinc, may be affected, side effects may ensue in the mother and therapy is a considerable financial burden on the National Health Service.

Until Inductively Coupled Plasma Mass Spectrometry (ICP-MS) became available, determination of stable isotope ratios was difficult with sample preparation and measurement being both complex and time consuming. Techniques such as neutron activation or thermal ionisation mass spectrometry require extensive sample treatment.

The work presented here describes the use of ICP-MS with sample introduction by electrothermal vaporisation without prior sample preparation. This enabled rapid determination of the 54/56 and 57/56 iron isotope ratios in serum from four normal non-pregnant women following simultaneous oral and intravenous administration of enriched ferrous sulphate. Serum samples were collected over 6 hours and the mean absorption of a 5mg oral dose of iron was 10.4 percent (95% confidence internal 5.2 to 20.4). Work is in progress to assess serial changes in absorption during pregnancy.

FAST ATOM BOMBARDMENT MASS SPECTROMETRY FOR THE MEASUREMENT OF ZINC ABSORPTION IN HUMAN NUTRITION STUDIES

J. Eagles, D.E. Portwood and S.J. Fairweather-Tait
AFRC Institute of Food Research
Colney Lane, Norwich NR4 7UA

A. Götz and K.G. Heumann
Institute of Inorganic Chemistry
University of Regensburg
Universitätsstraße 31, D-8400 Regensburg
W. Germany

The quantitative measurement of stable isotopes of zinc in biological samples is essential for the advancement of research in human nutrition, as exemplified by studies using thermal ionization mass spectrometry (TIMS)[1]. Following the initial demonstration that calcium could be analysed by fast atom bombardment (FAB) mass spectrometry[2], we used similar techniques to develop methods for the quantitative determination of stable isotopes of iron[3] and zinc[4]. More recently, improvements have been made in the sample preparation stage[5]. The objective of the present study was to directly compare results of FAB analysis with those of TIMS from samples relating to an investigation into the apparent absorption of zinc by human subjects from cereals.

The nutritional study was concerned with the effects of thermal food processing on mineral absorption[6]. Subjects were fed a 5.50 mg dose of enriched zinc (93.11 atom % ^{67}Zn ie 5.13 mg of ^{67}Zn) together with a bran-based cereal. Faecal collections were made over the next few days until all the unabsorbed isotope had been collected. The faecal material collected from each subject was combined, dried, homogenised and subsamples ashed in silica crucibles at 480°C for 48 hours. Portions of the ash (0.1 g) were warmed in 2 mL concentrated HCl ("Aristar", BDH Chemicals Ltd. UK) overnight in silica crucibles, a further 2 mL concentrated HCl added and the resulting solution transferred to a plastic scintillation vial by washing with 8 mL distilled water.

The diluted digest was added to a AG 1-X8 anion exchange resin, 200-400 mesh, chloride form (Bio Rad Laboratories, California, USA) previously prepared by swelling in water for 2 days, then stirring with a teflon magnetic bar, before packing into a short form glass disposable pasteur pipette. The 7 cm packing was plugged at the bottom with glass wool, washed, with 60 mL of 2 M HNO_3, using a LKB 2120 Varioperpex II pump operating at a flow rate of 1 mL min^{-1}, regenerated to the chloride form with 60 mL of the 0.5 M HCl. After addition of the sample, the column was washed with a further 30 mL of 0.5 M HCl and the zinc eluted with 20 mL of 0.04 M HCl collected as 1 ml fractions.

The first five were discarded and the remaining ten used for the mass spectrometric measurements. Each fraction was evaporated to dryness under a heat lamp and redissolved in 20 ml of 2 M HNO$_3$. The ^{64}Zn/^{67}Zn ratio was measured in 2 µl of the solution (containing approximately 1-3 µg of zinc in total) on a conventional organic KRATOS ANALYTICAL MS80 RFA mass spectrometer in the FAB mode. The measurement was carried out using the selected ion monitoring facility, repetitively measuring first the ^{67}Zn ion and then the ^{64}Zn ion and taken the mean of 75 measurement to obtain the result. The sample was analysed three times, interposed each time with bracketing standards, made from mixtures of standard zinc and enriched zinc, to correct the ratio. The ^{64}Zn/^{67}Zn ratio was also obtained on another fraction from the sample by TIMS on a FINNIGAN-MAT thermal quadrupole mass spectrometer[5].

From the 22 samples analysed, the average relative standard deviation for the measurement of the ^{64}Zn/^{67}Zn ratio was 0.5% for both FAB and TIMS. The average value obtained by FAB was 1.9% higher than TIMS, and although small, this difference is statistically significant ($p<0.01$). Using the two sets of values for ^{64}Zn/^{67}Zn ratios and the concentration of zinc in the faeces (obtained by atomic absorption spectroscopy), the weight of the enriched dose in the faeces and hence the apparent absorption can be calculated. The mean apparent absorption of the 22 samples was 20.1% by FAB and 18.6% by TIMS.

This study has shown that sample preparation using ion exchange followed by FAB mass spectrometry is a satisfactory method for zinc absorption studies giving the same precision as TIMS. Although it seems to have a bias when compared to TIMS the difference between the two methods is small when compared to other sources of error generally incurred in biological studies of this kind.

Acknowledgements

The authors thank Miss L.L. Symss and Mr A.J.A. Wright for technical assistance. Part of this work was funded by the Ministry of Agriculture, Fisheries and Food.

References

1.   M.J. Jackson, D.A. Jones, R.H.T. Edwards, I.G. Swainbank and
     M.L. Coleman, Br. J. Nutr., 1984, 51, 199.

2.   D.L. Smith, Anal. Chem., 1983, 55, 2391.

3.   J. Eagles, S.J. Fairweather-Tait and R. Self, Anal. Chem.,
     1985, 57, 469.

4.   D.E. Pratt, J. Eagles and S.J. Fairweather-Tait, J.
     Micronutrient Anal., 1987, 3, 107.

5.   A. Götz and K.G. Heumann, Fresenius Z Anal. Chem., 1986, 325,
     24.

6.   S.J. Fairweather-Tait, D.E. Portwood, L.L. Symss, J. Eagles
     and M.J. Minski, Am. J. Clin. Nutr., 1988, in press.

DETERMINATION OF ABSORPTION OF ZINC STABLE ISOTOPES UTILIZING FAST ATOM BOMBARDMENT SPECTROMETRY

L.V. Miller, K.M. Hambidge, K.M. Johnson, P.L. Peirce and P.V. Fennessey

Departments of Pediatrics and Pharmacology
University of Colorado Health Sciences Center
4200 East 9th Avenue, C232
Denver, CO 80262

Our experience with trace element stable isotope analysis by fast atom bombardment mass spectrometry (FABMS) using a standard organic mass spectrometer has demonstrated that, with minor modifications and common data acquisition techniques, levels of sensitivity and precision can be obtained that make this method a viable, accessible alternative to the more specialized, traditional inorganic mass spectrometry techniques.

After Smith's description[1] of calcium isotope analysis using FABMS, we began developing and applying stable isotope analytical methods for studies of zinc absorption. All work has been performed on a VG 7070EHF double focusing, sector mass spectrometer equipped with a standard VG FAB source and Ion Tech atom gun. Signal averaging is accomplished with a Tracor Northern TN-1710 Digital Signal Analyzer.

The use of magnet scanning has allowed us to monitor isobaric interferences and their subsequent elimination. This was invaluable during our early development work as significant isobaric and non-isobaric interferences were encountered. While unresolved isobaric species affect isotope ratio measurements, the presence of other atoms can affect ion current intensities. As zinc has a high ionization potential, it does not fare well against much more easily ionized atoms, e.g. Na and K, in the competition for ionization that is characteristic of FAB. We found that the presence of relatively small quantities of these elements significantly suppressed our zinc signal intensities. Interferences originating in biological matrices were eliminated to a great degree

38

by ashing and ion exchange chromatography procedures. A mass resolution of 3000 was sufficient to remove the remaining isobaric interference.

Biological matrices weren't the only source of interference. The stainless steel target, i.e. the components of the stainless steel and their oxides, proved to be a source of significant interference. Our initial response to this problem was to cover the standard sample target with gold foil.[2] We have since redesigned the target holder and are presently using sturdier targets made of pure silver rod.

We have routinely used this FABMS analytical technique in studies of zinc absorption utilizing faecal monitoring of ^{70}Zn isotope enrichment.[2] With two microgram samples on the target we obtain a precision of 1 to 3% RSD and a limit of detection of 0.04% enrichment; where enrichment is defined as the amount of isotopically enriched zinc divided by the total amount of zinc. In addition, we have measured isotope ratios of more than ten other metals and have confirmed for several of these that good sensitivity and precision can be attained. For example, we have recently examined copper and measured a precision of 0.8% RSD and a detection limit of 0.75% enrichment (^{65}Cu) for analysis of 100 nanogram samples. Other laboratories have successfully applied FABMS to stable isotope studies of nutritionally important metals.[3,4]

Even with magnet scanning we do not measure correct absolute isotope ratios. We consistently observe an isotope effect in which lighter isotopes appear relatively more abundant than predicted. As this was an unexplained phenomenon, we carried out a systematic investigation of instrument performance to determine the source of the isotope fractionation effect. It was determined that this effect is characteristic of the FAB desorption/ionization process.[5] In a further study we bombarded ten different elements with three different primary atoms.[6] We found isotope fractionation to be dependent on desorbed ion mass in a fashion similar to that described by researchers using secondary ion mass spectrometry (SIMS).[7]

During the isotope effect investigation, we discovered the presence of a significant and variable hydride component with most of the metals examined. A metal hydride signal was typically present at a level between a fraction and several percent of the metal signal. This finding has consequences for the selection of isotopes to be used in tracer studies. In the case of zinc, for instance, measurements of ^{67}Zn appear particularly vulnerable to interference from the hydride of ^{66}Zn.

As our trace element studies become more complex and demanding of our analytical methods, we recognize the need for increased productivity and sensitivity. To address these needs, we have recently modified our analysis process to take advantage of increased computer automation and selected ion monitoring. A personal computer-based system now acquires data directly from the mass spectrometer, and processes and reports the data with minimal operator assistance. Though scanning gives us valuable information on interferences, etc., it is a relatively inefficient data collection method. Therefore, we are developing selected ion monitoring techniques and have found that we can decrease sample size by a factor of twenty to fifty and suffer no decrease in precision.

This increase in sensitivity will be sufficient to meet the requirements of current tracer studies; but future studies will require even smaller samples sizes, larger number of samples, and streamlined cleanup and analysis procedures. We are, therefore, investigating the potential for further increases in sensitivity and productivity with FABMS. Exploratory projects being considered will examine target geometry, sample preconcentration, pulse counting signal detection, and different ionization techniques.

This work supported by NIH Clinical Mass Spectrometry Research Resource RR001152, General Clinical Research Centers RR69 and NIH Studies of Human Zinc Deficiency AM12432.

1. D.L. Smith, Anal. Chem. 1983, 55, 2391.
2. P.L. Peirce, et al., Anal. Chem. 1987, 59, 2034.
3. R. Self, et al., Anal. Proc. 1987, 24, 366.
4. X. Jiang and D.L. Smith, Anal. Chem. 1987, 59, 2570.
5. L.V. Miller, et al., ASMS 1986.
6. L.V. Miller, et al., ASMS 1987.
7. N. Shimizu and S.R. Hart, J. Appl. Phys. 1982, 53, 1303.

Isotope dilution techniques for the study of zinc bioavailability from whole diets

M.J. Jackson

Department of Medicine,
University of Liverpool,
P.O. Box 147,
Liverpool,
L69 3BX.

Zinc appears to play a crucial role in mammalian nutrition, being required in only 'trace' quantities in the diet, but essential for the normal functioning of many body systems. Experimental work suggests that zinc can be absorbed from most of the small intestine (1), but in practice it is likely that the vast majority of the absorption occurs from the duodenum. Many studies have demonstrated that various constituents of the diet can influence the amount of zinc absorbed from a test meal (2) although the net contribution of any one of these to overall zinc homeostasis does not appear to have been evaluated.

In particular zinc absorption rates appear to be reduced by phytate, fibre and polysaccharides in unrefined cereal products (2,3) and by excesses of other cations such as copper (4) or iron (5). In addition low molecular weight chelating agents (6) and various other compounds found in food stuffs (7) have been claimed to enhance zinc absorption. The rate of zinc absorption also appears to be very dependent on the zinc status of the individual with zinc depleted rats absorbing greater than 90% of a test dose of radioactive zinc compared to approximately 60% for zinc sufficient animals (8) while a normal human subject was found to decrease the proportion of zinc absorbed from approximately 60% to 20% as the zinc content of a standardised diet was increased from 110 to 470 mmoles/day (9).

It is therefore very difficult to evaluate the net effect different factors which may be acting in opposition in terms of

41

zinc absorption. Many diets high in unrefined cereal products (rich in phytate and other agents decreasing zinc bioavailability) may also be rich in citrates or some amino acids (reported to enhance zinc absorption) and the resultant total effect on zinc absorption is unknown. In addition dietary factors reducing zinc availability, and hence absorption, could produce a marginal zinc deficiency which would promote gastrointestinal zinc absorption although whether such a homeostatic adaptation would overcome the deleterious effects of the dietary constituents is unknown. There is therefore a need for methods of assessing zinc bioavailability/absorption from whole diets in order to examine the relative importance of these various factors in the maintenance of body zinc content.

Methods of assessment of zinc absorption from entire diets

Various different techniques have been used to provide a measure of the amount of zinc absorbed from a complete diet in man. These range from relatively simple metabolic balance studies to complex techniques utilising two separate isotopes of zinc.

1) Metabolic balance studies: Conventional metabolic balance techniques can provide information on the retention of zinc from any diet and several workers have combined this figure with the urinary zinc output to indicate a 'net absorption' value for zinc (10). In the case of calcium or some other elements this is likely to be a valid estimate of absorption but in the case of zinc this is unlikely to be true since the major portion of the zinc excreted from the body is secreted into the gut.

2) Isotopic techniques: Techniques using radioactive or stable isotopes generally involve extrinsic labelling of an individual dietary component with the isotope or oral administration of the isotope with a test meal (11). Considerable work has been undertaken to examine the validity of this approach in terms of whether exogenous zinc is handled in the same manner as the endogenous zinc within the food, but it is apparent that this approach will not offer a means of assessing zinc absorption from complete diets.

3) Isotope dilution techniques: The isotope dilution technique for the measurement of zinc absorption is essentially

a refinement of conventional metabolic balance studies to permit the simultaneous measurement of gastrointestinal zinc secretion. It has been validated in animals by Weigand and Kirchgessner (12) and by Evans and coworkers (13) and applied to man using enriched stable 67- zinc (9). In essence each subject receives an intravenous injection of the zinc isotope and at various times following this the plasma isotope enrichment and the faecal isotope enrichment are compared to provide a measure of zinc flux into the gut. The total dietary zinc, faecal zinc and urinary zinc are obtained from a concurrent metabolic balance study and hence true absorption of zinc can be calculated.

The disadvantages of the gastrointestinal isotope dilution technique in its present form are that: it is slow and tedious (in common with metabolic balance techniques); the limits to the time resolution is the minimum period in which reliable faecal collections can be made (in our experience this is 4 - 5 days) and therefore if there are variations in absorption rates with a greater frequency than this these would not be detected; the accuracy of the technique is limited by the accuracy of metabolic balance techniques which even in an ideal situation would never be better than $\pm$ 5% and values much greater than this are frequently seen; frequent blood sampling is required to carefully define the decay of isotope enrichment in the blood plasma; reabsorption of labelled zinc secreted into the gastrointestinal tract will negatively bias the calculated rate of zinc secretion.

We have recently utilised enriched 67-zinc and the gastrointestinal isotope dilution technique to examine zinc absorption in a chronically malnourished population in which cassava flour provided a major proportion of the food intake together with white bread and fish (14). Previous work with root-based crops such as cassava had indicated a deleterious effect of these materials on zinc bioavailability (2), but use of the gastrointestinal isotope dilution techniques has revealed that in these subjects absorption rates were high. Total dietary zinc of 5 lactating women in this population ranged from 7.2 - 11.1 mg/day, which is well below internationally recommended values, while results obtained showed a fractional absorption from these diets in the range 59-84%. It therefore apears that in this situation either the overall bioavailability of zinc from the whole diet was high or that homeostatic mechanisms had overridden the effects of the various factors in the diet inhibitory to zinc absorption.

References
1. A.H.Methfessel and H.Spencer. J. Appl. Physiol. 1973; 34: 58.
2. N.W.Solomons. Am. J. Clin. Nutr. 1982; 35: 1048.
3. A.Pecoud, P.Donzel and J.L.Schelling. Clin. Pharmacol. Therap.   1975; 17: 469
4. G.W.Evans, C.I.Grace and C.Hahn. Bioinorg. Chem. 1974; 3: 115.
5. N.W.Solomons and R.A.Jacob. Am. J. Clin. Nutr. 1981; 34: 475.
6. D.Oberleas, M.E.Muhrer and B.L.O'Dell. J. Nutr. 1966; 90: 56.
7. B.Lonnerdal, A.G.Stanislowski and L.S.Hurley. J. Inorg. Biochem.   1980; 12: 71.
8. M.J. Jackson, D.A. Jones and R.H.T. Edwards. Br. J. Nutr. 1981; 46: 15.
9. M.J. Jackson, D.A. Jones, R.H.T. Edwards, I.G. Swainbank and M.L.   Coleman. Br. J. Nutr. 1984; 51: 199.
10. M.J. Dauncey, J.C.L.Shaw and J. Urman. Paed. Res. 1977; 11: 991.
11. B.Sandstrom and A.Cederblad. Am. J. Clin. Nutr. 1980; 33: 1778.
12. E. Weigand and M. Kirchgessner. Nutr. and Metab. 1979; 22: 101.
13. G.W. Evans, E.C. Johnson and P.E. Johnson. J. Nutr. 1979; 109: 1258.
14. M.J. Jackson, R. Guigliano, L.G. Guigliano, E.F. Oliveira, R. Shrimpton   and I.G. Swainbank. Br. J. Nutr., 1988; 59: 193.

A DOUBLE LABEL STABLE ISOTOPE METHOD FOR MEASURING CALCIUM ABSORPTION FROM FOODS

S. J. Fairweather-Tait, A. Johnson, J. Eagles
AFRC Institute of Food Research, Colney Lane, Norwich.

M. I. Gurr, S. Ganatra
Milk Marketing Board, Thames Ditton, Surrey.

and H. Kennedy
Norfolk & Norwich Hospital, Norwich NR1 3SR

1 INTRODUCTION

Information on the bioavailability of calcium in different foods, known to be dependent on a number of dietary and physiological factors[1], is limited. Furthermore, it has been argued that there is a homeostatic mechanism which responds to variations in the level of calcium intake by altering the intestinal absorptive efficiency of calcium, but further research is required to substantiate this hypothesis. The recent advances in inorganic stable isotope methodology have facilitated investigations into these two aspects of calcium nutrition.

2 MATERIALS AND METHODS

Bioavailability Study

The absorption of calcium from skimmed milk was measured using a double label stable isotope technique[2,3] and compared with 'Vital', a commercial product comprised of skimmed milk fortified with calcium gluconate, and a non-dairy source of calcium, watercress soup. The calcium isotopes were measured by fast atom bombardment mass spectrometry (FABMS)[4].

Ten adult men were fasted overnight and given 250 g watercress soup (130mg Ca); on a separate occasion five were given 136ml skimmed milk (150mg Ca) and the other five 83ml Vital (154mg Ca). The calcium was labelled extrinsically with 30mg ^{44}Ca. After two to three hours each subject was given an I.V. injection of 3mg ^{42}Ca. Absorption from the oral dose was calculated from the measured isotopic ratios in plasma 24h later and also in urine samples collected on days 2 and 3 post-dosing as follows:

$$\text{Fractional absorption} = \frac{(^{44}Ca/^{40}Ca)_{na} \times {}^{42}Ca_{dose} \times \Delta\% \text{ XS } {}^{44}Ca}{(^{42}Ca/^{40}Ca)_{na} \times {}^{44}Ca_{dose} \times \Delta\% \text{ XS } {}^{42}Ca}$$

where $(^{44}Ca/^{40}Ca)_{na}$ = 0.021518 (naturally-occurring isotopic ratio)

$(^{42}Ca/^{40}Ca)_{na}$ = 6.6742×10^{-3}

$\Delta\% \text{ XS } {}^{44/42}Ca$ = amount of isotope in excess of natural abundance

Adaptation Study

All subjects consumed one pint of Vital daily (1000mg Ca) in addition to their normal diet for 4 weeks. The calcium absorption measurement from milk was then repeated.

3 RESULTS AND DISCUSSION

Percentage absorption calculated from isotopic ratios in 24h plasma was significantly correlated with day 2 (R = 0.86) and day 3 (R = 0.88) urine samples (P < 0.001).

Absorption of calcium from skimmed milk was significantly greater than from watercress soup (P < 0.05), but not different from Vital as shown in Table 1. The wide variation in absorption amongst the small number of subjects makes interpretation of the results difficult, and it cannot be concluded from this study that the bioavailability of calcium in Vital is similar to that in the skimmed milk. However, it is clear that calcium in watercress soup, was less well absorbed.

Increasing daily calcium intake by approximately 1000mg for 4 weeks did not reduce mean absorptive efficiency of calcium, as shown in Table 1. However, calcium absorption fell in seven subjects, remained constant in two and doubled in one. The lack of consistency in response makes it impossible to rule out the existence of an adaptive response based on the small number of results in this study.

Table 1   Calcium absorption (24h plasma) from skimmed milk, Vital and watercress soup (Mean ± SEM)

	% Ca absorption	P (paired t)	% Ca absorption after 1 pint Vital/d for 4 weeks
Skimmed milk	45.5 ± 1.9	< 0.001	39.0 ± 3.7
Watercress soup	26.3 ± 1.9		
Vital	35.7 ± 4.7	N.S.	33.2 ± 4.6
Watercress soup	28.5 ± 3.3		

4 CONCLUSIONS

Calcium absorption can be measured using a double label stable isotope technique. Isotopic ratios in urine collected 2 or 3 days post-administration, measured by FABMS, can be used to calculate % absorption from the oral dose. This technique is less invasive as it avoids the need to take blood samples.

Calcium was better absorbed from skimmed milk than watercress soup. The bioavailability of calcium in milk fortified with calcium gluconate (Vital) was not dissimilar to that of skimmed milk. Consumption of an additional 1000mg Calcium per day for 4 weeks, in the form of Ca-fortified milk (Vital), did not appear to significantly change the absorptive efficiency of calcium in adult men, although further work is required to confirm these preliminary results.

REFERENCES

1. L.H. Allen, Am. J. Clin. Nutr., 1982, 35, 783.
2. J.A. DeGrazia, P. Ivanovich, H. Fellows and C. Rich. J. Lab. Clin. Med., 1965, 66, 822.
3. A.L. Yergey, N.E. Vieira and D.G. Covell, Biomed. Env. Mass Spec., 1987, 14, 603.
4. D.L. Smith, C. Atkin and C. Westenfelder, Clin. Chim. Acta. 1985, 146, 97.

Analytical Techniques

METHODS OF INORGANIC ANALYSIS AND DETECTION. APPLICATION TO BIOLOGICAL PROBLEMS

R. Cornelis

Laboratory for Analytical Chemistry
Institute for Nuclear Sciences, Rijksuniversiteit Gent
Proeftuinstraat 86. B-9000 Gent   Belgium

1 INTRODUCTION

Many analysts must be wondering about the apparently limitless supply of innovating instrument developments for the determination of trace and major elements in biological materials. The progress goes on unabated, resulting in increasing sensitivity and specificity, speed and simplicity of analysis and computerised information retrieval. No wonder that potential users are tempted to manage a commercially available sophisticated instrument as a "black box". It goes without saying that it is unwarranted to do so. A highly skilled analytical chemist is an essential prerequisite to guarantee the accurate use of any given method.

The trace elements present in foodstuffs are either essential, toxic or without any known effect. Up to now routine work on trace analysis mainly dealt with toxic elements. The nutritive value of trace elements has hardly been considered outside the walls of academic laboratories. It is a virgin territory to be explored by the many field laboratories in the next decade. Trace elements of particular interest in nutrition are Cr, Se and Zn[1].

Methods currently used for the determination of trace elements will be briefly reviewed and their performances to the assay of nutrients for trace element contents will be considered. An interesting survey on the determination of minerals in food can be read in the critical review by Gross et al.[2] covering the literature from October 1984 to October 1986.

2 SAMPLE COLLECTING AND HANDLING PROCEDURES

There is some ambiguity in studying the trace element concentrations in foodstuffs. From a scientific point of view a researcher would like to pursue the authentic element concentrations. Then all manipulations have to be performed in non-contaminating conditions. Such an endeavour requires a special infrastructure and is time consuming. Considering that all food will be treated in trace element contaminating conditions, it may be over-doing things to sample and handle the specimens in the sanctuary of an ultra clean laboratory. It is an open question if normal analytical practice would not do sufficiently for this type of work.

Contamination of samples with measurable amounts of trace elements is a well publicised phenomenon. The problem is endemic in the field of the ultra trace analysis (i.e. <0.01 μg g^{-1}). This may be illustrated with trace element additions to liver cut with surgical blades. Table 1 compares the observed contamination to the in-trinsic concentrations of the elements. The additions are negligible for Mn, Fe, Co, Cu and Zn ($<5\%$). The same conclusions probably hold for Sc, Ag, Sn and Sb. For Au, a contamination of 10–25% is found. For Cr and Ni, the figures become very significant (order of magnitude 100%).

Table 1   Trace element additions in wedge biopsies of liver taken with surgical blades[3]

Element	Unit	Intrinsic concentration	Metal ion additions	
Sc	ng g^{-1}	≤ 0.4	<0.00072	– 0.010
Cr	ng g^{-1}	5.4	2.8	– 20
Mn	μg g^{-1}	1.41	0.00091	– 0.0035
Fe	μg g^{-1}	205	0.34	– 4.6
Co	ng g^{-1}	34	0.095	– 1.51
Ni	ng g^{-1}	33	2.3	– 64
Cu	μg g^{-1}	5.98	0.0034	– 0.018
Zn	μg g^{-1}	59.0	0.00044	– 0.01
Ag	ng g^{-1}	12.2	<0.0051	– 0.064
Sn	ng g^{-1}	476	<0.54	– <2.1
Sb	ng g^{-1}	11.0	0.072	– 1.1
Au	ng g^{-1}	≤ 0.155	<0.0025	– 0.015

The main logistics to avoid contamination bear on clean room conditions, cleaning of laboratory ware, pure chemicals and good practice[4].

3 SAMPLE PREPARATION

Most of the techniques require that samples be introduced in liquid form. The most conventional sample digestion procedures[5] are acid digestions (nitric acid, sulfuric acid, perchloric acid), possibly supplemented with hydrogen peroxide. These operations may occur in open beakers, in a reflux system to avoid loss of volatile compounds or in a sealed system (under pressure). Some researchers use dry-ashing procedures or oxygen combustion, followed by dissolution of the ash in acids.

Extraction of trace elements by leaching with concentrated acids was found to be as quantitative, simpler and faster than other techniques[6].

A revolution in sample digestion has occurred with microwave dissolution. It is found to be faster, more controlled, more elegant, and more amenable to automation than conventional open-beaker or closed-vessel techniques[7].

Separation of particular elements of interest by liquid extraction, ion exchange, electrodeposition, coprecipitation or other procedures, may still be necessary as a preconcentration step, if not to eliminate major matrix interferences.

Another trend is the growing popularity of solid sample introduction, either as a solid, slurry or suspension[8,9] in graphite furnace atomic absorption spectrometry (AAS) and atomic emission spectrometry (AES). It is plausible that in the near future the application may even be extented to inductively coupled plasma mass spectrometry.

4 ANALYTICAL TECHNIQUES

The most popular techniques are those based on optical phenomena[10] such as absorption (spectrophotometry, fluorometry, AAS), and emission (arc and spark source emission spectrometry, inductively coupled plasma AES, X-ray spectrometry). Electrochemical techniques (stripping voltammetry, pulse polarography) cover a minor share of the workload. More sophisticated techniques such as mass spectrometry (spark source mass spectrometry, isotope dilution mass spectrometry, inductively coupled plasma mass spectrometry) and neutron activation analysis are more often than not restricted to academic circles.

The principles of the different techniques can be learned in modern handbooks on analytical chemistry and in specialized journals.

Trends in the methodology continue to favour multielement techniques, such as continuum source atomic absorption spectrometry[11], inductively coupled plasma atomic emission spectrometry (ICP-AES) and the new-comer inductively coupled plasma-mass spectrometry (ICP-MS).

Atomic Absorption Spectrometry[12,13]

Atomic absorption spectrometry is based upon the measurement of the decrease of the power of electromagnetic radiation energy brought along by the analyte.

Both flame and graphite furnace atomic absorption spectrometry are used. The elements As, Se, Sb and Sn are preferably determined after hydride generation and introduction of the gaseous compounds in the flame or the oven. Hg is assessed by cold vapour AAS.

In their excellent review articles, Brown et al.[14,15,16] state that the technique most favoured for the determination of trace elements in food and beverages, is AAS which accounts for 70% of the papers they reviewed. The elements of greatest importance are Pb, Cd, As and Hg respectively. With respect to sample types, the two most discussed ones are milk and milk products and edible oils. Another topical application concerns the effect of food packaging on the trace element contents.

Atomic Emission Spectrometry

Atomic emission spectrometry is based on the spectral line radiation emitted by excited atoms.

ICP-AES[17] is gaining more and more ground in the field of trace element analysis in biological materials. The introduction of plasma sources for atomization-excitation significantly improved detection limits, accuracy, and precision of atomic emission procedures.

Neutron Activation Analysis[18]

Neutron activation analysis (NAA) is based on the measurement of the induced radioactivity of an element. Instrumental neutron activation analysis offers the advantage of involving a very simple sample preparation, without any requirement to dissolve the food. Although not labour intensive, it may take several months before all the data are available, as the technique uses the different half-lives and decay patterns of the induced radioisotopes. The additional application of radiochemical neutron activation analysis allows the determination of a total of about 30 elements.

Mass Spectrometry

In mass spectrometry the sample is transformed in a beam of gaseous ions which are sorted out according to their mass to charge ratio.

Inductively coupled plasma-mass spectrometry (ICP-MS)[19,20] is one of the most recently commercialised developments in mass spectrometry. Similarly to ICP-AES the samples are introduced with a conventional cross flow pneumatic nebuliser, followed by atomization in the inductively coupled plasma. It is advertised as a most promising method for fast trace elemental detection, suitable for routine analysis.

5 SPECIFICITY AND SENSITIVITY

A technique is specific if the detection signal can be unequivocally attributed to a particular element in the presence of many more. A specific detection is, for example, the gamma-ray energy of a radionuclide, the mass of an isotope,...

Sensitivity refers to the amount of the trace element detected which gives rise to an observable change in measurement. Ideally a method should be highly specific and very sensitive. There exist, however, many circumstantial factors, such as matrix effects, spectral interferences and so forth, which decrease the sensitivity substantially and even may affect the specificity. Therefore, it is only relevant to describe these characteristics for a particular matrix, as they will always be less advantageous than for the single element in ideal circumstances.

Sensitivity has been defined in many different ways. It may be appropriate to use the definitions proposed by the International Union for Pure and Applied Chemistry (IUPAC)[21]. The "limit of detection", LOD, indicates the lowest concentration level that can be determined to be statistically different from a blank. Let S_t represent the total value measured for the sample, S_b for the blank, and σ the standard deviations for the measurements. The analyte signal is then the difference between S_t and S_b. It can be shown that for normal distributions, $(S_t - S_b) > 0$ at the 99% confidence level when the difference $(S_t - S_b) > 3\sigma$. The recommended value of LOD is 3σ. Signals below LOD should be reported as not detected. The second notion "limit of quantitation", LOQ, is defined as the level above which quantitative results may be obtained with a specified degree of confidence. The recommended value is LOQ = 10σ, corresponding to an uncertainty of ± 30% in the measured value (10σ ± 3σ) at the 99% confidence level. The region of quantitation lies $>10\sigma$. It is most desirable that every series of analytical data be accompanied with their respective LOD and LOQ values.

6 QUALITY OF THE MEASUREMENT

Although the intrinsic quality of the trace element data took a change for the better during the last decade, much more concern is still requested about the precision and accuracy of the analytical results[22,23]. This fact often surfaces during interlaboratory collaborative studies. The state of the art of trace elements determinations such as As, Cd, Co, Cr, I, Mo, Ni, Sn, ... in foodstuffs seems very poor. This statement may be illustrated with a very restricted excercise on the iodide content of 2 solutions (with known concentrations) and the natural iodine content in 2 milkpowders. The results are given in table 2. The participants came from different countries and were supposed to be experts in this type of determination. Whereas 4 out of the 6 laboratories displayed sufficient analytical know-how to determine accurately the iodide in the solutions, far less agreement can be discovered between the analysis results for the milkpowders. During the discussion the main handicap for the electrochemical method was suspected to be inadequacy in achieving complete mineralization of the product. Lack of a rigorous standardization of the catalytic methodology was thought to be underlying reason for the bad performance of some of the catalytic procedures.

Table 2 Results of an intercomparison excercise of I
        determinations in 2 solutions and 2 milkpowders

Lab + Method	Sol 1 $\mu g\ ml^{-1}$	Sol 2 $\mu g\ ml^{-1}$	Milk 1 $\mu g\ mg^{-1}$	Milk 2 $\mu g\ mg^{-1}$
1 CAT	15.55 ±.45	16.47 ±.39	.531 ±.024	.378 ±.019
2 CAT	19.20 ±.22	15.30	.675 ±.135	.017 ±.007
3 CAT	15.62 ±.35	14.86 ±.42	.645 ±.023	.473 ±.016
4 CAT	14.73 ±.22	15.86 ±.50	.967 ±.125	1.300 ±.100
5 CSDPV	19.55 ±.68	19.85 ±.45	.545 ±.030	.389 ±.043
6 RNAA	15.27 ±.19	15.07 ±.06	.541 ±.019	.420 ±.006
real value	15.29	15.29		

CAT   : Sandell − Kolthoff
CSDPV: cathodic scanning differential pulse voltammetry
       of IO_3
RNAA : radiochemical neutron activation analysis

7 EVALUATION OF THE RESULTS

The correct way to evaluate the accuracy of the analytical results is to analyse standard reference materials,
certified for their trace element content. These are
available among others from the National Bureau of Standards (Washington, USA), the Bureau of Reference Materials of the European Communities (Brussels, Belgium)
and the International Atomic Energy Agency (Vienna,
Austria). A survey of currently available reference
materials has been published by Muramatsu and Parr[24].

An outstanding reference material for trace element
determination in foodstuffs was the mixed diet reference
material, RM 8431, available to the scientific community
through the above mentioned National Bureau of Standards' Office of Reference Materials[25]. It has been
characterized for 17 elements (K, P, Na, Ca, Mg, Fe, Zn,
Mn, Al, Cu, As, Ni, Mo, Se, Cr, Cd, Co). This reference
material fulfills all the essential requirements of
similar matrix effects, analyte concentrations and chemical form as the real world samples for which it will
serve as a control. The exhausted RM 8431 has been
replaced by a similar interim product RM 8431a until a
new mixed diet standard reference material is available.

Another interesting reference material is the BCR

CRM single cell protein CRM 273 certified for Ca, Mg, K and Fe, and the CRM 274 certified for Mn, Co and Zn[26].

The participation in National or International Quality Control Assessment Schemes is a most useful endeavour[22]. Complemented with regular checks on certified material, the accuracy can be safeguarded on a long term basis.

8 SUMMARY

There is an increasing interest to learn the trace element content of foodstuffs. It will soon come to the point that reference values will be put forward, not only for toxic but also for nutritive trace elements. However, many difficulties may be anticipated when exploring the ultra-trace element levels.

REFERENCES

1. E. Garfield, Current Contents, Life Sciences, 1988, 31, no 28, 3.
2. A.F. Gross, P.S. Given,Jr. and A.K. Athnasios, Anal. Chem., 1987, 59, 212R.
3. J. Versieck, F. Barbier, R. Cornelis and J. Hoste, Talanta, 1982, 29, 973.
4. R. Cornelis, J. Radioanal. Nucl. Chem., 1987, 112, 141.
5. T.T. Gorsuch,'The destruction of Organic Matter'. Pergamon Press, Oxford, 1970.
6. R.F. Puchyr and R. Shapiro, J. Assoc. Off. Anal. Chem., 1986, 69, 868.
7. H.M. Kingston and L.B. Jassie, 'Introduction to Microwave Sample Preparation:Theory and Practice', American Chemical Society, Washington, USA, 1988.
8. Fresenius' Z. Anal. Chem., 1985, 322, 653 (complete edition 7).
9. Fresenius' Z. Anal. Chem., 1987, 328, 315 (complete editions 4 & 5).
10. J.A. Holcombe and D.A. Bass, Anal. Chem., 1988, 60, 226R.
11. J. Marshall, B.J. Ottaway, J. M. Ottaway and D. Littlejohn, Anal. Chim. Acta, 1986, 180, 357.
12. D.L. Tsalev and Zaprianov, 'Atomic Absorption Spectrometry in Occupational and Environmental Health Practice', Volume I+II, CRC Press, Inc. Boca Raton, Fla, 1983+1984.
13. B. Welz, 'Atomic Absorption Spectrometry', 2nd ed.,

Verlag Chemie, Deerfield Beach, Fla., 1985.

14. A.A. Brown, D.J. Halls and A. Taylor, J. Anal. At. Spectrom., 1986, 1, 29R.
15. A.A. Brown, D.J. Halls and A. Taylor, J. Anal. At. Spectrom., 1987, 2, 43R.
16. A.A. Brown, D.J. Halls and A. Taylor, J. Anal. At. Spectrom., 1988, 3, 45R.
17. M. Thompson and J.N. Walsh, 'A Handbook of Inductively Coupled Plasma Spectrometry', Blackie, Glasgow, 1987.
18. R. Cornelis and J. Versieck, 'Treatise on Analytical Chemistry', 2nd ed., I, vol 14, B., Biological Materials, Ed. P. J. Elving, John Wiley & Sons Inc., New-York, 1986.
19. A.L. Gray , Spectrochim. Acta, 1985, 40B, 1525.
20. R.S. Houk, Anal. Chem., 1986, 58, 97A.
21. G.L. Long and J.D. Winefordner, Anal. Chem., 1983, 55, 712A.
22. K.W. Boyer, W. Horwitz and R. Albert, Anal. Chem., 1985, 57, 454.
23. J.K. Taylor, 'Quality Assurance of Chemical Measurements', Lewis Pub., Michigan, 1987.
24. Y. Muramatsu and R.M. Parr, 'Survey of currently available reference materials for use in connection with the determination of trace elements in biological and environmental materials', IAEA/RL/128, Vienna, 1985.
25. N.J. Miller-Ihli and W.R. Wolf, Anal. Chem., 1986, 58, 3225.
26. K. Vercoutere and R. Cornelis, J. Trace Microprobe Tech., 1987, 5, 191.

MICROSCOPIC AND ENERGY DISPERSIVE X-RAY
MICROANALYSIS OF OAT BRAN COMPONENTS
BEFORE AND AFTER *IN VIVO* DIGESTION

S. H. Yiu

Food Research Centre
Agriculture Canada
Ottawa, Ontario K1A 0C6
Canada
(FRC Contribution No. 779)

1 INTRODUCTION

Oat bran, which is rich in soluble dietary fibre and
phytate, can lower serum cholesterol levels in humans
and rats (1). However, it may decrease the bioavailability of certain nutrients because phytate and some
dietary fibres have mineral binding properties (2).
Knowledge of how these components are degraded in the
body helps in the understanding of their interactions
with other nutrients. The microscope provides a powerful detection method for assessing the digestive break-
down of food components. The present study aims at
demonstrating how microscopic techniques can be applied
to analyse structural and chemical changes of the above
components after they have passed through the digestive
system of the rat.

2 METHODS AND MATERIALS

Digesta containing oat bran remnants were obtained from
the large intestines of rats fed a balanced diet rich
in oat bran (3), and were prepared for fluorescence,
and scanning electron microscopic (SEM) examinations as
well as energy dispersive X-ray (EDX) microanalysis
according to previously described methods (3).

3 RESULTS

Using Calcofluor White as a microscopic marker, (1-3)-
(1-4)-linked β-D-glucan (β-glucan) was located in most
of the subaleurone and the inner aleurone cell walls of

60

oat bran (Fig. 1). The distribution of the subcellular phytin-containing structures (phytin globoids) within the aleurone and scutellum cells was revealed by another fluorescent dye, Acriflavine (Fig. 2). SEM-EDX analysis revealed their elemental content to be rich in phosphorus (P), potassium (K) and magnesium (Mg).

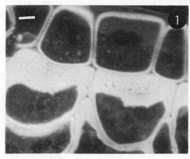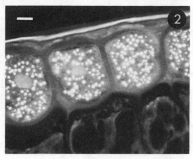

Figs. 1 & 2. Glycol methacrylate-embedded sections of oat bran stained with Calcofluor White and Acriflavine revealing its β-glucan-rich cell walls and phytin globoids, respectively. (Scale bars represent 10 μm)

Acridine orange, a metachromatic fluorochrome, was also useful as a staining reagent for revealing structural changes in the oat bran components before and after the *in vivo* digestion. The microscopic examination showed little subaleurone and aleurone cell wall materials. Oat bran remnants present in the digesta were composed almost entirely of the pericarp and seed coat layers. They could be identified based on the fluorescent characteristics of their lignin and phenolic contents. In addition to the undigested fibres, many crystalline clusters and some partially digested phytin globoids were revealed among the rest of the digesta. SEM-EDX microanalysis of these structures revealed two distinctly different elemental profiles (Figs. 3 & 4). It also showed that there was a slight increase in the calcium content of the partially digested phytin globoids (Fig. 4).

4 DISCUSSION

The analytical capability of fluorescence microscopy was demonstrated by examples given in the present study. The technique enables structural and chemical analyses to be conducted simultaneously. The detection of β-glucan-rich cell walls and phytin globoids

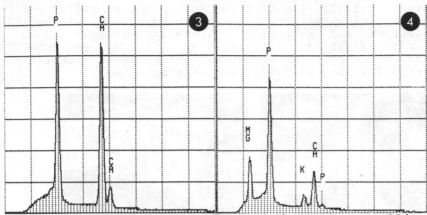

Figs. 3 & 4. EDX spectra of the undigested crystalline structures and phytin globoids, respectively.

in the structural components of oat bran indicated that both were not greatly affected by the impact of commercial processing. The absence of the former structures in the rat digesta suggested that most of their β-glucan content was degraded. Microscopic evidence indicated that the above degradation took place through the passage between the small and the large intestines of the rat (3). The detection of phytin globoids in the digesta implied poor digestibility of the former and the observation supported results of a previous study (4). Similarly, the detected crystalline structures probably represented unabsorbed minerals present in the diet. The present study has demonstrated the potential application of the techniques of SEM-EDX microanalysis which have the same advantage as that of fluorescence microscopy. The ability of the former techniques to determine the elemental composition of a given structure should prove to be a valuable tool for studying mineral and nutrient interactions in food.

REFERENCES

1. J.W. Anderson and W.J.L. Chen, Oats: Chemistry and Technology', AACC, Minnesota, 1986, 309.
2. W. Frølich and N.-G. Asp, Cereal Chem., 1985, 62,238.
3. S.H. Yiu and R. Mongeau, Food Microstruc., 1987, 6,143.
4. R.A. McCance and E.M. Widdowson, Biochem. J. 1935, 29,2694

DETERMINATION OF MOLYBDENUM IN PLASMA BY GRAPHITE FURNACE ATOMIC ABSORPTION SPECTROPHOTOMETRY

P.C. Morrice, Anya McNiven, W.R. Humphries and I. Bremner

Rowett Research Institute, Greenburn Road, Bucksburn, Aberdeen, AB2 9SB

1 INTRODUCTION

Molybdenum is present as a co-factor in several enzymes, including xanthine oxidase and sulphite oxidase, and is essential for optimum growth and performance in animals. However problems of molybdenum deficiency have rarely been encountered in animal husbandry and interest in this element has centred mainly on its toxicity, particularly with regard to its antagonistic effects on copper metabolism in ruminants. In recent investigations we have shown that growth and reproduction in cattle are severely impaired when copper deficiency has been induced by dietary molybdenum but not by iron or sulphur[1]. This suggests that identification of copper-deficient animals that are likely to benefit from copper supplementation requires some assessment of molybdenum exposure. Unfortunately current methods for the analysis of molybdenum in blood samples lack the necessary sensitivity or are subject to interference effects. In this report, a graphite furnace atomic absorption method (GF-AAS) for the analysis of molybdenum in plasma is described.

2 METHODS

Atomic absorption spectroscopy was carried out on a Pye Unicam PU 9000 instrument fitted with a PU 9095 Video Furnace Programmer and Auto-Sampler. All reagents were Analar grade. Plasma samples were obtained from cattle and sheep which had received diets with varying molybdenum contents.

Plasma samples (1 ml) were acid-digested with a mixture of conc. HNO_3:$HClO_4$:H_2SO_4 (2:1:0.5 ml) on an electric heating rack. Excess acid was then carefully boiled off and the residue was transferred with 10 ml distilled water to a Liddex Mixxor liquid-liquid extraction unit. Cresol red indicator was added and the pH adjusted to about 1.6 by the addition of 8M NH$_3$, whereupon 200 µl of a 5% solution of 8-hydroxyquinoline in 2M acetic acid was added.   After mixing,   the molybdenum-hydroxyquinoline complex was extracted into chloroform (5 ml).

An aliquot (2.5 ml) of the extract was removed and evaporated to dryness under N$_2$.   The residue was redissolved in 0.05M Tris-HCl,   pH 7.95 (0.5 ml),   allowing at least 2 hours for complete dissolution of the molybdenum.   The solution was then analysed for molybdenum by GF-AAS, using the conditions described in Table 1.

Table 1 Operating conditions for GF-AAS

Stage	Temp. (°C)	Time (sec)	Ramp
Dry	130	40	5
Ash	1000	20	2
Atomise	2800	3	0
'Burn off'	3000	3	0

3 RESULTS AND DISCUSSION

Although standard solutions of molybdenum can be analyzed directly by GF-AAS,   unsatisfactory results are obtained with ovine and bovine plasma,   with poor and variable recoveries for internal standards.   These ranged from 15-120%,   with a mean value ($\pm$ SEM) of 74 $\pm$ 18%.   Equally poor recoveries were obtained with dry ashed plasma samples,   indicating that the interference factors were of inorganic composition.   The extraction procedure obviated this problem and recoveries increased to 94 $\pm$ 1% when plasma samples were spiked with 50 ng molybdenum/ml.   The relationship between absorbance values and molybdenum concentrations is shown in Fig. 1.   The coefficient of variation for plasma molybdenum estimations was 8% and the limit of detection was 4 ng/ml.

Care was needed during the acid digestion procedure to prevent volatilisation of molybdenum-chlorine derivatives.   In extreme cases, when the acid was boiled off over a bunsen burner, as much as 80% of the molybdenum could be lost.   The temperature of the acid digest was therefore kept below 300°.

Effective atomisation of the molybdenum during GF-AAS required a rapid heating step in which a temperature of 2800° was attained.   No ramp mode was therefore used in the atomisation step.   Since a small amount of molybdenum remained on the rod after this step, a final "burn-off" at 3000° was essential before application of the next sample.

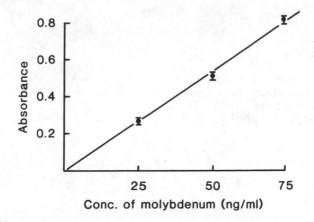

<u>Figure 1.</u>   Standard curve for analysis of molybdenum by GF–AAS.

The precision and accuracy of the method was confirmed by analysis of an NBS standard reference bovine serum with an authenticated molybdenum concentration of 16 ± 4 ng/ml.   The concentration determined by this method was 19 ± 1 ng/ml.

The value of the method is evident from the changes in plasma molybdenum levels in sheep which were given for one week a diet containing supplements of 0, 2, 5 or 10 mg molybdenum/kg. The concentrations in plasma were 4 ± 1,   32 ± 7, 87 ± 11 and 211 ± 35g ng/ml respectively.

REFERENCES

1.   I. Bremner, W.R. Humphries, M. Phillippo, M.J. Walker and P.C. Morrice, <u>Anim. Prod.</u>, 1987, <u>45</u>, 403.

NBS STANDARD REFERENCE MATERIALS FOR VALIDATING DETERMINATIONS OF MICRONUTRIENTS AND TOXIC SUBSTANCES IN FOODS

R. Alvarez

National Bureau of Standards
Office of Standard Reference Materials
Rm. B316 Chemistry Bldg.
Gaithersburg, MD 20899, U.S.A.

1 INTRODUCTION

Instrumental methods for determining nutrients and potentially hazardous substances in foods and other biological materials have generally replaced older, more time-consuming procedures. Because the instruments are usually calibrated with laboratory synthetic standards the accuracy of the results depends on the reliability of the standards. If the constituents of interest and matrix components are of questionable purity, the analytical determinations, especially of trace nutrients, and hazardous constituents will be suspect. In addition to instrument calibration problems, inaccurate data may result from faulty experimental techniques. The difficulty in obtaining accurate data is evident from discrepant data obtained when a homogeneous milk powder was analyzed by a number of laboratories[1]. One approach towards validating experimental data is through the use of certified reference materials (CRM's) issued by a number of national and international organizations. In the United States, the National Bureau of Standards is responsible for issuing CRM's which are called Standard Reference Materials (SRM's) for historical reasons.

2 NBS FOOD STANDARD REFERENCE MATERIALS

Inorganic Constituents

NBS issues approximately 900 SRM's most of which are certified for chemical composition. Table 1 lists elements for which a certified concentration is given in the Certificate of Analysis of at least one of the SRM's.

Table 1   Certified Elemental Concentrations in the NBS Food SRM's

Element	Non-Fat Milk Powder, SRM 1549	Wheat Flour, SRM 1567a	Rice Flour, SRM 1568a	Bovine Liver, SRM 1577a
Aluminum	(2)	5.7	4.4	(2)
Arsenic	(0.0019)	(0.0006)	0.29	0.047
Cadmium	0.0005	0.026	0.022	0.44
Calcium	1.30%	0.0191%	0.0118%	120
Chlorine	1.09%	(565)	(300)	0.28%
Chromium	0.0026	----	----	----
Cobalt	(0.0041)	(0.006)	(0.018)	0.21
Copper	0.7	2.1	2.4	158
Iodine	3.38	(0.0009)	(0.009)	----
Iron	1.78	14.1	7.4	194
Lead	0.019	(<0.020)	(<0.010)	0.135
Magnesium	0.120%	0.040%	0.056%	600
Manganese	0.26	9.4	20.0	9.9
Mercury	0.0003	(0.0005)	0.0058	0.004
Molybdenum	(0.34)	0.48	1.46	3.5
Phosphorus	1.06%	0.134%	0.153%	1.11%
Potassium	1.69%	0.133%	0.1280%	0.996%
Rubidium	(11)	(0.7)	6.14	12.5
Selenium	0.11	1.1	0.38	0.71
Silver	(0.0003)	----	----	0.04
Sodium	0.497%	6.1	6.6	0.243%
Strontium	----	----	----	0.138
Sulfur	0.351%	0.165%	0.120%	0.78%
Uranium	----	(0.0003)	0.0003	0.00071
Zinc	46	11.6	19.4	123

1. Concentrations in μg/g or, where noted, in percent by weight.
2. Values in parentheses are not certified.
3. SRM 1568a is the renewal for SRM 1568, which is presently being issued.

    Certified concentrations are based on the results of either two or more independent analytical methods or, in the case of SRM 1577a, also on the results of definitive methods. A definitive method is the highest accuracy method available for a constituent. Methods based on isotope dilution mass spectrometry are examples of such methods. These IDMS methods were used for the determination of lead, rubidium, strontium, uranium, and vanadium.

In addition to the food SRM's in Table 1, a Brewer's
Yeast (SRM 1569), certified for its Cr content is available. An oyster tissue (SRM 1566a) is being analyzed for
issue later this year. Analysis of a Total Diet (SRM
1548) for inorganic and organic constituents is also in
progress. A Corn Kernel (SRM 8413) is available.

Organic Constituents

    The certificate of analysis for Cholesterol and Fat-
Soluble Vitamins in Coconut Oil, SRM 1563, provides
certified concentrations of cholesterol, retinyl acetate,
ergocalciferol, and dl-α-tocopheryl acetate in a fortified coconut oil.
    Whole Egg Powder, SRM 1845, is being analyzed for
its cholesterol content by an isotope dilution mass
spectrometric procedure.

3 SRM's FOR METABOLIC STUDIES

    Bovine Serum, SRM 1598, which is similar to human
serum, has been analyzed and the data is being evaluated.
At present, 13 elements are proposed for certification.
They are: Al, Cd, Co, Cr, Cu, Fe, Mg, Mn, Mo, Ni, Rb,
Se, and Zn.
    A Freeze-Dried Urine, SRM 2670, certified for a
number of elements at two different levels is available.

4 MISCELLANEOUS FOOD REFERENCE MATERIALS IN PROGRESS

    Twelve food materials have been processed under the
direction of Milan Ihnat, Agriculture Canada, for analysis
by cooperating laboratories for distribution by NBS.

5 RECOMMENDATIONS

    The certificates for the SRM's provide certified
total concentrations for constituents. The miscellane-
ous food RM's should be considered for collaborative
bioavailability analyses. Please write M. Ihnat or
R. Alvarez.

    REFERENCES

1. R. Dybzynski, A. Veglia, and O. Suschny, Report on
    the Intercomparison run A-11 for the determination of
    inorganic constituents in milk powder, 1980, Inter-
    national Atomic Energy Agency, Vienna, Austria.

TRENDS IN THE DAILY DIETARY INTAKE OF MINOR AND TRACE ELEMENTS BY HUMAN SUBJECTS: AN ANALYTICAL APPRAISAL

C. V. Iyengar

NBS/USDA
Gaithersburg, MD 20899
United States of America

1   INTRODUCTION

Food analysis laboratories have been slow in recognizing
the role of reference materials (RM) for analytical
quality control (QC), and even commonly available biological RMs are not frequently used for QC in such
laboratories.   In turn there is slow progress in generating specific RMs of dietary matrices[1].   Most of the QC
of inorganic analysis of food materials has been carried
out only recently.   The periods before 1970, from 1970
to 1980, and from 1980 onwards represent three phases in
the analysis of foods;   unresolved analytical problems,
improvements in analytical techniques, and a better
analytical insight coupled with the use of certified RMs,
respectively.

2   DIETARY INTAKE DATA

Dietary inorganic analysis data from selected sources are
presented in Table 1.   The ICRP-23[2] evaluation, which may
be regarded as a check point for earlier intake estimations,
summarizes the data recorded until the late sixties.
Subsequent studies carried out in the U.K.[3] and in Finland[4]
illustrate the efforts undertaken in the seventies.
These reflect an improved understanding of the analytical
techniques applied for food analysis, supported by efforts
to evaluate their precision and accuracy by analyzing
biological RMs.   Thus, several gross over-estimations
in earlier studies were exposed.

The review[5] in 1982 serves as another check point
of daily dietary intakes on a global basis. In the seventies, analytical improvements contributed to the

quantification of an increased number of trace elements.
However, a valid comparison of analytical data even for
diets derived from similar geographical background[5] was
restricted to a few elements such as Cu, Fe, Zn and Mn.
Not surprisingly, the problem related to several trace
elements occurring at ppb level remained controversial.

The examples chosen as a model for recent investigations in this area[6,7] represent a combination of
established analytical procedures and stringent steps to
ensure QC by frequent analysis of "appropriate dietary"
reference materials.   This phase highlights the understanding of specific matrix related problems in dealing
with different kinds of foods[8] by way of developing single
and composite type of dietary RMs[9] and the development of
several element-specific assays. For example, the use of
neutron activation analysis in conjunction with mass
spectrometry (NAA-MS), a recently developed technique[10],
has shed more light on the intake of Li, indicating
further improvements over 1979 estimates. Further, consistent dietary intake data are emerging for Al, As, Cd,
Cr, Mo, Si and Sn, among others.

Among the minor elements Ca, Cl, K, Mg, Na, P and S,
only S shows an elevated value for the example reflecting
U.S. diet in Table 1(6). This is due to the high protein
content which amounts to about 105 g in the daily diet of
a 25 to 30 year old American male.

3 GENERAL COMMENTS

The above examples have been chosen to reflect analytical
considerations only.   The results from Ref. 6 are from a
single collection, prepared with great care.   Extensive
QC procedures were adopted to set guidelines for preparing
total mixed diet samples.   Several analytical methods
have been used to cover the range of elements shown in
Table 1 under the column reference 6. A detailed evaluation of all the results and associated analytical uncertain-
ties is in progress.   The ICRP-23 listing has been used
as a basis for grouping the elements under g, mg and μg
as shown in Table 1.   Gross errors in some earlier
estimations can be readily noticed as they differ from
recent assessments by orders of magnitude.

On the whole, this survey revealed several trends.
In contrast to the earlier estimates in daily dietary
intakes of trace elements, decreases by factors of 2 for
Cu, 2 - 5 for Cr, 5 - 10 for Cd, Hg and Pb, and $>$10 for Ag,
As, Co, Li, Sb and V could be identified. In specific
cases, the decline of total intake can partly be linked

Table 1   Dietary Intake of Minor and Trace Elements:
Examples reflecting analytical improvements

El.		1975(1)	1979(2)	1980(3)	1982(4)	1987(5,6)
Ca	g/d	1.1	1.4	1.5	1.1(0.4-1.4)	0.84
Cl		5.2	5.4		5.8(5.2-6.6)	4.62
K		3.3	2.8		3.3(1.6-4.1)	3.12
Mg		0.34	0.25	0.44	0.4(0.2-0.74)	0.31
Na		4.4	4.6		4.5**(2.5-6.7)**	3.20
P		1.4	1.87		1.4(1.2-1.9)	1.63
S		0.85	0.94		0.9(0.85-1.2)	1.40
Al	mg/d	45	2.33	6.7	10(1-45)	14.3
As		1	<0.05	0.06	0.1(0.01-1.0)	0.05
B		1.3	2.82	1.7	1.3(0.4-2.8)	1.52
Br		7.5	8.4	4.2	4(0.8-8.4)	6.80
Cu		3.5	3.1	1.7	2.5(1.0-5.8)	1.50
F		1.8	0.5	0.56	2(0.4-4.5)	*
Fe		16	23.3	19	16(9-23)	15.7
Li		2.0	0.11		0.1(<0.1-2.0)	0.03
Mn		3.7	2.7	6.1	4(2-8.7)	2.70
Rb		2.2	4.35	5.6	2(1.6-4.4)	2.80
Si		3.5		29	?(18-46)	26.5
Sr		1.9	0.86		1.5(1-4)	1.40
Sn		4.0	0.19		1(0.2-4.0)	2.00
V		2.0			?(0.<01-0.02)	0.01
Zn		15	14.3		13(8-15)	16.3
Zr		4.2				<0.005
Ag	µg/d	70	27		20(2-70)	4.5
Au			<7		0.1(0.01-2)?	0.5
Ba		750	603		500(440-1600)	58
Cd		150	64	13	40(10-150)	15.5
Ce					?(16-240)?	<15
Cs		10	13		13(10-31)	9.5
Cr		150	320		50(10-320)	37
Co		300			20(10-300)	18
Hg		15	<16		10(3-60)	3
I		200	220		200?	300
Mo		300	128	120	200(70-300)	130
Ni		400	<300	130	400(200-600)?	170
Pb		440	320	66	300(60-550)	52
Sb			34		15(2-34)	5
Sc					0.1(0.04-1.0)	<0.5
Se		150	200	30	150(30-560)	130
Th		3	<0.5			1.0
Ti		850	800			*
Tl		1.5	<2			<2
U		1.9	1		1.5(1-4.5)	1.8
W			<1		10(<1-34)?	6

*
not determined, diet handled with teflon and titanium

Table 2   Some Biological and Dietary RMs for Zinc

Matrix	Code	Con.[a]	Error(%)[b]
Oyster tissue	NBS-SRM-1566	852	1.6
Aquatic plant	BCR-CRM-061	566	2.3
Pepperbush	NIES-CRM-1	340	5.9
Aquatic plant	BCR-CRM-060	313	2.6
Horse kidney	IAEA-H-8	193	3.1
Lobster	NRCC-TORT-1	177	5.6
Human hair	NIES-CRM-5	169	5.9
Copepod	IAEA-MA-A-1	158	1.3
Mussel tissue	IAEA-MA-M-2	156.5 (R)	4.4
Bovine liver	NBS-SRM-1577a	123	6.5
Mussel	NIES-CRM-6	106	5.6
Animal bone	IAEA-H-5	89	5.9
Animal muscle	IAEA-H-4	86	3.9
Tomato leaves	NBS-SRM-1573	62	9.7
Milk powder(spiked)	BCR-CRM-151	50.4 (NC)	
Spinach	NBS-SRM-1570	50	4.0
Milk powder(spiked)	BCR-CRM-150	49.5 (NC)	
Milk powder	NBS-SRM-1549	46.1	4.8
Milk powder	BCR-CRM-063	42 (NC)	
Milk powder	IAEA-A-11	38.9	5.9
Fish flesh	IAEA-MA-A-2	33	3.0
Corn stack	NBS-RM-8412	(32) (I)	
Kale	Bowen's kale	32.3	8.5
Citrus leaves	NBS-SRM-1572	29	6.9
Mixed human diet	IAEA-H-9	27.5	6.4
Orchard leaves	NBS-SRM-1571	25	6.0
Hay powder	IAEA-V-10	24	13
Chlorella	NIES-CRM-3	20.5	4.9
Rice flour	NBS-SRM-1568	19.4	4.9
Mixed human diet	NBS-RM-8431	17 (R)	3.5
Olive leaves	BCR-CRM-062	16	4.4
Korn kernel	NBS-RM-8413	(15.7) (I)	
Albacore tuna	NBS-RM-50	13.6 (I)	7.4
Animal blood	IAEA-A-13	13	7.7
Wheat flour	NBS-SRM-1567a	11.6	3.5
Rye flour	IAEA-V-8	2.5	13
Serum	KL-146-II	2.1 (R)	25
Serum	KL-146-I	1.5 (R)	15
Bovine serum	NBS-RM-8419	1.1	9
Serum	NYE-164	0.72	

a)   b)
   mg/kg or mg/L   at 95 % confidence interval

to environmental regulations, e.g., depletion of Pb from gasoline. A reversal is seen in the case of Si, with recent estimations being higher than the ICRP value (Table 1). This may be attributed to the analytical improvements in the determination of Si in biological materials, especially after the introduction of Inductively Coupled Plasma Atomic Emission Spectrophotometry.

4 CONCLUSIONS

There is a need for developing carefully prepared and well characterized certified dietary RMs, e.g., individual food matrices with varying fat, starch, protein, phytate and fiber contents, as well as a few mixed diet combinations of these foods.

Importantly, food analysis laboratories should use the available biological and dietary reference materials on a regular basis to demonstrate the reliability of the analytical findings. Unless the QC component is answered satisfactorily, the data generated have very little use in answering questions on mineral nutrition and environmental contamination aspects of public health.

REFERENCES

1. G.V. Iyengar, Sci. Total Environ. 1986, 53, 1.
2. 'The Reference Man', ICRP-23, Pergamon Press, New York, 1975.
3. E. I. Hamilton, 'The Chemical Elements and Man', Charles C. Thomas, Springfield, IL, 1979.
4. P. Koivistoinen, Acta Agriculturae Scandinavica, 1980, Supplement 22.
5. H.J.M. Bowen, Environmental Chemistry, Special Publication of the Royal Society of Chemistry, London, 1982, Vol.2, 70.
6. G.V. Iyengar, J.T. Tanner, W.R. Wolf, R. Zeisler, Sci. Total Environ., 61, 235 (1987), and unpublished additional results, 1988.
7. R.M. Parr, IAEA Co-ordinated Project on Daily Dietary Intake of Minor and Trace Elements by Human Subjects, IAEA, Vienna, 1988.
8. G.V.Iyengar, Clin. Nutr., 1987, 6, 105.
9. W.R.Wolf, 'Biological Reference Materials' Wiley & Sons, New York, 1985.
10. W.B.Clarke, M.Koekebakker, R.D.Barr, R.G.Downing, R.F.Fleming, Appl. Radiat. Isot., 1987, 38, 735.

EDITORIAL NOTE: This extended paper covers 2 conference presentations.

DEVELOPMENT OF AN ENZYME-LINKED IMMUNOSORBENT ASSAY FOR METALLOTHIONEIN

A. Ghaffar, P.J. Aggett and I. Bremner

Rowett Research Institute, Greenburn Road, Bucksburn, Aberdeen, AB2 9SB

1 INTRODUCTION

Metallothionein (MT) plays important roles in the homeostatic control of zinc and copper metabolism. It is mainly an intracellular protein but is present also in plasma and urine, in amounts that are related to tissue MT concentrations. It has been suggested that assay of MT in these fluids, or in blood cells, can be used in the assessment of trace element status and particularly in the diagnosis of zinc deficiency[1]. The concentrations of MT in these fluids are relatively low and at present can only be measured by immunoassay. The radioimmunoassay developed in these laboratories for rat MT-I has a detection limit of 1-2 ng/ml, is suitable for all metalloforms of MT but is specific for the isoprotein MT-I from rat[2]. It cannot be used to measure any isoform of human MT.

Although the radioimmunoassays for MT are generally very sensitive, they have the disadvantage that they are time-consuming and require regular production of radioactive tracers. A fluorimetric enzyme-linked immunosorbent assay (ELISA), which takes only one day to complete and has similar sensitivity to the radioimmunoassays, has recently been reported[3]. In this paper we describe an alternative colorimetric ELISA, which requires only a few hours and is suitable for measurement of MT in tissues and fluids from most animal species, including man.

2 MATERIALS AND METHODS

The antiserum used in the ELISA was raised in sheep immunized with a conjugate of rat liver MT-I and rabbit IgG[2]. Rabbit anti-sheep immunoglobulin-peroxidase conjugate was from Dako Ltd. Microwell modules (NUNC immunoplates) were obtained

74

from Gibco Europe Ltd.

Plate sensitization.   The wells in the microwell modules
were sensitized with 50 μl of a solution of human MT in 100 mM
$Na_2CO_3/NaHCO_3$ buffer,   pH 9.6 (100 ng MT/ml).   Plates were
incubated at 4° overnight whereupon the solution was decanted and
the wells washed three times with 10 mM phosphate buffer, pH 7.4,
containing 0.15 M NaCl and 0.05% Triton X-405.   A solution of
bovine serum albumin (200 μl;   5% w/v) was then added to each
well and left for 30 min at room temperature before decantation.
Plates were dried at 37°, sealed and stored.

ELISA procedure.   Dilutions of samples and standards were
made in 200 mM phosphate buffer, pH 7.2, containing 0.15 M NaCl,
0.01% merthiolate and 1% BSA.   To each well was added 50 μl of
MT solution (standard or sample) and 50 μl of primary antibody
(1:8000 dilution).   After mixing and incubation for 30 min, the
solutions were decanted, the wells were washed 5 times and then
treated with 100 μl of secondary antibody-peroxidase conjugate
(1:1000 dilution) in 20 mM phosphate/150 mM NaCl (pH 7.2)
containing 0.1% BSA and 0.05% 8-anilino-1-naphthalene sulphonic
acid.   After a further incubation for 30 min, decantation and
repeated washing, each well was treated with 100 μl of
2',2''-azino-bis-3-(ethylbenzthiazoline)-sulphonic   acid   in
citrate buffer, pH 4.0 (0.6 mg/ml).   After incubation for 15 min
reaction was stopped by the addition of 1.5% NaF and the
absorbance at 405 nm was measured on a microplate reader.

3 RESULTS

A typical standard curve for the ELISA is illustrated in
Figure 1.   The working range for the assay was from 10 to 500
ng/ml and equivalent responses were obtained for zinc- and
cadmium-MT, and for both main isoforms, MT-I and MT-II.
Complete cross-reactivities were also obtained with rat, pig and
dog MT, confirming that the ELISA was less specific than the RIA,
even though the same antiserum was used in both assays.   That
the ELISA was suitable for the measurement of MT in biological
samples was confirmed by setting up standard curves for MT in
samples of urine, plasma and lysates of erythrocytes (Figure 2).
The coincidence of the standard curves suggests that the
cross-reactivity was not affected by components in these fluids.
In addition excellent recoveries were obtained for internal
standards, the values for plasma and urine being 93-106 and
88-98% respectively.

Typical MT concentrations in plasma and erythrocyte
lysates from adult females were 75 ± 7 ng/ml and 234 ± 12 ng/g
haemoglobin respectively.

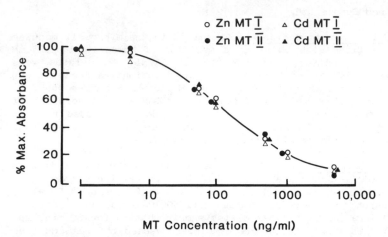

Figure 1.   Standard curve for assay of human MT.   The maximum absorbance is from wells containing no added MT.

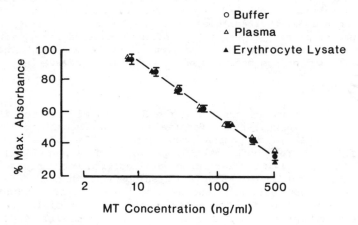

Figure 2.   Dilution curves for human MT solutions in buffer, plasma and blood cell lysates.

REFERENCES

1.   I. Bremner and J.N.   Morrison, in 'Essential and Toxic Trace Elements in Human Health and Disease' (A.S.   Prasad, ed.), Alan R. Liss, Inc., New York, 1988, p. 365.
2.   R.K. Mehra and I. Bremner, Biochem. J., 1983, 213, 459.
3.   D.G. Thomas, H.J. Linton and J.S. Garvey, J. Immunol. Methods, 1986, 89, 239.

Evaluation of the Vitamin B₆ content in foods by HPLC analysis.*)

R. Bitsch and J. Moeller

Department of Home Economics, Nutrition Section,
University of Paderborn,
D-4790 Paderborn, W.-Germany

INTRODUCTION

Since the existing data on Vit.B₆ content of foods are based mainly on microbiological analyses these are not too much reliable. The recommendations for the daily required Vit.B₆ intake of man founding on these data are, therefore, uncertain up to now.

The lack of reliable data on Vit.B₆ content of food is also remarked by the US Food and Nutrition Board in the recommended dietary allowances (RDA) 1980.

Thus, there is need for a new evaluation of the data on the Vit.B₆ content in food tables by using improved assay methods which lead to a safer basis of the RDA. HPLC methods enable a fast and quantitative separation of B₆ vitamers.

Objectives

A modified HPLC method was used in order to evaluate the content of B₆ vitamers in several foods and to quantify their turnover under varying conditions of storing and processing. The method is based on a ion-pair elution technique on reversed phase following fluorescence detection after derivatisation by bisulfite as first described by (1) and (2). Modifications relate to the elution technique and the extraction procedure. Details of the method are communicated elsewhere (3).

*) Supported by Deutsche Forschungsgemeinschaft, grant
   Bi 218/5-1

.esults and Discussion

By the used HPLC procedure a complete separation of phosphorylated and nonphosphorylated B_6 vitamers as well as the inactive pyridoxic acid is achieved except pyridoxolphosphate (PNP).

In food samples with complex matrices, however, the resolution of PLP having the shortest retention time near to the elution front may be inadequate. For better verification a sample duplicate can be treated with alkaline phosphatase leading to a disappearance of phosphorylated and an enhancement of unphosphorylated derivatives as to be seen in liver (fig. 1).

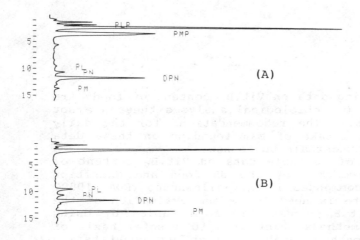

Fig. 1 chromatogram of raw pork liver before (A) and after (B) treatment with alkaline phosphatase

Heating of milk leads depending on the duration to a partly drastic decrease of the whole B_6 content (table 1).

In the rather long heated sterilized milk the B_6 content has diminished to about 50% as compared with the raw product. Processing of milk generally seems to reduce the B_6 content since there are no distinct differences between the 3 commercial products. Regarding the single vitamers heating leads mainly to a decrease of PL, PLP and PNS, whereas PMP is even increasing and PN as well as PM remain nearly unchanged.

Table 1: content of B₆ vitamers in milk (µg/100 g)

B₆ derivatives	raw milk	pasteurized milk	UHT milk	sterilized milk
pyridoxalphosphate (PLP)	9,63	5,83	1,15	0
pyridoxaminphosphate(PMP)	3,02	2,86	4,14	9,34
pyridoxal (PL)	30,23	19,64	19,70	10,15
pyridoxamin (PM)	4,00	3,04	3,33	4,55
pyridoxol (PN)	2,09	1,18	1,18	1,31
pyridoxic acid (PNS)	18,28	12,02	11,34	9,31
total B₆ activity	67,25	44,57	40,84	34,66

When comparing to data given in food tables the total B₆ content is corresponding to our results only after the inactive pyridoxic acid is added.

On the other hand the main B₆ components of banana are PN and PM, exceeding the content of PL and PLP by 3 to 4 times, PMP and PNS are negligible or totally absent. Ripening of the fruits during storage enhances the vitamin content by about 13% obviously caused by de novo biosynthesis of PN since no major changes appear among the other derivatives (table 2).

Table 2: content of B₆ vitamers in banana (µ/100g)

B₆ derivatives	banana unripe	banana ripened	banana overripe
pyridoxalphosphate (PLP)	31,23	25,01	23,16
pyridoxaminphosphate (PMP)	2,30	0	0
pyridoxal (PL)	37,13	34,71	36,71
pyridoxamin (PM)	122,11	130,17	132,96
pyridoxol (PN)	103,60	147,25	145,02
pyridoxic acid (PNS)	0	0	0
total B₆ activity	296,37	337,14	337,85

The used HPLC method seems to be suitable for investigating the alteration of B₆ derivatives in foods under varying conditions leading to a more valid basis for the RDA of man.

REFERENCES
1. S.P. Coburn and J. D. Mahuren, Methods in Enzymol., 1986, 122, 102
2. F.F. Gregory and D. Feldstein, J. Agric.Food Chem. 1985, 33, 359
3. J. Moeller and R. Bitsch, Lebensmittelchem. Gerichtl. Chem. 1988, 42, 71

Analysis of Cis-Beta-Carotenes in Food and Colorant Additives

S.J. Schwartz and G.L. Catignani

Department of Food Science, Box 7624
North Carolina State University
Raleigh, North Carolina 27695   USA

The naturally occurring configuration of beta-carotene in plant foods generally occurs as an all-trans isomer. As a provitamin A nutrient, the all-trans compound possesses the highest bioavailability relative to the cis configurations in rats (1) and presumably humans. The cis isomeric composition increases with food processing particularly heating and the quantity formed appears related to the severity and extent of heat treatment . The structures of the predominate cis-isomers found in foods are the 13 and 9-mono-cis isomers (2,3).

The widespread use of processed foods as a part of daily diets implies that the consumption of cis- beta-carotene isomers is prevalent. The biological significance and metabolism of these compounds in humans and animals is largely unknown. Moreover, the presence of cis-beta-carotenes in plant foods suggests that consumption of other cis-carotenes and carotenoids possessing altered bioactivity are also abundant. Lack of analytical data, however, precludes the use of this information in both food composition tables and nutrition labels.

Compositional studies in our laboratory are based on HPLC methodology developed by Tsukida et al (4) using calcium hydroxide stationary supports with detection at 436 nm. This wavelength is used since it is close to an isobestic point for the predominate isomers, thus allowing for quantitation of cis-forms based on the molar absorbtivity of the all-trans compound. The moisture content, type and particle size of calcium hydroxide is critical in order to obtain packed columns with satisfactory resolution. Reversed phase HPLC on a commercially available columns (Vydac TP201) can be used to resolve cis isomers (5), however, better resolution can be achieved on properly prepared calcium hydroxide columns. The identity and geometrical configuration of the isomers were confirmed in this study by mass spectral and 250 MHz NMR analysis after isolation by preparative HPLC. Typical chromatograms as well as conditions for the preparation of HPLC columns and chromatographic separation are published elsewhere (2,3,5).

Table 1 lists the composition of isomers found in selected plant foods, naturally derived and synthetic colorant preparations. Beta-carotene derived from Dunaliella algae contained a relatively high content of isomers. Presumably, the formation of these high levels of isomers arise via a photochemical mechanism but their formation may be biosynthetic (6). The fact that multiple cis-isomers co-exist with the all-trans compound suggests that some cis forms arise via post harvest handling of the algae. The food colorant preparations (beadlets and oil based) are both derived from synthetic all-trans beta-carotene. As shown in Table 1, marked differences in isomeric composition were found dependent upon the carrier medium. This study demonstrates that processed vegetables and food colorants may contain a significant portion of their beta-carotene in a form that is less bioavailable than would be indicated by current assay procedures.

Table 1.   Isomeric composition (percent) of beta-carotene
           preparations.

	13-cis	trans	9-cis
Sweet potato (raw)	5	95	-
Processed sweet potato (canned)	15	75	9
Beta-carotene beadlets (water dispersible)	34	35	31
Beta-carotene (in oil)	7	93	-
Algae extract (Dunaliella species)	28	30	42

References

1. S.J. Sweeney and A.C. Marsh, J. Am. Diet. Assoc., 1971, 59,
    238.
2. L.C. Chandler and S.J. Schwartz, J. Agric. Food Chem., 1988,
    36, 129.
3. L.C. Chandler and S.J. Schwartz, J. Food Sci., 1987, 52, 669.
4. K. Tsukida, K. Saiki, T.Takii and Y. Koyama, J. Chromatogr.,
    1982, 245, 359.
5. F.W. Quakenbush, J. Liq. Chromatogr. 1987, 10, 643.
6. A. Ben-Amotz, A. Katz and A. Mordhay, J. Phycol., 1982, 18,
    529.

BIOSPECIFIC ANALYSIS OF VITAMINS

M. R. A. MORGAN, P. M. FINGLAS, S. ALCOCK, H. C. MORRIS and R. M. FAULKS

AFRC Institute of Food Research
Norwich Laboratory
Colney Lane
Norwich, NR4 7UA
U.K.

1 INTRODUCTION

The widespread adoption of nutritional labelling has created a substantial demand for vitamin analysis. Unfortunately, independent assessment has found that fully validated and accepted methodology for the determination of a number of vitamins is not available[1]. We have, therefore, been involved in the development of more acceptable methods.

The use of biospecific methods of analysis such as non-isotopic immunoassays (employing antibodies) or protein binding methods (employing natural binding proteins) can offer a number of advantages to the food analyst. These have clearly been demonstrated already in a number of areas, notable examples being the trace analysis of mycotoxins[2] and the determination of soya protein in meat products[3]. At the forefront of the benefits are the specificity and sensitivity, the rapid through-put of large numbers of samples and the comparatively low cost of equipment associated with the technical simplicity of the procedures.

We have now developed and validated methods in a variety of foods for the quantification of biotin,[4] pantothenic acid,[5,6] folate,[7] B_6 group and vitamin B_{12}. These procedures are all based on the microtitration plate format using enzymes as markers.

2 CONVENTIONAL VITAMIN ASSAYS

Conventional methods of routine analysis are most commonly of the microbiological type, dependent on the degree of stimulation of growth of specific organisms in the presence of vitamin in the food extracts. Such methods are invariably lengthy, can be subject to interferences and high variability, and in some instances are known to be of doubtful quantitative value. In addition, microbiological methods often require careful, subjective interpretation.

HPLC methods have been adopted in certain instances (e.g. for the determination of thiamin and riboflavin[8], and the B_6 group[1]) and can provide a powerful analytical tool, though initial capital and recurrent costs are high.

3 COMPARISON OF BIOSPECIFIC AND CONVENTIONAL METHODS

As part of the validation programme for the biospecific methods of analysis that we have developed, results have been compared with those obtained by conventional procedures and with data presented in U.K. Food Tables[9]. Agreement has been extremely good. For example, the results obtained by the immunoassay for pantothenate content of six foods gave a correlation coefficient, r, of 0.999 compared to those obtained by microbiological assay, and also Food Table values[6]. A binding protein assay for folate applied to 14 types of raw and cooked vegetables produced results that gave a correlation coefficient of 0.940 with those obtained by microbiological assay[7].

In these and other examples, the antibody/binding protein assays possessed higher sensitivities and specificities, were more rapid and showed potential for high sample through-puts compared to conventional procedures.

4 CURRENT RESEARCH

Primary aims of the current work are to widen the range of vitamins covered and to increase their use by undertaking collaborative trials and ring tests. Research applications already undertaken using the methodlogy include investigations into the effects of conventional cooking of pantothenate content of chicken[10] and cook-chill on folate content of hospital meals[11]. Future work will include investigations into vitamin stability during other types of food processing (such as microwave cooking and irradiation) and during food storage.

5 FUTURE DEVELOPMENTS - BIOAVAILABILITY

The nutritional value of vitamins in foods depends both upon the concentration of biologically active forms present, and upon their availability for absorption and utilisation by normal metabolic pathways.

At present the developed methods have been designed to assay comparable vitamin forms to the conventional procedures. For example, a "total" amount is usually determined following enzymic hydrolysis of covalently bound material. These determinations are often carried out with little or no information on the likely bioavailability of such material, or its potential contribution to vitamin levels in the body.

It is hoped that the high sample through-put, combined with sensitivity and specificity of the biospecific techniques will enable the appropriate experiments to be performed to add to our knowledge in this important area.

REFERENCES

1. G. Brubacher, W. Muller-Mulot and D.A.T. Southgate "Methods for the Determination of Vitamins in food", Elsev. App. Sci. Publ., London, 1985.
2. M.R.A. Morgan, A.S. Kang and H.W.-S. Chan, J. Sci. Food Agric., 1986, 37, 908.
3. J.H. Rittenburg, A. Adams, J. Palmer and J.C. Allen, J. Assoc. Off. Anal. Che., 1987, 70, 582.
4. P.M. Finglas, R.M. Faulks and M.R.A. Morgan, J. Micronutr. Anal., 1986, 2, 247.
5. H.C. Morris, P.M. Finglas, R.M. Faulks and M.R.A. Morgan, J. Micronutr. Anal., 1988, 4, 33.
6. P.M. Finglas, R.M. Faulks, H.C. Morris, K.J. Scott and M.R.A. Morgan, J. Micronutr. Anal., 1988, 4, 47.
7. P.M. Finglas, C. Kwiatkowska, R.M. Faulks and M.R.A. Morgan, J. Micronutr. Anal., 1988, in press.
8. P.M. Finglas and R.M. Faulks, Food Chem., 1984, 15, 37.
9. A.A. Paul and D.A.T. Southgate, McCance and Widdowson's "The Composition of Foods", 4th Ed., HMSO, London, 1978.
10. G. Bertlesen, P.M. Finglas, J. Loughridge, R.M. Faulks and M.R.A. Morgan, Human Nutr.: Food Sciences and Nutr., 1988, in press.
11. V. Beamish, P.M. Finglas, M.R.A. Morgan and R.M. Faulks, unpublished results.

The Importance of Speciation

THE SIGNIFICANCE OF SPECIATION FOR PREDICTING MINERAL BIOAVAILABILITY

W. van Dokkum

TNO-CIVO Toxicology and Nutrition Institute
Zeist
The Netherlands

1 INTRODUCTION

It is well documented that various factors may influence mineral bioavailability. Of particular interest are those factors that play a
role during the pre-absorptive stage, i.e. during the digestion process. Various intraluminal interactions occur, such as adsorption of
minerals to macro-nutrients, binding of minerals to other components
and inclusions. In addition, reduction and oxidation reactions will
take place. The net result of all these interactions is decisive for a
mineral to be available for the actual absorption process. Knowledge
of the valence state and the chemical "environment" of any mineral may
contribute to the understanding and prediction of the (bio)avail-
ability of minerals and trace elements. The term (element) "speciation" has been introduced for the determination of the chemical form
of a mineral, including the valence state, the metal-ligand complexes
and mineral compounds. Although speciation seems particularly meaningful for the elements present in food and in the gastrointestinal contents, knowledge of the biochemical nature of minerals and trace
elements in the post-absorptive stage may be relevant for predicting
the metabolic behaviour of a certain metal. For the latter case the
term **"biochemical** speciation" has been suggested[1]. Even the term
"metabolic speciation" might be used, indicating to which extent a
metal can be biotransformed into a metabolically active species.
The significance of speciation of metals in food has been recognized
during the past decades for toxic elements, such as mercury, tin and
lead, of which the organometallic derivatives are more toxic than the
inorganic species. Regarding the essential elements, speciation of
iron (haem iron versus non-haem iron) is the best known example. However, in many cases knowledge of the chemical form of any metal in
food is of limited value since many determinants in the gastrointestinal tract may alter the "environment" considerably. The prediction of
the availability of a metal for absorption may, therefore, diverge

from that originally derived from metal speciation in food. Thus the
(bio)availability of metals largely depends on the species formed in
the gastrointestinal tract. Still the form in which many metals occur
in foodstuffs and in the gut is largely unknown. Moreover, many determinants of metal species interact in a complex way, making the bioavailability of a metal hard to predict. The relevance of metal
speciation in the gut is indicated when an emphasis is put on the determination of soluble and/or absorbable metal ions or metal complexes. It should be borne in mind that mineral and trace element
solubility and "hence" availability for absorption cannot easily be
predicted from the solubilities of metals in individual foodstuffs or
from other determinants; these determinants are multifactorial and in-
terdependent. Data should be interpreted with care: the fact that a
metal complex is available for absorption does not necessarily mean
that absorption will take place or that the absorbed complex will release the metal in a biologically active form.
From these general considerations it should be clear that metal
speciation is an important and challenging matter, but also a rather
new and very complicated area of mineral and trace element analysis.

2 METAL SPECIES IN FOOD

The (essential) minerals and trace elements in foods from animal origin are mainly present as organic complexes, very often metalloproteins having functional properties. In vegetable foods the metals are
mostly bound to structural or storage components such as fibre and
phytate, but also various enzymes may be the "carrier" for minerals
and trace elements. The exact structure of many metal complexes is,
however, not known. In this brief review only the predominant classes
of metal compounds in foodstuffs are mentioned. (For more details reference is made to the review of Hazell[2]).
Regarding the toxic trace elements the organometallic species such as
tetraethyl lead, triethyl tin and methyl mercury compounds are much
more toxic than the inorganic derivatives. This is mainly caused by
the apolar nature of these compounds which enhances their ability to
cross membranes. These organometallic species may be present in foods
contaminated with residues of xenobiotics of industrial or other origin. The naturally occurring form of **arsenic** (As^{5+}) is much less toxic
than As^{3+}; in fish products the predominant forms of arsenic are
arsenobetaine and arsenocholine[3], which are probably not hazardous.
The major portion of **cadmium** in (animal) foods is present as a heat-
stable metallothionein[4]. **Tin** may be present in foods as a result of
contamination with this metal in canned products. **Nickel** will be bound
to albumin or other proteins in animal foods, in vegetable foods probably to phytate or to phenolic groups such as tannins in tea or coffee. The most important forms of **selenium** are Se analogues of the S-
containing amino acids methionine and cysteine; other Se compounds in-

clude selenates, selenites and selenides (in vegetable foods and in fish). Calcium in dairy products is mainly bound to casein-phosphate complexes, in vegetable foods complexed with either phytate, phosphate and sulphate or carboxyl and hydroxyl groups of dietary fibre. For **magnesium** similar complexes are applicable as mentioned for calcium in vegetable foods. In addition, magnesium in leafy vegetables is mainly present as a Mg-chlorophyll complex. Cobalt exists in foods from animal origin in various forms of cobalamins, such as methyl cobalamin in eggyolk and cheese. Chromium may be present as Cr-amino acid chelate or as inorganic Cr salt. Of particular interest is the presence of chromium in the "glucose tolerance factor" with Cr as the central element surrounded by compounds such as cysteine and nicotinic acid. Cr^{6+} salts are toxic. Iron in plant foods is mainly present as inorganic salts or phytates (cereals), but also in various metalloproteins. In animal foods iron is found in various forms of haem compounds or proteins (lactoferrin in milk, ferritin and transferrin in meat and fish). Copper may be present in the less soluble Cu+ valence state or as a Cu^{2+} complex; in meat Cu may be bound to protein, probably partly as a metallothionein such as superoxide dismutase. For **zinc**, proteins will be the predominant "carrier" in animal foods, phytate and phosphate in vegetable foods. Protein (casein, lactoferrin), phytate and fibrous substances are probably important ligands for **manganese** and **molybdenum** as well.

The determination of metal species in food is even more complex for two reasons. First of all, the conformation of the ligand may play an important role as can be illustrated for phytic acid. The phytic acid molecule can exist in two chair conformations; that with a single phosphate group in the axial position (5 eq./1 ax) will be more stable than the conformation with the single phosphate group in the equatorial position (5 ax/1 eq.). Factors such as pH and the metal ion present will change the ratio of the two conformations. The binding of some metals is proposed to occur mainly *via* the phosphate group in the equatorial position of phytate (Cu, Co, Zn), the binding of some other metals *via* the phosphate group in the axial configuration (Ca, Ni, Mn)[5,6]. In general, the ligand must have the proper steric and electronic configuration in relation to the metal being complexed; in addition, factors such as pH, ionic strength and solubility are important for complex formation as well. A second factor complicating metal speciation in food is the fact that food processing (heat treatment such as baking or cooking, fermentation or the action of enzymes such as phytase) may contribute to either enhanced or reduced availability of a mineral or trace element; new compounds may be formed, the food environment may be altered and new external factors may be introduced.

In conclusion, knowledge of metal speciation in foodstuffs may provide valuable information facilitating prediction of mineral bioavailability in only a limited number of cases; the best known example is haem iron versus non-haem iron. Apart from the organometallic compounds, speciation of most metals in food is a challenging matter from a scientific point of view, but of limited value with regard to the prediction of the availability for absorption.

3 METAL SPECIES IN THE GASTROINTESTINAL TRACT

Although metal speciation in the gastrointestinal contents is generally more meaningful for predicting mineral availability than the determination of the metal species in food, the analytical aspects are particularly complex in the former case, both from a theoretical and a practical point of view. The ultimate species at the site of absorption (for most elements the duodenum) will be decisive for any mineral or trace element to be at least taken up by the mucosal cell. Before this stage is reached many factors may interfere with the ingested metals and these factors determine to which extent the species are finally becoming available for absorption. The solubility of metal species can increase or decrease during digestion and is highly pH–dependent. However, the influence of pH will be different for various metals as is described by Crews et al.[4]. Lead in wholemeal bread is completely soluble after peptic digestion, but not at pH 7; on the contrary, cadmium in wholemeal bread is soluble at both acid and neutral pH, but the solubility decreases during pancreatic digestion, probably due to differences in behaviour between phytate complexes of both metals. Enzymes and (partly digested) food items may as well be responsible for a change of the metal species from a soluble into an insoluble form, or conversely, for example by releasing ligands which may form soluble metal complexes from insoluble species. For copper it is postulated that after peptic digestion ionic copper passes through the proximal duodenum and is then complexed in the less acid upper duodenum by ligands of alimentary or enzyme origin; so a species–change may occur by enzymolysis[4]. Calcium–zinc–phytate precipitates may be dissolved by EDTA; picolinate can act as an important intestinal chelating agent for zinc, cadmium and copper by desorbing the metals from calcium phytate at neutral pH[7]. Also various amino acids are capable of dissolving metal–phytate precipitates and hence making the metals more available for absorption[4,7]. The molecular weight of proteins is probably an important factor for the formation of either soluble or insoluble metal species, as is discussed for iron by Berner and Miller[8]; during digestion peptides are released which may enhance the availability of metals by forming soluble complexes that prevent metal precipitation. But availability of metals may also be inhibited when peptides form insoluble complexes or even soluble complexes which do not release the metal to a mucosal receptor. In general, the strength of a bond of a ligand with a metal may contribute to either enhancement or inhibition of metal availability. For enhancement the ligand must bind the metal securely enough to maintain the stability through the gastrointestinal tract; yet the bond must not be so strong that the metal cannot be released to an acceptor in the intestinal mucosa. In certain cases metal chelates can be absorbed intact as has been shown for EDTA complexes, but the metal may be so tightly bound that it cannot be utilized by the body and the complexed metal is excreted in the urine. Apart from the molecular weight, the particle size of any precipitate formed will influence the extent to which a metal species changes into a soluble form as is illustrated for phytate by Wise[7]: the larger the particles of, for example, a metal–phytate precipitate, the slower the precipitate will be dissolved. This may cause that the action of phytase to "digest" large phytate crystals is less effective. Moreover, the factor "time" should not be underestimated; a neutral liquid containing a precipitate of an iron complex that is acidified may take up to one hour to convert the iron from its crystalline form into a soluble form[9]. However, many reactions are so slow that the transit time through the stomach is too short for any change in metal solubility. So the rate of gastric emptying, partly influenced by the composition of the food ingested, largely determines which metal species are formed during digestion. Regarding the oxidation state of minerals and trace elements it can be remarked that different valence states of the same metal will cause a different behaviour of a metal as to availability. This is mainly due to a difference in solubility of the two (or more) oxidation states. Ferrous compounds show a greater solubility at the pH of the intestinal contents than do ferric compounds, cupric species are more soluble than are cuprous species. The influence of various factors on the oxidation state, and hence the solubility, of metals can be illustrated by the action of ascorbic acid. It is well known that vitamin C may enhance iron availability by reducing ferric iron to ferrous iron, but copper availability may be decreased because of the reduction to cuprous species; for this conversion an oxygen–free environment is necessary, which may well be the condition of the intestinal lumen[10]. Generally the oxidation potential in the gastrointestinal tract will determine which valence state of a certain metal species will be predominantly formed.

The prediction to which extent a certain metal species is formed in the gastrointestinal contents is difficult from a theoretical point of view because so many factors may be involved. Moreover, the dynamic behaviour of the metal ions during all stages in the gastrointestinal tract makes any prediction of availability difficult. For these and other reasons the actual analysis of metal species (speciation), with the aim of predicting metal availability for absorption, is an arduous task. It is, therefore, not surprising that speciation of minerals and trace elements is still at an early stage of development.

    4 METHODS OF SPECIATION (models for predicting metal availability)

Many **in vitro digestion** procedures have been described to simulate the

processes that take place in the stomach and small intestine. Results
are often expressed in terms of solubility of a certain metal (ligand)
under the conditions of the test, such as pH, the enzymes applied and
the food items examined, because solubility is considered to be an important determinant for metal availability. Still the (quantitative)
extrapolation from in vitro studies to the in vivo situation is debat-
able, partly because of the dynamic changes that take place in biological systems which cannot easily be simulated. In vitro experiments
may result in "stability constants" of metal complexes. The determination of stability constants is, however, an arduous task and the experimental conditions must be similar for meaningful comparisons to be
made. This is illustrated by the different orders of stability reported for metal–phytate complexes[4,7]. In complex food systems containing numerous interfering components, stability constants are of
limited value[11]. Moreover, the dynamic changes that occur in the
gastrointestinal tract (pH and the environment of the metal) add to
the uncertainty as to the usefulness of applying stability constants,
which are derived from in vitro tests, for predicting mineral and
trace element availability. A computerized approach of in vitro simulation experiments as described by Robb et al.[12] is, however, challenging. For valid comparisons to be made, standardization of in vitro
methods seems a prerequisite.
For the species analysis in food or in the final solution/precipitate
after in vitro digestion, various methods are described by
Schwedt[13,14] and Sabbioni et al.[1]. These include preconcentration/
separation techniques such as centrifugation, dialysis, ion exchange
and various chromatographic separations, and methods for the final
analysis such as atomic absorption spectrometry, neutron activation
analysis and spectrophotometric or electrochemical methods (see also
the contribution of Cornelis in this volume.) A special practical
problem is the fact that the concentration of the metal ions is often
low. Contamination during the different analytic steps should also be
taken into account and, finally, there is a risk that the chemical
equilibrium in foods or the analyte after in vitro digestion is
altered, possibly resulting in false predictions of either the
structure of the metal species or the availability for absorption[14].
Changes during the analytic stage are particularly hazardous for the
determination of the oxidation state of a metal. Various precautions
have to be made to prevent any oxidation or reduction of a metal
during detection and measurement. Methods include nuclear magnetic
resonance (NMR), electron–nuclear double resonance (ENDOR), electron
spin echo (ESE), electron paramagnetic resonance (EPR) and Mössbauer
spectrometry[1].
Direct analysis of the gastrointestinal content could be considered
through in vivo experiments with human subjects.
We have applied the technique of analysis of **gastric** fluid to a project on determination of nitrosamine formation after consumption of

nitrate-rich vegetables. A nasogastric tube was inserted by the subjects, and a gastric fluid sample was taken at intervals. Relevant results of *in vitro* studies could be checked by these *in vivo* experiments, although the same disadvantages as mentioned above for *in vitro*
tests are applicable such as the problem of standardization and the
aspect of dynamic changes during digestion. Sampling of the **intestinal**
content will be more of a burden for the subjects from a practical
point of view.

5 CONCLUSIONS

The main objective of this paper was to discuss in what way and to
which extent speciation of minerals and trace elements might contribute to a better understanding of the processes that take place prior
to absorption and, as a consequence, to a better prediction of metal
availability. It was stated that, to this end, metal speciation in
foods only seems relevant in a few cases. The importance of the determination of metal species could, however, be increased if at the same
time various (known) enhancing and/or inhibitory factors for metal
availability are analysed in the food (mixtures), such as phytate,
oxalate, dietary fibre and ascorbic acid. In vitro techniques could be
used to estimate the relative importance of the factors mentioned for
metal availability and to determine various solubility/stability constants of metal species. But standardization of methods and analytical
procedures is essential. These types of experiments will generally
yield many results, so that some form of computerized approach seems
necessary. The advantage of such a model is that at least foods or
mixtures of food components can be ranked into broad classes of metal
availability taking the contents of minerals and trace elements as
well as the enhancing/inhibitory factors into account. It is then
challenging to predict the reactions that can take place in the gastrointestinal tract from the specific composition of the food as mentioned above. Questions may be answered such as to what extent
ascorbic acid can compensate the inhibitory action of phytate, polyphenols, oxalate, *etc*. In reality, however, these reactions strongly
depend on pH and (transit) time; it is therefore not clear whether all
reactions that are possible from a theoretical point of view (as calculated from the *in vitro* model) will take place during digestion.
Probably the thermodynamic most stable situation will not be reached
but the real situation will be more under kinetic control. Relevant
predictions of metal availability through *in vitro* data can be checked
by animal or human experiments, either by *in vivo* studies as discussed
in section 4 or by controlled metabolic balance studies (e.g. with
stable isotopes). It is beyond the scope of this paper to go into details with regard to this type of human experiments. For the ultimate
determination of the individual metal species in food or in the gastrointestinal fluids various methods have been suggested. Most data
collected in this way, however, seem to be more relevant from a scientific point of view than that they can be used for predicting metal
availability.

The prediction of the availability of minerals and trace elements for absorption will particularly be more valid when a combination of methods and techniques will be applied.

6 REFERENCES

1. E. Sabbioni, J. Edel and L. Goetz, Nutr.Res., 1985, Suppl.1, 32.
2. T. Hazell, Wld.Rev.Nutr.Diet., 1985, 46, 1.
3. J.B. Luten, G. Riekwel—Booy and A. Rauchbaar, Environm.Health Persp., 1982, 45, 165.
4. H.M. Crews, J.A. Burrell and D.J. McWeeny, Z.Lebensm.Unters.Forsch., 1985, 180, 221.
5. A.N. Egbewatt and K. Dill, Inorg.Chim.Acta, 1987, 136, L37.
6. C.J. Martin and W.J. Evans, J.Inorg.Biochem., 1987, 30, 101.
7. A. Wise, Nutr.Abstr.Rev., 1983, 53, 791.
8. L.A. Berner and D.D. Miller, Food Chem., 1985, 18, 47.
9. K.T. Smith, Food Techn., 1983, 37, 115.
10. J.A. Rendleman, 'Interactions of Food Components', Elsevier, London, 1986, Chapter 5, p.63.
11. T.E. Furia, 'Handbook of Food Additives', CRC Press, Cleveland, 1972, p.271.
12. P. Robb, D.R. Williams and D.J. McWeeny, 'Trace Elements in Man and Animals — TEMA 5', Commonwealth Agricultural Bureaux, Slough, 1985, p.630.
13. G. Schwedt, Trends in Anal.Chem., 1983, 2, 39.
14. G. Schwedt, Lebensmittelchem.Gerichtl.Chem., 1988, 42, 36.

MODELLING BIOAVAILABILITY AS A FUNCTION OF SPECIATION USING PHYSICOCHEMICAL DATA AND COMPUTERS

M.I.Barnett*, J.R.Duffield, D.A.Evans, J.A.Findlow,
B.Griffiths, C.R.Morris, J.A.Vesey and D.R.Williams

School of Chemistry & Applied Chemistry, and Welsh
School of Pharmacy,* University of Wales College of
Cardiff, Cardiff CF1 3XF

1 INTRODUCTION

The availability of trace elements to normal biochemical and metabolic processes will be a function of the
chemical speciation of the trace element(s) in question. Here, the term chemical speciation denotes all
of the different chemical forms of an element occurring
in a given aqueous system. It will include an analysis
in terms of percentage formation of cationic, anionic
and neutral species and indicate that fraction prone to
precipitation/dissolution, all factors involved in
either reducing or increasing uptake. In addition, and
of particular importance with respect to bioavailability, will be the changes in speciation occurring in different body compartments as this will be a reflection
of the chemical availability of the trace metals.
     In general, speciation analysis is experimentally
very difficult. Total concentrations of trace metals
in vivo are at, or near, their limits of detection, and
speciation analysis requires sub-totals. Furthermore,
biological systems are complicated mixtures of components which tend to perturb instrument sensitivity,
precision and accuracy, whilst the very act of measurement, which is generally invasive, alters the steady
state or equilibrium conditions. Paradoxically, however, it is this latter difficulty which provides a
solution to the determination of speciation analysis,
as will be discussed and illustrated with examples
below.
     The aforementioned difficulties regarding specia-
tion analysis can be circumvented by modelling the
metal-ligand interactions occurring under steady state
conditions using large computer simulation programs, in

conjunction with thermodynamic databases. The latter
contain the formation constants and solubility products
which describe the aqueous processes[1].

2   EXAMPLES ILLUSTRATING SPECIATION MODELLING AND BIOAVAILABILITY

2.1 The bioavailability of tin

Although tin occurs in trace amounts in most
natural foods, the main dietary source is canned food.
Little is known of the form in which the tin occurs
and, therefore, using computer modelling, an attempt
has been made to characterize the obviously complicated
speciation of tin in canned foodstuffs, both before and
following ingestion. The calculations suggest that
much of the tin in a soluble form is bound in complexes
of organic acids, particularly citrate, and in order to
improve the model, formation constants of stannous
citrate complexes were determined by glass electrode
potentiometry. Stannous salts have also found applications in dental therapy for many years[2], and the speciation study has, therefore, been extended to consider
the dissolution of a tin-containing dentifrice in water
and in saliva.

2.2 The bioavailability of aluminium

Aluminium has been implicated in a number of
neurodegenerative disorders such as Alzheimer's disease
and recent publicity has underlined the ubiquitous
nature of Al in the environment and foodstuffs. A
knowledge of Al bioavailability is thus essential in
assessing likely risks to the population at large who
are continually exposed to low levels of Al.
Computer-aided speciation analysis is being used
to assess these problems and it is found, for example,
that in human and bovine milk the presence of citrate
greatly reduces the formation of neutral Al species
which would be subject to absorption across the duodenal mucosal cells[3]. In addition, presence of phosphate and silicate will lead to the formation of Al
solids under pH conditions found in the gastrointestinal tract and these would be excreted rather than
absorbed.

2.3 Bioavailability of the actinides

As is the case for aluminium, there is currently
much public concern over the fate of actinides in the

biosphere, particularly with regard to plutonium uptake in areas around the nuclear fuel reprocessing plants at Dounreay and Sellafield[4]. Here, speciation analyses have shown that, if both chemical- and bio-availabilities are taken into account, less than 0.1% of the total plutonium in a given foodstuff would be absorbed. Studies such as this, coupled with the very low levels of Pu in the environment, give some reassurance as regards risk factors associated with plutonium and the incidence of childhood leukaemias.

2.4 Stability of total parenteral nutrition solutions

An increasing number of patients are being kept alive by intravenous feeding of TPN solutions which contain all of the necessary components to sustain life including trace elements, amino-acids and lipids. In some cases, treatment lasts for many years and it is important to ensure that the components are presented in a form which is both stable and bioavailable[5].

Chemical speciation simulation is of great value in this context as it allows prediction of likely solid formation (e.g. $CaHPO_4$) under different pH and concentration conditions. Such knowledge aids manufacturers and pharmacists in their formulations so that undesirable phenomena like precipitation can be avoided.

3   CONCLUSIONS

The studies above illustrate the breadth and power of computer speciation analysis. The method can be used to predict, understand and guide experimentation and to allay unnecessary fears. As with all modelling exercises, it is important to consider the assumptions made and to validate and verify the predictions against experimental data, wherever possible.

REFERENCES

1. J.R.Duffield and D.R.Williams, Chem.Soc.Rev., 1986, 15, 291.
2. S.J.Blunden, P.A.Cusack and R.Hill, "The Industrial Uses of Tin Chemicals", Royal Society of Chemistry, London, 1985.
3. J.A.Findlow, J.R.Duffield, D.A.Evans and D.R.Williams, Rec.Trav.Chim., 1986, 106, 403.
4. J.R.Duffield, D.P.Raymond and D.R.Williams, Inorg. Chim.Acta, 1987, 140, 369.
5. B.Shine and J.A.Farwell, Brit.J.Parent.Ther., 1984, p.42.

A STABLE ISOTOPE STUDY OF THE DEGREE OF EXCHANGE BETWEEN
EXTRINSIC ENDOGENOUS ZINC DURING IN VITRO ENZYME DIGESTION OF FOOD

Helen M Crews*, Robert M Massey*, Kevin C Jones+,
Linda M Owen+

* Ministry of Agriculture, Fisheries and Food, Food
Science Division, Norwich

+ Department of Environmental Science, University of
Lancaster

1.   INTRODUCTION

Dietary zinc bioavailability may be investigated by
labelling food with an enriched stable isotope of zinc
for subsequent detection in faeces, tissue or blood.
Labelling may be intrinsic (incorporated within the
food during growth) or extrinsic, whereby the inorganic
isotope is added to prepared food prior to consumption.
In the latter case, the important assumption must be made
that the extrinsic label completely exchanges with the
endogenous zinc. Comparisons of intrinsic and extrinsic
labelling[1,2] have not so far confirmed the exchangeability
of extrinsic and endogenous zinc. This project
investigates the exchangeability of an extrinsic label
of enriched ^{68}Zn with endogenous zinc in cooked chicken
leg and wholemeal bread, following an in vitro
enzymolysis procedure designed as a simplified model of
human gastric digestion.

2.   METHOD AND MATERIALS

Cooked chicken leg and fresh wholemeal bread were
homogenised. The stable isotope label, a 50:50 mixture
of normal zinc and ^{68}Zn enriched to 97.58% (obtained
from the stable Isotope Unit, Chemistry Division,
Harwell Laboratory), was added as an aqueous spike
(0.5ml) prior to enzymolysis. The total amount of
extrinsic zinc (98.9µg) was of a similar order of magnitude to the total amount of endogenous zinc from wholemeal bread (120µg) and chicken leg (150µg). The enzymolysis procedure was modified from that previously
described[3]. Briefly, samples (10g wet weight) were
incubated (4 hr at 37°C) with pepsin (10mg ml^{-1}, 20ml)
in deionised distilled water acidified to pH1.5 with
HCl. Samples and reagent blanks were taken through the

enzyme digestion, then ultracentrifuged and filtered
(0.22 μm). The supernatants were analysed using ICP-MS
(Plasmaquad; VG Elemental, Winsford, Cheshire, UK).
Sample introduction was by flow injection (500 μl sample
look; carrier deionised distilled water; flow rate
(1ml min^{-1}). Isotopes were measured in the scanning
mode (number of scan sweeps 800; dwell time 150 μs;
number of channels 1024; number of runs/sample = 5).
Aqueous standards of normal zinc and the stable isotope
label were also analysed. Total zinc and the $^{66}Zn/^{68}Zn$
ratio were calculated.

3. RESULTS AND DISCUSSION

Table 1

$^{66}Zn/^{68}Zn$ ratios for Gastric Supernatants (pH1.5)
and the Ratio of Soluble Endogenous Zinc
to Soluble Extrinsic Zinc

GASTRIC SUPERNATANTS

Sample	$^{66}Zn/^{68}Zn$ (range, n=4)		% soluble endogenous Zn/ % soluble extrinsic Zn
	Unlabelled	Labelled*	
Chicken leg	1.451 (1.425–1.463)	0.220 (0.191–0.245)	1.17
Wholemeal bread	1.448 (1.431–1.470)	0.271 (0.252–0.297)	1.01
Reagent blank	1.415 (1.393–1.428)	0.248 (0.246–0.251)	1.08¥
Expected#	1.448 (1.437–1.457)	0.247 (0.245–0.250)	–

* $^{66}Zn/^{68}Zn$ calculated by subtracting counts for
unlabelled supernatant from counts for labelled
supernatant.

¥ assumes all endogenous zinc is soluble.

measured ratios for standards of natural zinc and
the extrinsically added zinc.

The results in Table I show that for the unlabelled
gastric digests of chicken leg and wholemeal bread the
$^{66}Zn/^{68}Zn$ ratios are in good agreement with the value
of 1.45 obtained for a standard solution of zinc
(0.5mg/litre) in 1% hydrochloric acid. As shown in

Table I the mean ratio of % solubility (endogenous: extrinsic) was 1.17 for the gastric digest of the chicken leg and 1.01 for the wholemeal bread digest. For complete exchange of the endogenous and extrinsic zinc a ratio of 1.00 would be anticipated. For the chicken tissue there was an indication that the endogenous zinc was slightly more soluble than the extrinsic label, however this difference was not statistically significant (P < 0.05). In the case of the wholemeal bread it was apparent that the endogenous and extrinsic zinc partition identically between the supernatant and the solid residue remaining after gastric enzymolysis. In fact under the acidic conditions of the digest (pH = 1.5) the % solubility of the endogenous and extrinsic zinc was essentially 100% in each of the two food matrices.

In conclusion it has been established that after simulated gastric digestion the % solubility of extrinsic zinc is very similar to that of the endogenous zinc in both wholemeal bread and chicken tissue. It should however be noted that this does not necessarily mean that the extrinsic and endogenous atoms have completely exchanged from a chemical standpoint. To assess this requires a more detailed knowledge of the degree of exchange of both forms for all of the zinc species in the digest. HPLC studies using the ICP-MS as detector are to commence shortly to assess whether the expected ratio of the extrinsic and endogenous forms of the metal is in fact present in the chromatographically separable zinc containing species in the digest supernatant.

References

1.   M. Janghorbani, W.I. Nawfal, J.O. Pagournes, F.H. Steinke, and V.R. Young: *Amer. J. Clin. Nutr.*, 1982, *36*, 537.

2.   J.R. Hunt, P.E. Johnson, and P.B. Swan: *J. Nutr.* 1987, *117*, 1913.

3.   H.M. Crews, J.A. Burrell, and D.J. McWeeny: *Z Lebensm. Unters. Forsch.* 1985, *180*: 221.

CHEMICAL FORMS OF METAL ELEMENTS IN RICE BRAN

Akemi Yasui and Masumi Tanaka

National Food Research Institute, Ministry of Agriculture, Forestry and Fisheries
2-1-2 Kannondai, Tsukuba-shi, Ibaraki-ken 305, Japan

1 INTRODUCTION

Rice bran is known to contain a lot of minerals and phytic acid. Phytic acid is generally considered to bind minerals and have adverse effects in bioavailability of minerals[1]. In order to know existing forms of metal elements in rice bran, magnesium, calcium, zinc, manganese, iron and copper were studied in aspects of correlations with phytic acid, proteins and other components.

2 EXPERIMENTAL

Total amounts of metal elements and phosphorus in full-fat bran of rice (Oliza sativa japonica) were determined by atomic absorption spectrometry (AAS) and inductively coupled plasma - atomic emission spectrometry (ICP-AES), respectively, after dry ashing at 550°C. Total nitrogen was determined by coulometric titration after Kjeldahl digestion. Rice bran was extracted at 20°C for 3 hrs with different pH buffers (pH 2 - 11) to study solubility characteristics. Metal elements, phosphorus and nitrogen in extracts were determined.

Extract by pH 8 buffer (0.05M Tris - 0.025M HCl) was separated with gel chromatography using Sephadex G-15, 25, 50 and 100 and Toyo Pearl HW 40, 55 and 60 to seek a suitable gel material for separation of chemical species of metal elements. Eluate was fractionated. Metal elements, phosphorus and protein in fractions were measured by AAS, ICP-AES and absorbance of UV (254 and 280 nm), respectively. Extract by pH 8 buffer was separated also with ultrafilters (fractional molecular weight: 1×10^4, 3×10^4 and

1×10^5). Extract by pH 2 (0.05M KCl - 0.01M HCl) and 11 buffer (0.1M Borax - 0.05M NaOH) were also separated with Sephadex G-50 and Toyo Pearl HW 55.

Rice bran was three times extracted successively at 5°C for 1 hr with water, 5% NaCl, 60% EtOH and 0.4% NaOH for frationation of protein. Metal elements and phosphorus in each protein extract were determined.

Binding ratio of metal element to phytic acid was studied with gel chromatography using mini-column directly coupled with atomic absorption spectrometer as detector.

3 RESULTS AND DISCUSSIONS

Maximum solubility of phosphorus was observed at pH 3-5. Solubility of nitrogen increased according as pH heightened. Correlation of phosphorus and nitrogen was not found. Solubility of calcium, magnesium and manganese was increased according as pH lowered. Correlation among these three elements and phosphorus was very high in solubility. They are considered to exist mainly as phytate, which is insoluble in rice bran. Solubility of zinc had minimum value at pH 6-7. Above and below pH 6-7, solubility of zinc increased. In alkaline condition, there was a high correlation between zinc and nitrogen in solubility. Solubility of copper had minimum value at pH 4. Above and below pH 4, solubility of copper increased. Solubility of iron had maximum value at pH 5.

Sephadex G-50 and Toyo Pearl HW 55 were found to be suitable for separation of chemical species of metal elements. Twenty-five, 20, 25 and 70% of total zinc, manganese, iron and copper, respectively, was soluble in extract with pH 8 buffer. Soluble zinc was eluted in void volume, which existed in correlation with high molecular weight component. Another zinc containing peak was not related to phytic acid. Soluble manganese was eluted as one peak at the same position as mono-manganese phytate. Soluble iron existed in mono-ferric phytate and in correlation with high molecular weight component. Soluble copper existed in correlation with high molecular weight component and in inorganic form. In extract with pH 2 buffer, most of manganese and zinc and 35-50% of iron and copper was soluble. They are considered to exist in correlation with chloride ion. In extract with pH 11 buffer, zinc in correlation with high molecular weight component increased. Alkaline soluble protein (glutelin) is considered to bind zinc in neutral and alkaline conditions. Metal elements changed

<u>Table 1</u> Metal Elements, Phosphorus and Nitrogen in Rice
          Bran (on dry basis)

K	Mg	Ca	Zn	Mn	Fe	Cu	P	N
(			μg/g				)	(%)
18000	10700	520	70	107	101	4.4	32400	2.72

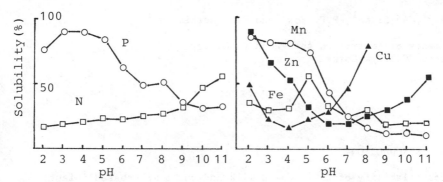

<u>Figure 1</u> Solubility Characteristics of Metal Elements,
          Phosphorus and Nitrogen in Rice Bran

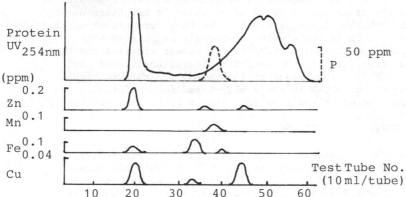

<u>Figure 2</u> Gel Chromatogram on Sephadex G-50 Column for
          Separation of Chemical Species of Metal Elements
          in Extract of Rice Bran with pH 8 Buffer

existing forms according to pH conditions.

        REFERENCE

1. M.Cheryan, <u>CRC in Food Science and Nutrition</u>, 1980,
    <u>13</u>, 297

IMPROVED BIOAVAILABILITY OF ZINC IN COLLOIDAL CALCIUM PHOSPHATE-FREE INFANT FORMULAE

J. Kiely[1], A. Flynn[1], P.F. Fox[2] and P.A. Morrissey [1]

Departments of [1]Nutrition and [2]Food Chemistry
University College Cork
Ireland

1 INTRODUCTION

The bioavailability of Zn in cow's milk and cow's milk-based infant formulae is lower than in human milk[1]. While the reasons for this remain unknown, it has been suggested that it is related to differences in the distribution of Zn between different Zn-binding ligands in the milks and in the fate of these Zn complexes during passage through the digestive tract. We have recently shown that over 60% of the Zn in cow's milk is strongly associated with colloidal calcium phosphate (CCP) in the casein micelles and that CCP removal significantly improves the bioavailability of Zn in cow's skim milk[2]. The object of this study was to investigate the binding of Zn to CCP in cow's milk-based infant formulae and to determine whether the bioavailability of Zn is affected by CCP.

2 MATERIALS AND METHODS

Bulk cow's milk (unpasteurized) was defatted by centrifugation at 3000g for 20 min at room temperature. Three cow's milk-based infant formulae were used: (A) SMA White Cap (Wyeth Laboratories), a skim-milk based formula containing 1.5% protein on reconstitution; (B) Progress (Wyeth Laboratories), a skim milk/whey protein-based formula containing 2.9% protein; (C) Premium (Cow and Gate Ltd), a modified formula with a casein:whey ratio of 40:60, containing 1.5% protein. The formulae were reconstituted in distilled water according to manufacturers' instructions. CCP-free milk and formulae were prepared by the method of Pyne and McGann[3]. Ca and Zn were determined by atomic absorption spectrophotometry and inorganic phosphorus was determined by the AOAC method.

Zn bioavailability was determined in rat pups by a modification of the method of Sandstrom et al[1]. Sixteen day-old rat pups, fasted overnight, were intubated with 0.2 ml milk or formula, extrinsically labelled with ^{65}Zn (1μCi ml^{-1}), and liver uptake of isotope determined after 6h by counting in a well gamma counter. As there was significant variation between litters in the response of liver ^{65}Zn uptake from milks, comparisons of ^{65}Zn uptake were made only within the same experiment where paired littermates were used.

3 RESULTS AND DISCUSSION

Removal of CCP from cow's skim milk reduced the Zn content from 3.81 to 2.39 mg l^{-1}, indicating that $\sim$63% of the Zn was associated with CCP. Of the total Ca and P$_i$ in cow's milk, 626 mg l^{-1} (55%) and 230 mg l^{-1}(37%), respectively, were associated with CCP. In the formulae 40–56% of total Ca and 39–45% of total P$_i$ was associated with CCP (Table 1). Thus, all three formulae contained significant amounts of CCP and the CCP contents were in the same order as the total Ca and P$_i$ contents, i.e., Formula B > Formula A > Formula C. Of the total Zn in the infant formulae (4.68 – 6.75 mg l^{-1}) 65–73% was associated with CCP, indicating that, like cow's milk, CCP-Zn is the major Zn fraction in these formulae.

Removal of CCP significantly improved the bioavailability of Zn in cow's skim milk and in each of the infant formulae (Table 2). This did not appear to be due to the lower Zn concentrations in the CCP-free milk or formulae, as the bioavailability of Zn in CCP-free cow's skim milk with added Zn as $Zn(NO_3)_2$ ($21.8 \pm 1.0\%$ of dose, n = 7) was also significantly greater ($p < 0.01$) than in skim milk ($18.5 \pm 0.6\%$, n = 17).

Thus, the presence of CCP in cow's skim milk and cow's milk-based infant formulae reduces the bioavailability of Zn. This could be due to the effect of CCP on the digestion of casein. It has been proposed that the formation of hard casein curds in the

TABLE 1   Total and CCP-bound Ca, P$_i$ and Zn in infant formulae

Formula	Ca/mg l^{-1}		Pi/mg l^{-1}		Zn/mg l^{-1}	
	Total	CCP	Total	CCP	Total	CCP
A	595	336(56)[1]	307	137(45)	6.75	4.62(68)
B	805	352(44)	445	175(39)	5.20	3.80(73)
C	580	230(40)	160	71(44)	4.68	3.04(65)

[1]values in parentheses give CCP-bound as % of total

TABLE 2   Effect of CCP removal on the bioavailability of Zn
           (liver uptake, % dose) in cow's skim milk and infant
           formulae

		milk			CCP-free milk		
	n	$\bar{x}$	SE	n	$\bar{x}$	SE	p value
Skim milk	17	18.5	0.6	17	21.6	0.5	< 0.01
Formula A	11	21.4	0.5	10	24.6	0.4	< 0.01
Formula B	6	18.1	0.9	6	20.7	0.6	< 0.05
Formula C	6	21.7	0.6	6	25.7	0.7	< 0.01

stomach when cow's milk is fed could lead to the formation of
undigested casein-Zn complexes in the small intestine, which could
render Zn unavailable for absorption[4].   Reduction of the CCP
content reduces the rennet curd tension of cow's milk[5], and may
thus improve casein digestibility. Alternatively, the effect of
CCP on Zn bioavailability could be due to the precipitation of
insoluble calcium phosphate-Zn complexes in the small intestine.
There is evidence[6] that insoluble calcium phosphate occurs in the
small intestine, and studies in vitro have shown[7] that Zn co-
precipitates with Ca and P_i at intestinal pH.

Acknowledgement The financial support of the Development Fund
University College, Cork, is gratefully acknowledged.

REFERENCES

1.   B. Sandstrom, C.L. Keen and B. Lonnerdal, Am. J. Clin. Nutr.,
      1983, 38, 420.

2.   J. Kiely, A. Flynn, H. Singh and P.F. Fox, Trace Elements in
      Man and Animals - TEMA-6, Plenum Publishing Co., New York,
      1988 (in press).

3.   G.T. Pyne and T.C.A. McGann, J. Dairy Res., 1960, 27, 9.

4.   P. Blakeborough, M.I. Gurr and D.N. Salter, Br. J. Nutr., 1986,
      55, 209.

5.   G.T. Pyne, J. Dairy Res., 1962, 29, 101.

6.   R. Van Der Meer and H.T. De Vries, Biochem. J., 1985, 229, 265.

7.   T.C.A. McGann, W. Bucheim, R.D. Kearney and T. Richardson,
      Biochem. Biophys. Acta, 1983, 760, 415.

DISTRIBUTION OF MOLYBDENUM IN HUMAN MILK

Clare E. Casey

Department of Medicine & Therapeutics
University of Aberdeen
Aberdeen   AB9 2ZD

1   INTRODUCTION

Essential trace elements such as zinc and copper are
distributed in milks according to the relative amounts
and affinities of the various binding ligands in the
major milk compartments.[1] Differences in bioavailability
of trace elements from various milks and formulas arise
largely from differences in trace element distribution
and binding. In the case of Zn, the difference in bioavailability from various milks is large enough to be of
practical significance in infant nutrition, with
absorption from human milk being higher than from some
formulas, including cows' milk.[2] Other essential trace
elements have received little attention, in part because
of the analytical problems associated with measuring very
low concentrations in the complex milk matrix. This report
presents the concentration and distribution of Mo in
human milk samples from the first 6 weeks post-partum.

2   MATERIAL AND METHODS

Milk samples were obtained from healthy women living in
Denver, Colorado, who were fully breast-feeding their
infants. They collected samples (2-5 ml) by manual
expression at mid-feed, during their mid-morning feed.
Milk was defatted by centrifugation at 1000 g and Mo was
analyzed in whole and defatted milk by graphite furnace
atomic absorption spectrometry (Perkin-Elmer Corp, Norwalk
CT). Appropriate precautions were taken to minimize
contamination. Molybdenum analyses were carried out on
untreated, liquid milk, using the method of standard
additions: 100 µl of milk was mixed with 200 µl standard

solutions containing 0, 1.0, 2.0 ng Mo/ml in 0.03M HNO_3;
40 µl was applied to the pyrolytically coated tube. The
spectrophotometer was set in peak height mode and
deuteurium background correction was used. Details of the
furnace program have been published.[3] Day-to-day coefficient of variation for Mo in a stock milk was 8%;
recovery of added Mo was 99 + 8%. The value for Mo in
NBS 1549 Nonfat Bovine Milk (Department of Commerce,
Washington DC), after dry ashing was 329 + 26 ng/g,
compared with the certificate value of 340 ng/g.

3   RESULTS

Molybdenum was analyzed in a total of 62 milk samples.
The overall concentration range was 0.69-26.7 ng/ml with
a marked decline with time post-partum up to about 3
weeks (Figure).

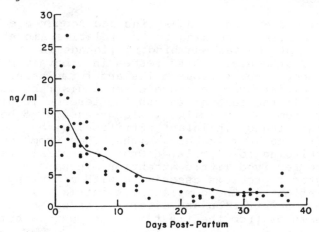

Figure   Concentration of molybdenum in human milk
         (individual samples with mean)

Whole and skim milk were analyzed separately in
samples from 6 women; the Table gives individual results
with the calculated concentration of Mo in the milk fat.

4   DISCUSSION

The fall in the average level of Mo in milk during the
first weeks of lactation, from 15.0 + 6.1 ng/ml on day
1 to 4.5 + 2.9 ng/ml on day 14, is similar to the
declines seen in Zn and Cu levels.

Table Concentration of molybdenum in human milk fractions

		Molybdenum			
		whole	skim	fat	fat
	Days	milk	milk		
Subject	post-partum	ng/ml	ng/ml	ng/g	% total
V1	15	2.4	0.9	63	63
V2	15	6.2	4.3	76	34
V3	45	2.7	1.6	18	44
V4	8	3.9	2.2	53	46
V5	14	6.9	5.1	59	29
V6	23	3.2	2.0	30	41
mean		4.2	2.7	50	43
(SD)		(1.9)	(1.6)	(22)	(12)

Xanthine oxidase (XO), a major molybdoenzyme, is present in human milk with an apparent molecular weight of about 700,000,[4] and containing 1 atom Mo per molecule FAD co-factor.[5] Higher activities of XO have been reported in colostrum compared with milk obtained later in lactation.[6] Levels of XO protein do not appear to have been documented for human milk, but as in cows' milk, it is mainly present in the milk fat globule membrane, of which it comprises about 10% of the protein. Thus the expected level of XO in milk fat is about 1-2 nmol/g fat, the same order as the average level of molybdenum, 0.52 nmol/g fat, found in the present study.

Supported by contract no. 01 HD 22801 and grant no. HD-19547 from the National Institutes of Health and Grant no. RR-69 from the General Clinical Research Centers Program of the Division of Research Resources.

REFERENCES

1. B. Lonnerdal, C.L. Keen and L.S. Hurley, Ann.Rev. Nutr. 1981, 1, 149.
2. P.A. Walravens and K.M. Hambidge, Am.J.Clin. Nutr. 1976, 29, 1114.
3. C.E. Casey and M.C. Neville, Am.J.Clin.Nutr., 1987, 45, 921.
4. I.H. Mather, K. Weber and T.W. Keenan, J. Dairy Sci., 1977, 60, 394.
5. L. Zeise and J.P. Zikakis, J. Agric. Food. Chem., 1987, 35, 942.
6. J.P. Zikakis, T.M. Dougherty and N.O. Biasotto, J. Food Sci., 1976, 41, 1408.

SPECIATION OF SELENIUM IN BOVINE WHEY.

P. VAN DAEL and H. DEELSTRA

Laboratory of Food Sciences, Dept. Pharm. Sciences
University of Antwerp (UIA), B-2610 Wilrijk.

G. VLAEMYNCK and R. VAN RENTERGHEM
Government Dairy Research Station, B-9230 Melle

Belgium.

1 INTRODUCTION

Since it was demonstrated in 1957 that selenium prevents liver necrosis in rat (1), the essentiality of selenium has been proved for a variety of mammals (2) . Strong evidence for the essentiality of selenium in human beings comes from its presence in the enzyme glutathione peroxidase, protecting cells against oxidative damage by peroxides (3). Further selenium deficiency has been associated e.g. with Keshan disease, which could be eliminated by sodium selenite supplementation (4).

Babies can be more susceptible to selenium inadequancy because of their increased demands for growth and their almost exclusive dependency on milk or milk formulas, with low selenium content, as sources of food. However the total selenium content does not give information on the overall utilisation or bioavailability of the element (5). The chemical forms and the distribution in food are important parameters of the selenium availability.

This study was designed to determine the selenium content of the different protein fractions of bovine whey.

2 MATERIALS and METHODS

Milk samples

Fresh mature bovine milk was collected at a local farm in acid washed containers . Major protein fractions of bovine whey were purchased from Sigma Chemical Co., St-Louis (USA).

Fractionation procedure

Skimmed milk was prepared by centrifugation at 1500 x g
for 30 min. at 4°C. The pH of the skimmed milk was
adjusted to 4.6 to precipitate the caseins. The major
whey proteins were prepared by selective precipitation
using the method of Aschaffenburg and Drewry (6). The
protein fractions were freeze-dried and stored at - 20°C
prior to purity control and selenium analysis.

Purity control

The purity of the isolated protein fractions was checked
by FPLC analysis on a Mono Q column (7). Only protein
fractions resulting in a purity of 80 % or more were
used for selenium determination.

Selenium analysis

Samples were digested with a mixture of nitric and
perchloric acids (8). The digests were analysed for
selenium by hydride generation atomic absorption
spectrometry (Perkin-Elmer 372 with an MHS-20 unit).
Conditions for selenium determination were described
elsewhere (9).

3 RESULTS and DISCUSSION

The results of the selenium analysis of the whey proteins are summarized in Table 1.

The results obtained for the commercial whey fractions show that especially β-lactoglobulin is a
selenium-rich protein, contributing up to 80 % of the
total selenium content of bovine whey. A possible explanation of this phenomenon could be the presence of a
large quantity of sulphur-containing amino-acids in this
protein (11). However the β-lactoglobulin prepared by a
selective precipitation method has a much lower selenium
concentration, for the other isolated fractions this
difference is not so extreme. This could be due to the
precipitation technique using high salt concentrations
and pH-changes, which could disturb chemical equilibria
(12). Otherwise it might be reasonable to assume that
the commercial β-lactoglobulin is prepared from milk of
a selenium-rich area.
Further research upon this matter is in progress.

Table 1.   Se-content of the different proteins of bovine
           whey.

	ppb Se (ng/g)	ng Se/100 ml milk(*)
Whey proteins	490 - 660	245 - 462
Selective precipitated whey protein fractions		
α-lactalbumin	74 - 105	7 - 16
β-lactoglobulin	115 - 120	23 - 48
immunoglobulins and proteose-peptones	175 - 190	21 - 40
Commercial whey protein fractions		
α-lactalbumin	180 - 250	18 - 37
β-lactoglobulin	797 - 831	159 - 332
serum albumin	140 - 160	1 - 6
proteose-peptones	200 - 245	12 - 44

(*) after recalculation (10).

REFERENCES

1. K. Schwarz and C.M. Foltz, J.Am.Chem.Soc., 1957,
    79, 3292.
2. R.J. Shamberger, 'Biochemistry of Selenium', Plenum,
    New York,1983.
3. H.E. Ganther, D.G. Hafeman, R.A. Lawrance, R.E.
    Serfass and W.G. Hoekstra, 'Trace Elements in Human
    Health and Disease', Academic, New York, 1976.
4. X. Chen, G. Yang, J. Chen, X. Chen, Z. Chen and K.
    Ge, Biol.Trace Elem.Res., 1980, 2, 91.
5. A.R. Alexander, P.D. Whanger and L.T. Miller,
    J.Nutr.,1983, 113, 196.
6. R. Aschaffenburg and J. Drewry, Biochemistry, 1957,
    65, 273.
7. B. Manji, A. Hill, Y. Kakuda and D.M. Irvine, J.Dai-
    ry Sci,1985, 68, 3176.
8. H.J. Robberecht, R.E. Van Grieken, P.A. Van Den
    Bosch, H. Deelstra and D. Vanden Berghe, Talanta,
    1982, 27, 1025.

9. M. Verlinden, PhD Thesis, University of Antwerp (UIA), 1981.
10. H.I. Swaisgood, 'Development in Dairy Chemistry', Elsevier Applied Science Publisher, London, 1982.
11. J.L. Maubois and G. Brule, <u>Lait</u>, 1982, <u>617</u>, 485.
12. B. Lönnerdal and E. Forsum, <u>Am.J.Clin.Nutr.</u>,1985, <u>41</u>, 113.

DIETARY ADDITIVES OR CHELATING AGENTS FOR REDUCING METAL ABSORPTION AND RETENTION IN SUCKLINGS

B. Kargačin and K. Kostial

Institute for Medical Research and Occupational Health, University of Zagreb, M. Pijade 158, 41000 Zagreb, Yugoslavia

1 INTRODUCTION

In conditions of environmental exposure ingestion is the main route of metal and radionuclide entry into the body. In early life absorption of cations is known to be much higher than in later life[1]. This is partly due to milk diet and also to the immaturity of the intestinal tract. We previously found that this high absorption and retention can be reduced by some dietary additives[2] or oral administration of chelating agents[3]. The purpose of this work was to evaluate the comparative efficiency of these treatments in reducing cadmium, mercury and cerium retention.

2 MATERIALS AND METHODS

Experiments were performed on six-day-old suckling albino rats (about 11 g body weight).

    <u>Radionuclide administration</u>. Animals received ^{115m}Cd (260 kBq), ^{203}Hg (74 kBq) or ^{141}Ce (111 kBq) in milk or rat diet ingredients.

    <u>Dietary additives</u>. Rats were artificially fed over 8 h with either cow's milk (0.4 ml) or with rat food ingredients (0.2 g). The following mixture of ingredients was used: fish meal 37%, sunflower meal 28%, alfalfa 20%, cane molasses 12% and premix (vitamin-mineral mixture) 4%.

    <u>Chelating agents</u>. Animals receiving chelating agents were divided into two groups: the first one received Zn-DTPA on the first and second day (early treatment) and the second during the second and third day after radionuclide administration (delayed treatment). Zn-DTPA (Heyl and Co., Berlin) was administered at a dose of

3.64 mmol/kg b.w. to rats that received ^{115m}Cd or ^{141}Ce and Na-DMPS (Heyl and Co., Berlin) at a dose of 150 μmol/kg b.w. to those that received ^{203}Hg. Sucklings were returned to their dams each day after the end of the artificial feeding or chelating agent administration. Whole body (WB) retention was determined after the end of artificial feeding and six days later. Radioactivity was also determined in the gastrointestinal tract and organs. The results were corrected for radioactive decay and expressed as percentage of the control values (100%). They are presented as arithmetic mean and standard error of the mean of 10-18 animals in each group.

3 RESULTS AND DISCUSSION

Both treatments were very effective in reducing the retention of radioactive cadmium, mercury and cerium. Ingredients reduced Cd, Hg and Ce whole body retention to 60, 9 and 13% of control values mostly due to reduced gut retention (Figure). Early administration of chelation therapy reduced Cd, Hg and Ce whole body retention to 15, 46 and 5% of controls. Delayed chelation therapy was almost equally effective. Both treatments were also effective in reducing organ retention. Ingredients reduced Cd, Hg and Ce organ retention to 50, 20 and 50% of control. Early chelation therapy reduced radionuclide organ retention to 30-70% of control. Delayed chelation therapy caused increased Cd retention in liver, kidneys and femur and increased Hg retention in kidneys and brain. Delayed chelation therapy however, very effectively reduced cerium organ retention (to 30-70% of control). Chelation therapy was for Cd and Ce more effective than ingredients while for Hg ingredients were more effective than chelating agents.

It should be mentioned that early oral chelation therapy increases radionuclide and metal absorption from the intestine in adult experimental animals[4] while we found it very effective in reducing retention in sucklings. This difference in efficacy deserves attention. Dietary additives as nonspecific means were also very effective in reducing retention in sucklings and should be therefore taken into consideration when evaluating the toxicity as well as therapy in cases of exposure.

4 REFERENCES

1. J.C. Barton, "Age-related factors in radionuclide me-

tabolism and dosimetry", Martinus Nijhoff Publishers, Dordrecht, 1987, pp 1.
2. B. Kargačin and K. Kostial, "Speciation of fission and activation products in the environment", Elsevier Applied Science Publishers, London, 1986, pp 184.
3. K. Kostial, B. Kargačin and M. Landeka, <u>Int. J. Radiat. Biol.</u>, 1987, <u>52</u>, 501.
4. M.F. Sullivan and P.S. Ruemmler, <u>Health Phys.</u>, 1986, <u>51</u>, 641.

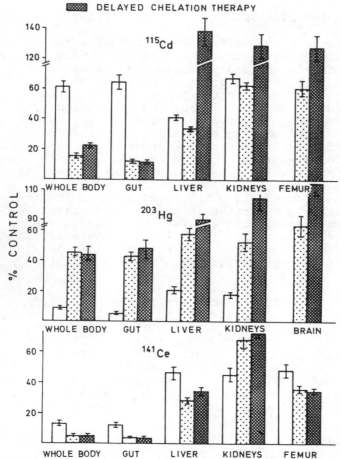

The influence of diet and oral chelation therapy on retention of gavaged ^{115m}Cd, ^{203}Hg and ^{141}Ce in rats.

ALUMINUM RELEASE FROM PHOSPHATE-BINDING AGENTS:
INFLUENCES OF DIGESTION PROCESS AND FOODSTUFF.
AN IN VITRO STUDY.

S. Treier, R. Kluthe.

Section of Nutritional Medicine and Dietetics,
Medical University Hospital Freiburg i. Br., FRG.

1 INTRODUCTION

Since the early observations of BERLYNE et al.[1] and ALFREY
et al.[2], many publications suggest that aluminum (Al)
accumulation in the human body is an essential factor in
the etiology of osteomalacia and encephalopathy. Drugs with
an high Al content were found to be the main source of
Al [3,4]. They are widely used as phosphate (P) binders in
patients with chronic renal failure (CRF) for the prevention and therapy of secondary hyperparathyroidism. Because
of their diminished renal function, these patients have a
high risk for Al accumulation. Since there is a lack of
therapeutic alternatives, a great demand exists for high
efficiency phosphate binders with low Al release.
Winterberg et al.[5] have demonstrated that agents with
nearly equal Al content may result in quite different Al
body burdens. To evaluate the therapeutic risk of phosphate
binders it is very important to know how they act in
stomach and gut.

2 METHODS AND MATERIALS

In order to estimate the fate of such drugs in the gastrointestinal tract, we used a three step in vitro digestion
model, which simulates the physiological conditions of the
digestion process very closely (pH, foodstuff, enzymes,
bile etc). Using this model we examined:

1   Aluminum release from several Al containing compounds
2   The influences of digestion procedure and the type of
     foodstuff
3   The P-binding capacity of the drugs

119

Gastric phase. Foodstuff (= 10 mg P) + Drug incubated
with pepsin-HCl solution, rotating frequency 50 rpm, pH
3.0, incubation time 1 h.
     Duodenal phase. Same task incubated with pancreatin-
bile-bicarbonate-solution, rotating frequency 50 rpm, pH
7.8, incubation time 3 h.
     Dialysis phase and centrifugation. Separation of
soluble and non-soluble Al, determination of P-binding
capacity.

As phosphorus sources we used skim milk powder (10 mg P/g),
whole rye bread (3 mg P/g) or a mixture of both with
phosphorus content shared 50:50.

     3 RESULTS AND DISCUSSION

As expected from the clinical data, P-binding capacities
varied enormously between the drugs, as did the releases of
Al. Evaluating the P-binding of different drugs in relation
to the Al release at the "50 % P-binding point" a rank
order balancing P-binding as well as Al release became
apparent. Despite the fact that the dosage of the substance
C (Al Hydroxide pharmaceutical grade) was three times
higher than the dosage of Substance A (Al Hydroxide
Chloride), Al release was lowest in substance C (table 1).
Any combination of Al Hydroxide and other salts seemed to
increase Al release in comparison with pure Al Hydroxide.
Statistics were evaluated on the basis of the confidence
belts of the regression lines of the Al releases. The null
hypothesis was rejected at $p < 0.05$.

Table 1 Al release from different P-binders

agent	C(P) (mg)	R(Al) (mg)	(* p<0.05)
A Al-Hydroxide-Chloride compound	47	2.36 ± 0.08	
B Al Hydroxide (chemical grade)	93	1.69 ± 0.16	
C Al Hydroxide + aux. (pharmaceutical grade)	151	1.47 ± 0.11	
D Al Hydroxide + Ca Carbonate	118	2.08 ± 0.12	

P-source: 1 g skim milk powder (10 mg P; 7.6 mg P avail.)
C(P): amount of drug needed for 50 % P-binding (3.8 mg).
R(Al): mg Al released at 50 % P-binding point

Table 2   Al release from Al Hydroxide (C) tested with
          different P sources at the 50 % P-binding point.

P-source	R(Al) mg	
buffer solution	6.81 ± 0.23	*
skim milk powder	1.47 ± 0.11	*
whole rye bread	0.53 ± 0.05	*
mixture	0.94 ± 0.10	*

Drug: Agent C (Al Hydroxide pharmaceutical grade)
* = statistically significant, $p < 0.05$.

Usually, P-binders are taken three times a day, mostly
associated with food intake but without regard to the food
composition. To study the eventual influences of food composition itself on Al release, we used a buffer solution,
then skim milk powder, ground rye wholemeal bread and a
mixture of both as different sources of P in combination
with the agent C (Results listed in table 2). Al release
from the drug was highest in aqueous buffer solution followed by skim milk powder, the mixture and rye wholemeal
bread. In each case, the differences were statistically
significant.

The results suggest that the type of the Al containing drug
as well as the type of food ingested have to be taken into
consideration when prescribing the efficacy and the therapeutic risk of different phosphate binders.

4   REFERENCES

1   R. Kluthe (ed.), "Medikamentöse Therapie bei Nieren-
     erkrankungen", Thieme Stuttgart, 1971, pp 171.
2   A. C. Alfrey et al., New Engl J Med, 1975, 294, 184.
3   A. C. Alfrey, Kidney International, 1986, 29, Suppl.
     18, 8.
4   H. Raidt et al., Trace elements in medicine, 1987,
     4, 107.
5   B. Winterberg et al., Nieren- und Hochdruckkrankheiten
     1986, 15, 183.

A PEPTIDE DEPENDENT INTESTINAL PATHWAY FOR THE ABSORPTION OF ESSENTIAL MINERALS

H. DeWayne Ashmead

Albion Laboratories, Inc.
101 North Main Street
Clearfield, Utah   84015
U.S.A.

Intestinal absorption of most mineral salts generally occurs in the duodenum where the acid pH enhances their solubility. As the cations descend into the jejunum and thence to the ileum, the elevated pH precipitates them, negating further absorption.[1] Such a model fails to assess absorption of minerals chelated to organic molecules such as amino acids.

Chelation occurs when a cation is held by ionic and coordinate covalent bonds from the same molecule (ligand). The ligand backbone isolates the cation from reactions with other compounds. Two amino acids can chelate a single polyvalent cation resulting in a bicyclic, dipeptide-like structure which resists gastric acid hydrolysis and intestinal enzyme cleavage.[1] The metals in these chelates are typically absorbed by active transport at jejunal dipeptide absorption sites. When such a chelate is ingested, intestinal uptake is significantly greater than for corresponding amounts of ingested inorganic metal salts as shown in Table 1.

Table 1 Mean ppm mineral uptake in rat jejunum *in vitro*

Mineral	Chelate	SO_4	O_2	CO_3	Control
Cu	35	8	11	6	trace
Mg	94	36	23	51	7
Fe	298	78	61	82	53
Zn	191	84	66	87	14

Following intestinal absorption, utilization is also significantly improved. Isotope studies *in vivo* indicate the dipeptide-like chelates generally enter the bloodstream intact, resulting in higher mineral retention and utilization than from equivalent amounts of metal salts. The 48 hour whole body counts from animals receiving radioactive metals from amino acid chelates <u>versus</u> inorganic salts revealed the following mean increases: 303 % Fe, 146 % Zn, 140 % Ca and 126 % Mn. The individual tissues are shown in Table 2.[1,2]

Table 2   Mineral metabolism in animal tissues from various sources. (corrected counts/minute)

Tissue	^{45}Calcium		^{65}Zinc		^{59}Iron		^{54}Manganese	
	CaCl$_2$	AAC	ZnCl$_2$	AAC	FeCl$_2$	AAC	MnCl$_2$	AAC
Bone	3682	5772					350	780
Muscle	614	1206	2.41	3.88	2	54	800	660
Heart	642	932	6.42	6.32	63	151	370	1190
Liver	664	742	5.15	8.65	136	243	760	1070
Brain	698	804	1.22	2.41	31	130	620	1170
Kidney	686	730	5.45	8.55	2	327	470	600
Lung	676	648					720	330
Blood Serum	8	31			700	1797		
RBC	18	13			742	2076		
Whole Blood	27	44	.90	1.64	1335	4215		

In spite of greater chelated mineral absorption, LD-50 tests confirm a greater tolerance to the metals when compared to respective inorganic salts.[2,4] This may result from bonding the minerals to biologically essential amino acids. Morbidity studies (gross pathology, histopathology, teratogenology, <u>etc</u>.) have shown no differences between treated and control groups.[5]

Greater bioavailability of essential minerals absorbed at intestinal dipeptide sites frequently results in significant physiological responses not seen when equivalent amounts of metal salts are ingested. Gestating sows were administered 600 mg of Fe as either the chelate or as ferrous fumarate 30 days prior to expected farrowing. Dosages were doubled 1 week before farrowing and continued 21 days into lactation. Upon farrowing and for the next 4 weeks, hemoglobin, hematocrit and serum ferritin were measured in all piglets. During this period, these parameters remained significantly higher (P<0.02, P<0.01 and P<0.05, respectively) in the chelate group.[2] Isotope studies reveal that due to its small molecular size (298), the chelate crossed the placental barrier intact, while serum Fe from salts was bound to high molecular weight (>56,000) carrier molecules which could not cross the barrier.[1,3]

In another study, 50 % of the cows in a university herd were given these chelates, while the controls received equivalent amounts of metals as salts. In the treated group, embryonic mortality was reduced 45 % and the period of estrous increased from 26 to 38 days. Periglandular fibrosis occurred in only 10 % of the treated group, as compared to 58 % in the controls (P<0.005).[4]

When pigs were given chelated Mn in their feed at the rate of 20 ppm, backfat was reduced from 15.1 mm to 13.6 mm (9.9 % <). Control animals fed equivalent amounts of Mn as salt with or without equivalent amounts of free amino acids found in the chelate, did not result in backfat reduction.[5] This reduction is believed to be due to Mn stimulation of the hypothalamus to secrete thyrotropin releasing factor (TRH) to promote the release of thyrotropin (TSH) from the pituitary. TSH stimulates the thyroid to release thyroxine. Isotope studies have demonstrated that when [54]Mn was chelated to specific amino acids, approximately 200 % more [54]Mn was found in the pituitary, and thyroid glands than was found when [54]MnCl$_2$ was given, with corresponding increases in thyroid activity.[5]

Primary dysmenorrhea in women has been successfully treated using a specific Mg amino acid chelate.[6] Also, patients afflicted with angina increased their physical work capacity by 20 % with a corresponding 22 % reduction of nitroglycerin intake after ingesting 50 mg of Mg per day as the amino acid chelate for 14 days.[5]

In summary, bioavailability of essential minerals is enhanced when they are chelated with amino acids to form stable dipeptide-like compounds. In this molecular configuration the mineral is absorbed in the jejunum as a peptide-like molecule in significantly greater amounts than occurs for metal ions in the duodenum. Once the chelates are absorbed, the benefits manifest themselves through superior physiological and anatomical performance.

REFERENCES

1. H.D. Ashmead, D.J. Graff and H.H. Ashmead, 'Intestinal Absorption of Metal Ions and Chelates', Thomas, Springfield, IL, 1985.
2. D. Ashmead, 'Chelated Mineral Nutrition in Plants, Animals and Man', Thomas, Springfield, IL, 1982.
3. D. Ashmead and D. Graff, Proc. IPVS, July 1982, p. 207.
4. J.E. Manspeaker, M.G. Robl, G.H. Edwards and L.W. Douglas, Vet. Med., Sept. 1987, p. 951.
5. Personal communication
6. G. Abraham, Clin. Ob. Gyn., 1978, 21, 139.

RELATIVE BIOAVAILABILITY OF TRACE ELEMENTS AND VITAMINS FOUND IN COMMERCIAL SUPPLEMENTS

J. A. Vinson, P. Bose, L. Lemoine* and K. Hsiao

Chemistry Department
University of Scranton
Scranton, PA 18510   USA

*Faculté de Médecine
Université de Reims
Reims, 50195   France

Commercial supplements of trace elements are available in a wide variety of forms. These include the isolated compounds such as inorganic salts, organic salts, amino acid chelates and a yeast form. The yeast form is made from a brewer's yeast grown in a nutrient media containing the inorganic salt. After several generations of yeast cell division the cell walls are removed by proteolytic enzymes and the yeast is then spray dried.

Vitamins are commercially available in two forms for human supplementation; a synthetic or isolated form and a natural form in which the synthetic vitamin is reacted with a natural yeast or plant extract containing proteins, carbohydrates, lipids and other natural substances.

Bioavailability of vitamins and trace elements has been determined in long-term animal supplementation (3-4 weeks) studies by measuring the vitamin or trace element in liver, blood, serum or plasma and comparing the slope of the dose-concentration plots. A preliminary depletion is usually performed using vitamin or trace element deficient food. In short-term experiments the area under the blood, serum or plasma concentration-time curve is used to compare bioavailabilities after a single dose of the test substance is given to either animals or humans.

Results of the trace element and vitamin studies are shown in Tables 1 and 2 on the following page.(1)

Examination of the blood concentration-time curves for the short-term human experiments involving selenium, zinc and copper revealed that the yeast form was more

Table 1.   Relative Bioavailability of Different Forms of Trace
           Elements.

Element	Animal	Length of Study	Analysis	Relative Bioavailability %[a]
Se	Rat	Long	Blood	100I, 60C, 122Y
Se	Rat	Long	Liver	100I, 146C, 226Y
Se	Human	Short	Auc[b]	100I, 122C
Mn	Rat	Long	Blood	100I, 111C, 156Y
Mn	Rat	Long	Liver	100I, 142C, 163Y
Zn	Rat	Long	Blood	100I, 101C, 172Y
Zn	Rat	Long	Liver	100I, 129C, 187Y
Zn	Human	Short	Auc	100I, 1110, 175Y
Fe	Rat	Long	Blood	100I, 57C, 101Y
Fe	Rat	Long	Liver	100I, 72C, 121Y
Cu	Rat	Long	Blood	100I, 930, 124Y
Cu	Rat	Long	Liver	100I, 1300, 195Y
Cu	Human	Short	Auc	100I, 1010 144Y
Cr	Human	Short	Glucose[c] (2)	100I, 356Y

[a]Relative bioavailability for long-term studies is determined from
the slope of the dose-concentration curve. For short-term experiments, it is calculated from the area under the concentration-
time curve. For all studies, the Inorganic Salt is defined as
100% bioavailable.
I = Inorganic Salt, C = Amino Acid Chelate, 0 = Organic Salt,
Y = Yeast.
[b]Auc = Area under Blood, Serum or Plasma Concentration-Time Curve.
[c]Percent of Fasting Serum Glucose Decrease.

Table 2.   Relative Bioavailability of Synthetic and Natural Vitamins.

Vitamin	Animal	Length of Study	Analysis	$\frac{\text{Natural}}{\text{Synthetic}} \times 100$
A	Rat	Long	Blood	149%
B1	Rat	Short	Auc[a]	138%
B2	Rat	Long	Serum	149%
B6	Rat	Long	Serum	254%
B6	Rat	Long	Liver	156%
B12	Rat	Long	Serum	256%
B12	Rat	Long	Liver	159%
Niacinamide	Rat	Short	Blood	394%
Niacinamide	Rat	Short	Liver	170%
C	Guinea Pig	Short	Auc	148% (3)
C	Human	Short	Auc	135%
E	Rat	Short	Liver	260%
Folic Acid	Rat	Long	Serum	107%
Folic Acid	Rat	Long	Liver	213%

[a]Area under Blood Concentration-Time Curve.

slowly absorbed, i.e. took longer to reach its maximum concentration than the other forms of trace elements. This is analogous to the situation of trace elements in foods which have been shown to be more slowly absorbed than the isolated salts of the trace elements. The peptides and free amino acids present in the yeast may associate or bind with the trace element and slow its absorption. As an example it was found for copper that the average time for maximum concentration in the blood of humans was 1.3 hours for copper sulfate, 1.7 hours for copper gluconate and 3.7 hours for the copper yeast. In comparing the area under these curves it was found that the yeast produced the greatest area and thus was the most bioavailable form. The long-term animal experiments also showed that the yeast was the most bioavailable form of the trace elements tested both in the blood and in the liver where many trace elements are stored.

Short-term vitamin experiments were done for vitamin B1 in rats and for vitamin C in guinea pigs and humans. The natural form of the vitamin was found to be more slowly absorbed than the synthetic form. For vitamin C in guinea pigs, ascorbic acid reached a maximum concentration in the plasma after 1.0 hours and after 1.6 hours with the natural vitamin C. In humans ascorbic acid at a dose of 500 mg reached its maximum after 2.9 hours and the natural vitamin C after 4.1 hours. In comparing the areas under the concentration-time curves it was found that the natural vitamin produced the greatest area. The long-term animal supplementations demonstrated that the natural form of the vitamin was more bioavailable in both the blood and liver.

In summary, yeast trace elements and natural vitamins are more slowly absorbed in animals and man; are more bioavailable; and are therefore the preferred form for supplementation.

REFERENCES

1.   J.A. Vinson and P. Bose, 'Proceedings of Mineral Elements 80', Helsinki, 1981, p. 615.
2.   J.A. Vinson and K.H. Hsiao, Nutr. Repts. Intl., 1985, 32, 1.
3.   J.A. Vinson and P. Bose, Nutr. Repts. Intl., 1983, 27, 875.

The Bioavailability of the Trace Minerals Iron and Zinc

FOOD AND DIETARY FACTORS INFLUENCING LEVELS AND BIOAVAILABILITY OF TRACE ELEMENTS

Bo Lönnerdal

Departments of Nutrition and Internal Medicine
University of California, Davis
Davis, California 95616 U.S.A.

INTRODUCTION

Essential trace elements are required for various biological functions in the human body. Deficiencies of iron, zinc and copper are known to occur in vulnerable populations such as pregnant women, infants and children. In order to avoid such deficiencies, an adequate supply of trace elements that can be utilized for biological functions is needed. This amount of trace elements is determined by the dietary supply and the degree to which they can be absorbed from the diet and retained by the body, i.e., their bioavailability. Individual components of the diet as well as the trace element status of each individual will affect this bioavailability. This overview will focus on different types of foods and the dietary factors that can enhance or decrease trace element bioavailability.

Dietary intake of trace elements

A primary consideration when assessing the bioavailability of trace elements is the quantity provided by the diet. Meats, particularly organ meats, are excellent sources of iron, zinc and copper and they are also a reasonable source of manganese. Besides being a good source of trace elements, meat is known to contain several factors that enhance trace element absorption. Milk and dairy products, however, are low in iron, copper and manganese, but are a relatively good source of zinc. This food group contains some factors that stimulate trace element uptake while some have a negative effect. In a global perspective, it should be recognized that the

consumption of meat and dairy products is very low in many
populations. An exception is milk and formulas used for
infants. In a large part of the world, the diet consists
largely of cereals, legumes, fruits and vegetables. Cereals and legumes are fairly good sources of trace elements
but they contain several factors that have an inhibitory
effect on trace element absorption. Fruits and vegetables
are low in trace element content but often contain constituents that will affect trace element bioavailability
positively when combined with other food items. This
latter consideration emphasizes the need to study the bioavailability of trace elements in the form they are consumed, i.e., as parts of composite meals.

Meats

It has been recognized for a long time that meat consumption is positively correlated to iron status. Part of
this is due to the high bioavailability of heme-iron in
meat (1). In addition, dietary factors that can negatively affect uptake of trace elements in general have little
effect on heme-iron absorption. This is explained by the
high stability of heme-iron and the fact that it is absorbed intact and via another pathway than non-heme iron.
Protein in general has a positive effect on trace element
intake. Since trace elements rarely are found in free
form, they are usually found associated to protein. Thus,
it has been shown that the intake of zinc is closely correlated to protein intake (2).

Another constituent of meat is known to have a positive effect on the absorption non-heme iron and has been
called the "meat-factor." Recent work has suggested that
this factor is likely to be the amino acid cysteine. When
iron absorption was studied in the presence of various
amino acids, cysteine was shown to be the most efficient
one (3,4). In addition, when cysteine was added to
legume-based meals from which iron originally was poorly
absorbed, a significant increase in iron absorption was
found (4). It was recognized, however, that cysteine in
free form easily becomes oxidized during cooking and
needed to be protected. Therefore, it was suggested that
cysteine in smaller peptides produced by digestion could
exert this stimulatory effect. This was supported by the
finding that cysteine-containing peptides isolated from
meat after proteolysis enhanced iron absorption as compared to the same peptides that had been treated to
completely oxidize the cysteine residues (5). Cysteine,
histidine and other amino acids have also been shown to

have a positive effect on zinc absorption (6). This effect is largely due to the presence of chelating groups in
the amino acids, as side chain modification causes a reduction in zinc uptake (7). Their presence in dipeptides
has also been shown to stimulate zinc absorption (6).

Milk and dairy foods

Several factors in milk are likely to affect trace
element absorption. Casein, calcium, citrate and lactose
may all affect absorption and possibly in a counteractive
fashion. Zinc absorption from human milk has been shown
to be higher than from cow's milk and cow's milk-based
infant formula (8). This difference in bioavailability
was suggested to be due to the high casein content of
cow's milk and the higher proportion of citrate-bound zinc
in human milk (9). It has subsequently been shown that
bovine casein has a negative effect on zinc absorption
(10), while human casein has no negative effect. In addition, zinc absorption from casein-predominant formula was
significantly lower than from whey-predominant formula
(11). The negative effect of bovine casein may be due to
the presence of phosphorylated amino acids which in
incompletely digested peptides may limit zinc uptake (9).
Another possibility is that bovine casein contains colloidal calcium phosphate (CCP) and that this form of calcium interferes with zinc absorption. It has been shown
that removal of CCP can affect zinc absorption positively
and that calcium and phosphate as such do not exert this
effect (12). Similarly, it has been shown that calcium
added to human milk at a concentration similar to that of
cow's milk does not affect zinc absorption (11). The
effect of calcium on iron absorption, however, may be more
pronounced. When calcium was added to the test solution,
intestinal uptake of ^{59}Fe in the rat was decreased (13).
Furthermore, when calcium was added to human milk at the
concentration of cow's milk, iron absorption was similar
to that from cow's milk, while uptake from human milk as
such was higher.

Citrate is an effective chelator of trace elements
and is present in milk at a high level. Because of its
high concentration, citrate may aid in the absorption of
trace elements by removing them from less accessible
ligands and keeping them in a soluble form. It has been
shown that citrate at concentrations found in common diets
efficiently solubilizes iron from food (14). Furthermore,
since the daily intake of citrate often is around 1 g
while that of ascorbate is around 40 mg, the quantitative

influence of citrate as an effector of trace element absorption may be larger than that of ascorbic acid.
Another consideration is the general effect of citrate on
sodium and water transport (15). In human subjects, this
transport was found to be optimal at a citrate concentration of 5 mM, which is similar to that found in milk (9).
It has been shown in rats that water and sodium transport
is correlated to zinc transport (16); possibly increased
water and ion flux enhances the passive component of zinc
absorption.

Carbohydrates are known to affect iron absorption and
lactose has been shown to have a positive effect on iron
absorption (17). When glucose polymers in soy formula
were substituted with lactose, however, no stimulatory
effect on zinc absorption was found (11). This may be due
to the presence of strong inhibitory factors in soy and
that the effect of lactose is too weak to counteract these
negative effects.

Cereals and legumes

It is well known that phytate in cereals and legumes
can have a negative effect on trace element absorption.
The quantitative significance of phytate versus other inhibitory substances in these foods has rarely been evaluated. Since we found very low absorption of zinc (8) and
copper (18) from soy-based infant formula as compared to
cow's milk-based formula in human subjects, we studied the
effect of adding phytate to cow's milk formula (11). Addition of an equimolar concentration of sodium phytate
decreased zinc absorption from cow's milk formula to about
half and to the same level as from soy formula. Furthermore, addition of a higher concentration of phytate decreased zinc absorption to a level similar to that of an
experimental soy formula made from crude soy instead of
soy protein isolate. Thus, virtually all the negative
effect of soy formula on zinc absorption could be ascribed
to phytate. In addition, we have shown that removal of
phytate by phytase increases zinc absorption from soy formula to a level similar to that of cow's milk formula
(19).

Soy and other legumes have also been shown to have a
negative effect on iron absorption (20). In soy, however,
the negative effect may not only be caused by phytate but
also by protein. A protein in soy which is similar to
ferritin has been shown to inhibit iron absorption (21).

Although cereals contain reasonable levels of trace elements, their degree of absorption has been shown to be low. This may be due to the presence of both phytate and fiber in cereals. In several countries this has been considered with regard to iron and cereals are therefore often fortified with iron. The situation for zinc may be similar, but fortification with this element is not yet used. It has been shown that substitution of part of the daily intake of human milk or cow's milk with cereals results in a considerably lower amount of zinc absorbed (22). Zinc absorption from several types of cereals has been shown to be low in humans and the negative effect is largely correlated to the concentration of phytate in the cereal (23). The effect of fiber on trace element absorption needs to be studied further. Cook et al. (24) found that muffins baked from bran caused low iron absorption as compared to several other types of fiber. In an attempt to quantitate the effects of various factors, Hallberg et al. (25) added bran to muffins baked from white wheat. Iron absorption increased when phytate was hydrolyzed by phytase and further increased when phosphate (and calcium) was removed by dialysis. However, iron concentration was still lower than from the white wheat muffins, suggesting that another factor, possibly fiber, was still interfering with iron absorption.

Vegetables and fruits

Although vegetables and fruits contain low levels of trace elements, they do contain several organic acids that can stimulate the absorption of trace elements from other food items. Ascorbic acid is known to have a significant effect on iron absorption from composite meals (1). Citric acid, malic acid and succinic acid have also been shown to stimulate iron absorption when present in high concentrations (26). As mentioned previously, several food items such as vegetables, fruits and milk contain significant amounts of citrate and may therefore be quantitatively important when considering iron absorption from mixed diets. On the other hand, vegetables containing oxalic acid, which is known to have a negative effect on calcium absorption, may also inhibit trace element absorption (1).

Tea and coffee are frequently consumed with meals and contain substances that can inhibit trace element absorption. It has been demonstrated that iron absorption from tea and coffee is low and that addition of these drinks to breakfast meals decreases iron absorption (27). The exact nature of the inhibitory substances is not known, but tannic acid, chlorogenic acid and caffeine are likely to be involved. Besides a direct inhibitory effect on absorption, some of these compounds may also interfere with the metabolism of some trace elements. Coffee, for example, has been shown to cause lower hemoglobin values in lactating mothers that consumed coffee during pregnancy and lactation, and in their infants, than in non-coffee drinkers (28). This effect appears to be due to an impaired capacity to mobilize iron from the liver for hemoglobin synthesis (29). Thus, low absorption of iron from coffee as well as decreased utilization of absorbed iron may be a consequence of coffee consumption.

Processing of foods

During handling of food items, in the home or by the industry, the inhibitory or stimulatory effect of various dietary factors may change. Such processes include milling, heating, fermentation, refining and fortification. While milling is generally believed to remove inhibitors, such as phytate and fibers, that are part of the hull, it should be recognized that trace elements are also removed by this process. Thus, the bioavailability may be improved while the amount of trace elements is significantly reduced. The net effect of this may actually be, as has been shown for zinc and wheat breads (2), that the total amount of trace elements absorbed is higher from the whole cereal than from the white flour. The effect of heating may also be complex to evaluate; while it is known that heating destroys ascorbic acid and thus lowers iron absorption (30), extrusion cooking used for bran can increase zinc absorption by hydrolyzing some of the phytate present (31). It has recently been shown that removal of phosphate from phytate has a beneficial effect on zinc absorption in that zinc absorption from inositol penta-, and in particular, tetra- and triphosphate, is higher than from the hexaphosphate (32).

Other methods of refining food items, such as preparing protein isolates, may have a beneficial effect on trace element absorption. As discussed earlier, a crude soy flour formula inhibited zinc absorption more than a soy protein isolate formula. When phytate was removed from soy protein isolate by introducing another precipitation step, zinc absorption from soy formula increased to a level similar to cow's milk formula (19).

Food fortification - Dietary supplements

In order to cover the iron requirement of vulnerable groups, some food items such as formulas, cereals and flour are fortified with iron. Realization of this need has also increased the use of iron supplements. Recently, popular beliefs have also led to the use of zinc, copper and manganese supplements. It is rarely realized, however, that trace elements that have similar absorption pathways may interact with each other. Thus, indiscriminate use of one trace element can cause a decreased absorption of another one. Examples of such interactions include iron-zinc, zinc-copper and iron-manganese. That ratios between these elements can deviate substantially from what can be expected normally, was illustrated by a study of trace elements in infant formulas (33). In many formulas the trace element ratios were quite different from those found in human milk. Solomons and Jacob (34) have shown that high levels of ferrous iron can interfere with plasma uptake of a pharmacological dose of zinc. A study of infants fed either iron-supplemented or unsupplemented formula appeared to support such an interaction (35). Although zinc retention studies in humans fail to show a pronounced effect of this interaction when food is consumed at the same time as the supplement is taken (36), there may be long-term consequences of smaller differences in absorption. An effect of zinc on iron absorption in humans has also been shown (37), but this effect was also abolished when a meal was given. The negative effect of manganese on non-heme iron absorption in humans, however, is pronounced and not affected by food (37). Similarly, iron supplementation of infant formula significantly reduces manganese absorption in humans (38).

Concluding remarks

The complicated interrelationships between dietary factors and trace element bioavailability as well as between the trace elements themselves need to be investigated further. Such studies can start with delineating the effects of individual factors on trace element absorption but should be followed by systematic studies of their relevance as parts of meals, i.e., as consumed. For iron, this approach has been well explored by adding or excluding various food items to composite meals (19,39). Similar approaches can now be used for the other trace elements.

REFERENCES

1. L. Hallberg, Ann. Rev. Nutr., 1981, 1, 123.
2. B. Sandström, B. Arvidsson, A. Cederblad and E. Björn-Rasmussen, Am. J. Clin. Nutr., 1980, 33, 739.
3. D. Van Campen and E. Gross, J. Nutr., 1969, 99, 68.
4. C. Martinez-Torres, E. Romano and M. Layrisse, Am. J. Clin. Nutr., 1981, 34, 322.
5. P.G. Taylor, C. Martinez-Torres, E.L. Romano and M. Layrisse, Am. J. Clin. Nutr., 1986, 43, 68.
6. R.A. Wapnir, D.E. Khani, M.A. Bayne and F. Lifshitz, J. Nutr., 1983, 113, 1346.
7. R.A. Wapnir and L. Stiel, J. Nutr., 1986, 116, 2171.
8. B. Sandström, A. Cederblad and B. Lönnerdal, Am. J. Dis. Child., 1983, 137, 726.
9. B. Lönnerdal, A.G. Stanislowski and L.S. Hurley, J. Inorg. Biochem., 1980, 12, 71.
10. B. Lönnerdal, C.L. Keen, J.G. Bell and L.S. Hurley, In: C.F. Mills, I. Bremner, J.K. Chesters, eds. Trace Elements in Man and Animals (TEMA)-5, 1985, pp. 427-430, Commonwealth Agricultural Bureaux, Farnham Royal, United Kingdom.
11. B. Lönnerdal, A. Cederblad, L. Davidsson and B. Sandström, Am. J. Clin. Nutr., 1984, 40, 1064.
12. J. Kiely, A. Flynn, H. Singh and P.F. Fox, In: L.S. Hurley, C.L. Keen, B. Lönnerdal and R.B. Rucker, eds., Trace Element Metabolism in Man and Animals (TEMA)-6, 1988, Plenum Press, New York (in press).
13. J.C. Barton, M.E. Conrad and R.T. Parmley, Gastroenterology, 1983, 84, 90.
14. T. Hazell and I.T. Johnson, Br. J. Nutr., 1987, 57, 223.
15. D.D.K. Rolston, K.J. Moriarty, M.J.G. Farthing, M.J. Kelly, M.L. Clark and A.M. Dawson, Digestion, 1986, 34, 101.
16. F.K. Ghishan, J. Pediatr. Gastroenterol. Nutr., 1984, 3, 608.
17. E.K. Amine and D.M. Hegsted, J. Agric. Food Chem., 1975, 23, 204.
18. B. Lönnerdal, J.G. Bell and C.L. Keen, Am. J. Clin. Nutr., 1986, 42, 836.
19. B. Lönnerdal, J.G. Bell, A.G. Hendrickx, R.A. Burns and C.L. Keen, Am. J. Clin. Nutr., 1988, 48, (in press).
20. L. Hallberg and L. Rossander, Am. J. Clin. Nutr., 1982, 36, 514.
21. S.R. Lynch and A.M. Covell, Am. J. Clin. Nutr., 1987, 45, 866.

22. J.G. Bell, C.L. Keen and B. Lönnerdal, Am. J. Dis. Child., 1987, 141, 1128.
23. B. Sandström, A. Almgren, B. Kivistö and A. Cederblad, J. Nutr., 1987, 117, 1898.
24. J.D. Cook, N.L. Noble, T.A. Morck, S.R. Lynch and S.J. Petersburg, Gastroenterology, 1983, 85, 1354.
25. L. Hallberg, L. Rossander and A.-B. Skånberg, Am. J. Clin. Nutr., 1987, 45, 988.
26. M. Gillooly, T.H. Bothwell, J.D. Torrance, A.P. MacPhail, D.P. Derman, W.R. Bezwoda, W. Mills, R.W. Charlton and F. Mayet, Br. J. Nutr., 1983, 49, 331.
27. L. Rossander, L. Hallberg and E. Björn-Rasmussen, Am. J. Clin. Nutr., 1979, 32, 2484.
28. L. Muñoz, B. Lönnerdal, C.L. Keen and K.G. Dewey, Am. J. Clin. Nutr, 1988, 48, (in press).
29. L. Muñoz, C.L. Keen, B. Lönnerdal and K.G. Dewey, J. Nutr., 1986, 116, 1326.
30. M. Gillooly, J.D. Torrance, T.H. Bothwell, A.P. MacPhail, D. Derman, W. Mills and F. Mayet, Am. J. Clin. Nutr., 1984, 40, 522.
31. B. Kivistö, A. Andersson, G. Cederblad, A.-S. Sandberg and B. Sandström, Br. J. Nutr., 1985, 55, 255.
32. B. Lönnerdal, A.-S. Sandberg, B. Sandström and C. Kunz, J. Nutr. (in press).
33. B. Lönnerdal, C.L. Keen, M. Ohtake and T. Tamura, Am. J. Dis. Child., 1983, 137, 433.
34. N.W. Solomons and R.A. Jacob, Am. J. Clin. Nutr., 1981, 34, 475.
35. W.J. Craig, L. Balbach, S. Harris and N. Vyhmeister, J. Am. Coll. Nutr., 1984, 3, 1983.
36. B. Sandström, L. Davidsson, A. Cederblad and B. Lönnerdal, J. Nutr., 1985, 115, 411.
37. L. Hallberg, L. Rossander, M. Brune, B. Sandström and B. Lönnerdal, In: L.S. Hurley, C.L. Keen, B. Lönnerdal and R.B. Rucker, eds., Trace Element Metabolism in Man and Animals (TEMA)-6, 1988, Plenum Press, New York (in press).
38. L. Davidsson, A. Cederblad, B. Lönnerdal and B. Sandström, In: L.S. Hurley, C.L. Keen, B. Lönnerdal and R.B. Rucker, eds., Trace Element Metabolism in Man and Animals (TEMA)-6, 1988, Plenum Press, New York (in press).
39. L. Hallberg and L. Rossander, Scand. J. Gastroenterol., 1982, 27, 151.

MALNUTRITION, MALDIGESTION AND MALABSORPTION OF DIETARY HAEM/NON-HAEM IRON (-^{59}Fe) IN MAN

H. C. Heinrich, E. E. Gabbe and A. A. Pfau

Division of Medical Biochemistry, University-Hospital-Eppendorf,
University of Hamburg
Institute of Animal Breeding (FAL) Mariensee, Neustadt,
Fed. Rep. Germany.

If iron deficiency is not caused by increased gastrointestinal or urogenital blood losses it does mostly result from a long period of negative iron balance due to malnutrition, maldigestion or malabsorption of dietary iron. The amount of average daily iron absorption is then below the physiological whole body iron loss and requirement of 1.3 mg/day in males and non-menstruating females or 1.8 mg Fe/day in menstruating females. By using ^{59}Fe-labeled Fe(II) ascorbate and meat iron and measuring the whole body retention of absorbed ^{59}Fe with a large volume 4π-geometry whole body radioactivity detector the reliable and sensitive detection and quantification of food iron malnutrition, maldigestion or malabsorption and gastrointestinal or urogenital blood losses from the body is possible. Very small ^{59}Fe-doses of only 0.1 µCi are sufficient for iron absorption and about 1 µCi ^{59}Fe for blood loss measurements, so that the additional radiation burden is insignificant with about 0.69 and 6.9 mrem equivalent to 0.2 and 2% respect. of the natural radiation burden of (= 300 mrem/year).

1. High Bioavailability of Haem-Iron in Meat and Poor Bioavailability of Non-Haem Iron in Plant, Egg and Milk.

The bioavailability of dietary iron in normal man depends on the chemical form of the iron and the presence of inhibiting substances. Plants, eggs and milk contain only non-haem ferric iron (mostly in the presence of absorption inhibitors) with a poor bioavailability of only 1-7% which is improved in the presence of iron absorption promoters like ascorbic acid and/or meat. Meat iron on the other side contains 75% of its iron as haemoprotein ion (50% in myoglobin, 20% haemoglobin) and only 17% as non-haem iron (5% ferritin-, 8% transferrin-like- and 4% low molecular weight iron) with high bioavailability. From 2.5 mg Fe in 200 g pork 28 $\pm$ 9 $\pm$ 1% (XA $\pm$ SD $\pm$ SEM) are absorbed by healthy subjects with normal iron stores and 43 $\pm$ 15 $\pm$ 3.3% with depleted iron stores (prelatent/latent

iron deficiency without iron deficiency anaemia). Liver iron
contains about 5 mg Fe/25 g hog liver of which 95% are incorporated
into trivalent iron containing non-haem iron (90% ferritin-, 3% trans-
ferrin-like- and 3% low molecular weight iron) and only 2-5% into
haemoglobin iron. Liver iron bioavailability is therefore reduced
to 6.3 $\pm$ 4.2 $\pm$ 0.9% in subjects with normal iron stores and increases
with depleted iron stores to 24 $\pm$ 10$_{59}$ $\pm$ 3%. Due to the high bioavailability of its endogenous haem iron ^{59}Fe-labeled meat can be used for
the detection of food iron maldigestion.

2.   Food Iron Malnutrition in Vegans and Lacto-ovo-vegetarians

        Malnutrition causes iron deficiency without or with anaemia in
populations living on an animal protein free vegetarian diet (vegans)
and also in lacto-ovo-vegetarians as a result of the poor bioavailability of dietary non-haem iron in plants, eggs and milk. The
regular consumption of food iron absorption inhibiting components in
beverages (e.g. tannins in tea) can - if taken with the meals -
intensify the development of iron deficiency. Iron deficiency due
to malnutrition has to be suspected after the exclusion of food iron
maldigestion with the demonstration of normal ^{59}Fe absorption from
^{59}Fe-labeled meat, iron malabsorption by demonstrating increased
^{59}Fe-absorption from ^{59}Fe(II)ascorbate and increased gastrointestinal
or urogenital blood losses by the demonstration of a normal ^{59}Fe-whole
body elimination rate (0.1%/day).

3.   Maldigestion of Haem Iron in Meat but Normal or Increased
     Bioavailability of Ferrous and Haemoglobin Iron in Persons
     without Normal Gastric Secretion.

        Maldigestion of food iron seems to be more relevant for the well
absorbable meat iron. It can be diagnosed with ^{59}Fe-labeled meat in
patients with gastric corpus mucosa atrophy and after partial or total
gastrectomy since the normal peptic-HCl digestion of meat in the stomach
is required for the release of iron from meat before its absorption.
In subjects with normal iron stores the bioavailability of 2.5 mg Fe
in 200 g pork (-^{59}Fe) is reduced from 28 $\pm$ 1% (XA $\pm$ SEM) in healthy
subjects to 11 $\pm$ 1.5% in patients with gastric corpus mucosa atrophy
(and absolute intrinsic factor deficiency) and after partial (⅔)-
gastrectomy (Billroth II). With depleted iron stores the bioavailability of pork iron is reduced from 43 $\pm$ 3.4% in healthy subjects to
15 $\pm$ 2% in patients after partial (⅔) gastrectomy. The co-admin-
istration of 0.5 g amounts of hog gastric mucosa extract or hog
pancreatin did not normalize the reduced bioavailability of pork iron
in patients with gastric mucosa atrophy or partial gastrectomy. The
overnight predigestion of 200 g chopped port (-^{59}Fe) with 0.5 g pepsin
at pH 2.0 did however double the reduced iron bioavailability in
patients with normal iron stores and gastric mucosa atrophy or partial
(⅔) gastrectomy from 10 to 21%. That a maldigestion of pork iron and
not its malabsorption is responsible for the reduced bioavailability

of pork iron is also supported by the observed completely normal iron
availability from small diagnostic (0.56 mg) and large therapeutic
(100 mg) doses of ^{59}Fe(II) administered as Fe(II)ascorbate in patients
with gastric mucosa atrophy.   Because of the better solubility of
haem in neutral pH the bioavailability of haemoglobin-^{59}Fe was shown
to be twice as high in patients with <u>gastric corpus mucosa atrophy</u> and
normal iron stores (15 $\pm$ 4%) than in healthy subjects with normal iron
stores (7.5 $\pm$ 1.2%) and further increased with the depletion of iron
stores.   Normal gastric HCl, pepsin or Intrinsic Factor is not
required neither for Fe(II) nor for haemoglobin iron absorption and
oral Fe(II) therapy is equally effective also in patients without
gastric juice.

   <u>Total gastrectomy</u> which is followed by a considerable reduction
of the bioavailability of pork and liver iron does also not interfere
with haemoglobin-^{59}Fe availability which is twice as high as in
subjects with normal gastric secretion and digestion.   Inorganic
^{59}Fe(II) in ^{59}Fe(II) ascorbate solution and commercial oral iron
preparations (^{59}Fe-labeled by neutron activation) is available in
totally gastrectomized subjects to the same degree as in normal persons
and its absorption is regulated according to available iron stores
also without a stomach.   Iron deficiency can be treated therefore
also in partially or totally gastrectomized subjects with oral Fe(II)
preparations of proven bioavailability.

   The exocrine secretion of the <u>pancreas</u> does not affect inorganic
or food iron absorption and does neither contain an iron absorption
inhibiting nor promoting factor as was claimed earlier.   Patients
with complete exocrine pancreatic insufficiency due to cystic fibrosis
or after total pancreatectomy were shown to absorb inorganic, haemoglobin, liver and pork iron ($^{-59}$Fe) according to their iron stores and
to the same degree as normal subjects.   Iron deficiency can be treated
with oral Fe(II) preparations of proven bioavailability also in patients without a pancreas.

4.   <u>Malabsorption of Food and Ferrous Iron in Duodenal/Jejunal
     Villous Atrophy and Acute Infection</u>

   The partial to total <u>villous atrophy</u> in the duodenum and jejunum
(flat mucosa) causes malabsorption of food iron and also from diagnostic and therapeutic doses (0.56 and 100 mg respect.) of ferrous
iron which parallels folate malabsorption in such patients with gluten-
sensitive enteropathy (coeliac disease). ^{59}Fe-absorption from the
diagnostic 0.56 mg ^{59}Fe(II)-dose (normal 95%-range in prelatent to
manifest iron deficiency 51–100%, median 80–90%) is reduced to 0–47%
($\bar{X}A \pm SD = 18 \pm 14\%$) in infants or adults with untreated gluten-induced
enteropathy even with simultaneous iron deficiency anaemia.   The ^{59}Fe-
absorption from ^{59}Fe-labeled haemoglobin, pork and hog liver is also
severely reduced.   The diminished food iron absorption causes iron
deficiency anaemia after the depletion of iron stores in such patients.

Only 2-4 weeks on a gluten-free diet are required for the normalization of haem-/non-haem iron and folate absorption whereas 6-12
months on a gluten-free diet are necessary for the regeneration of
the gluten-induced flat mucosa.   This early normalization of the
reduced to interrupted intestinal bioavailability of haem-/non-haem
iron and/or folic acid is a reliable indicator for gluten as the
cause of the malabsorption and <u>villous atrophy</u> and justifies the
continuation of the gluten-free diet over a long period.

   <u>Acute infection</u> creates an only temporary iron malabsorption
which disappears immediately after the successful treatment of the
acute infection.

THE DAY-TO-DAY REGULATION OF IRON ABSORPTION

A.J.A. WRIGHT, S. SOUTHON and S.J. FAIRWEATHER-TAIT

AFRC Institute of Food Research, Norwich Laboratory,
Colney Lane, Norwich, NR4 7UA U.K.

1 INTRODUCTION

Iron homeostasis is primarily maintained by variations in
the amount of iron absorbed from the diet. One of the accepted methods for measuring iron absorption uses ^{59}Fe retention from labelled food, and although it is known that
the efficiency of absorption changes in response to significant alterations in iron status, there is no satisfactory explanation for the observed day-to-day fluctuations
in absorption which occur under conditions of constant body
iron status[1].
 Previous work from this laboratory[2] has shown that a
one day change in iron intake significantly alters the capacity of the rat to absorb a subsequent iron dose, whereby
whole-body ^{59}Fe retention from a labelled dose is inversely
related to previous dietary iron concentration. The effect
is particularly marked over the physiological range (0-100
mg Fe/kg diet). However, high dietary iron concentrations
may cause an increase in mucosal iron levels resulting in
radio-isotope dilution of the test dose and errors in the
estimation of absorption. The following experiment was
designed to investigate this possibility.

2 EXPERIMENTAL

Sixty male Wistar rats (100-120 g) were randomly allocated
to 4 groups. All rats were given a control semi-synthetic
diet (38 mg Fe/kg) ad libitum for 7 days. On day 8 rats
were given access to unrestricted amounts of food as a
single meal between 15.15 and 16.45 hours. At the same time
the following day rats from groups 1 and 3 received a meal
of control diet, while groups 2 and 4 received a meal con-

taining 500 mg Fe/kg. The next morning all rats were intubated with 2 ml of a freshly prepared solution containing
120 μg Fe as ferrous sulphate, extrinsically labelled with
18 kBq ^{59}Fe, and immediately counted in a whole-body
counter (NE 8112 Nuclear Enterprises) to determine the
exact dose of ^{59}Fe given to each animal. The fasted rats
were killed 6 h (groups 1 and 2) or 24 h (groups 3 and 4)
later. The small intestine was removed and gently rinsed
with cold saline, separated into duodenum, jejunum, and
ileum, and each segment analysed for ^{59}Fe and total iron.
The ^{59}Fe content of the carcass, minus caecum and large
intestine was also measured.

3 RESULTS

The amount of ^{59}Fe transported to the carcass was significantly lower in the high-iron groups, due mainly to a reduction in mucosal uptake (SI + Carcass), as shown below.

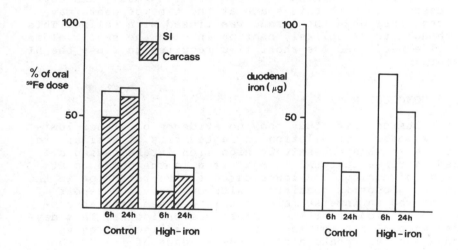

4 DISCUSSION

Mucosal cells are continuously shed into the intestinal
lumen, where they are broken down and their iron released.
This could in theory reduce the specific activity of an

oral ^{59}Fe labelled test dose. The duodenum is the major
site of iron transport and the difference in duodenal iron
loss between 6 and 24 h indicated that the maximum loss of
iron into the lumen of this region was 0.3 and 1.1 μg/h for
control and high-iron groups respectively. This is insufficient to cause significant isotopic dilution in the lumen.
    The possibility of isotopic dilution within the duo-
denal mucosal cells of the high-iron group must also be
considered. After deducting 10 μg 'basal iron' from duodenal iron contents, the loss of mucosal cell iron between
6 and 24 h for both control and high-iron groups was calculated to be no more than that which would be lost through
mucosal cell turnover (ca 30%). Because of this, and the
fact that the loss of radio-label was much greater (ca 80%)
over this period, it was concluded that most of the the
iron in the mucosal cells at the time of dosing in both
groups was in a non-exchangeable iron pool and as such
would not influence the specific activity of the ^{59}Fe
entering the cell.
    Finally, ^{59}Fe from the test dose could have undergone
dilution in the intervillous space of the high-iron group
by dietary iron remaining from the previous meal, and any
^{59}Fe associated with this space at the time of death may
have been lost when the tissue was rinsed with saline. This
was thought to be unlikely bearing in mind the small volume
of saline used, and the short time required to rinse the SI
segments.

5 CONCLUSION

The results of this study show no evidence of either luminal or mucosal ^{59}Fe dilution in fasted rats of similar iron
status, even when excessively high iron intake caused a
marked increase in total mucosal iron in the duodenum at
the time of dosing. The lower carcass ^{59}Fe retention in the
high-iron groups is consistent with our previous report[2]
which showed an inverse relationship between iron absorption and previous short-term dietary iron intake. This day-
to-day mucosal control appears to be exercised largely
through mucosal uptake and, in the absence of frank iron
deficiency, it is possibly a far more important regulator
of iron absorption than the level of body iron stores.

6 REFERENCES

1.   J.D.Cook, M.Layrisse & C.A.Finch, Blood 1969, 33, 421.
2.   S.J.Fairweather-Tait & A.J.A.Wright, Br. J. Nutr.,
      1984, 51, 185.

Sites of the intestinal mucosal cell where the interactions among Fe, Zn, and Cu occur affecting the bioavailability of these elements.

Dennis T. Gordon

Department of Food Science and Nutrition
Eckles Hall 221
University of Missouri
Columbia, MO   65211

1 INTRODUCTION

Interactions occur between each pair of the transition elements Fe, Zn, and Cu (1). A significant ($P \leq 0.05$) 3-way interaction has been shown among these elements affecting the hemoglobin concentrations in the growing rat (2). Significant ($P \leq 0.05$) 2-way interactions between Fe and Zn altering femur Zn concentrations and Fe and Zn, and Zn and Cu changing liver Cu concentrations were also observed in these same animals (3). The purpose of this study is to explore how the interactions among Fe, Zn, and Cu in the intestine alter the bioavailability of these elements.

2 MATERIAL AND METHODS

Thirty-six groups of male weanling rats (n=5) having equal weights per group were arranged in a randomized complete block design in which treatments were in a 3x4x3 factorial. Rats were fed semi-purified diets (AIN) ad libitum with the following amounts of dietary Fe: 18, 90 and 270 µg/g; Zn: 8.5, 10.5, 42.5 and 17.0 µg/g and; Cu: 2, 10, and 40 µg/g. After 21 days, the rats were killed and 10 cm of the proximal intestine were removed, rinsed with 0.9% NaCl solution, dried, digested in HNO_3-$HClO_4$, and analyzed for Fe, Zn, and Cu by atomic absorption spectrophotometry.

3 RESULTS AND DISCUSSION

Iron. Increasing concentrations of dietary Fe caused significant increases in duodenum Fe concentrations (Table 1). Zinc concentrations in the duodenum did not change, but Cu concentrations significantly ($P \leq 0.05$) decreased with added dietary Fe. Although other studies (4,5) including

Table 1. Effect of dietary Fe on duodenum concentrations
          of Fe, Zn, and Cu in the growing rat.

Dietary iron - μg/g -	n	Fe	Zn	Cu
		-μg/g duodenum[1] -		
18	60	96[c]	123	10.6[a]
90	60	254[b]	119	9.0[b]
270	60	485[a]	120	8.6[b]

[1]Mean pooled values (dry wt) for 12 groups of rats at all
 dietary concentrations of Zn and Cu. a≠b≠c (P≤0.05).

our own (3), have shown that Fe depresses Zn
bioavailability, the mechanism(s) must not cause a
reduction of Zn entry into the cell, but rather an
inhibition of Zn metabolism within the cell. Reduced Cu
entry into the cell with increasing concentrations of Fe
appears to occur at the cell membrane. Iron may also be
affecting Cu metabolism within the cell, the mechanism
being unknown.

Zinc. Zinc concentrations in the duodenum increase
with the level of dietary Zn (Table 2). High dietary Zn
will suppress cellular Cu concentrations and low dietary Zn
will allow more Cu to enter the cell. It has been shown
that Zn will enhance the production of metallothionein (MT)
which can subsequently retard Cu metabolism (6). It is
theorized that this impediment to Cu metabolism can have an
effect on Fe metabolism. Excess Zn is, therefore,
antagonistic to Cu and Fe at the mucosal cell membrane and
also within the cell, MT being involved in this latter
mechanism.

Table 2. Effect of dietary Zn on duodenum concentrations
          of Fe, Zn, and Cu in the growing rat.

Dietary zinc - μg/g -	n	Fe	Zn	Cu
		- μg/g duodenum[1] -		
8.5	45	296[a]	109[c]	9.2[b]
10.5	45	237[b]	107[c]	10.1[a,b]
42.5	45	319[a]	120[b]	10.3[a,b]
170.0	45	261[b]	147[a]	8.0[c]

[2]Mean pooled values (dry wt) for 9 groups of rats at all
 dietary concentration of Fe and Cu; a≠b≠c (P≤0.05).

Table 3. Effect of dietary Cu on duodenum concentrations of Fe, Zn, and Cu in the growing rat.

Dietary copper - μg/g -	n	Fe	Zn	Cu
		- μg/g duodenum[1] -		
2	60	316[a]	119	6.6[c]
10	60	265[b]	119	8.6[b]
40	60	254[b]	123	12.9[a]

[1]Mean pooled values (dry wt) for 12 groups of rats at all dietary concentrations of Fe and Cu; a≠b≠c ($P \leq 0.05$).

Copper. Duodenum Fe concentrations decrease and Cu concentrations increase with increasing amounts of dietary Cu and these changes were significant ($P \leq 0.05$) (Table 3). Copper had no effect on duodenum concentrations of Zn. The entry of Fe into the mucosal cell appears blocked by Cu but Cu does not affect Zn. Since Cu can also increase the amount of MT in the mucosal cell (7), the trapping of Zn by MT laden with Cu could explain how Zn metabolism is impaired, but not cellular uptake of this element. Significant ($P \leq 0.05$) interactions among elements were observed in this study, but are not discussed. Contribution from the Univ. of MO Ag. Exp. Station, No. 10640.

4 REFERENCES

1. D.T. Gordon. AIN Symposium Proceedings, Nutrition '87, Am. Inst. Nutr., Bethesda, MD, 1987, pg. 27.
2. D.T. Gordon, XIII Intl. Congress Nutr., pg 154 (abst.)
3. D.T. Gordon and M. Ellersieck. 'Trace Elements in Man and Animals-TEMA 6', Univ of CA, Davis, CA. 1988 (in press)
4. N.W. Solomons and R.A. Jacob. Am. J. Clin. Nutr., 1981, 34, 475.
5. B. Sandstrom, L. Davison, L. Cederblad and B. Lonnerdal. J. Nutr., 1985, 115, 411.
6. T.L. Blalock, M.A. Dunn and R.J. Cousins. J. Nutr., 1988, 118, 222.
7. P. Oestricher and R.J. Cousins. J. Nutr, 1985, 115, 159.

THE EFFECT OF PARENTERAL IRON ADMINISTRATION UPON ITS ABSORPTION IN YOUNG RATS

N. Gruden

Institute for Medical Research
and Occupational Health
University of Zagreb
41001 Zagreb, Yugoslavia

1 INTRODUCTION

Manganese absorption is greatly inhibited by the oral[1] and even more, by the intraperitoneal administration of iron[2]. The aim of the present study was to find out, under identical experimental conditions as in[2] to what extent intraperitoneally given iron affects its own metabolism.

2 ANIMALS AND METHODS

Three-week-old female albino rats were placed in groups according to the amount of iron they had received (in the form of sulphate) by intraperitoneal injection daily for four days: 0 (control) - 100 - 400 - 1600 µg Fe. On the fourth day all animals received iron-59 (37 KBq/rat) in 0.4 ml pasteurized cow's milk by the "drop-by-drop" feeding procedure[3]. Three days later radioiron was determined in the whole body, carcass and selected organs. From the beginning till the end of experiment all animals were bottle-fed cow's milk.

3 RESULTS AND DISCUSSION

The results were calculated as per cent of the iron-59 dose received. The Table 1 shows the retention data for the iron treated animals expressed as percentages of corresponding control values taken as 100 per cent. The lowest and next to lowest doses (100 and 400 µg Fe/rat/d) did not affect iron absorption but decreased its deposition in some parts of the small intestine, kidney and brain. Iron absorption and tissue distribution (with the exception of liver) were significantly lower (by

150

43-63 per cent) in animals on the highest iron dose (1600 µg Fe/rat/d) than in control rats. The comparison with previous results[2] suggests iron metabolism to be less sensitive to its parenteral administration, whereas manganese is less sensitive to oral iron administration[4].

Table 1   [59]Iron activity in different tissue of three-week-old rats given iron intraperitoneally*

Iron dose (µg)	Whole body	Intest. tract	Liver	Kidney	Brain
100	107.3 ±3.8	91.8 ±7.2	91.9 ±5.1	98.8 ±4.6	79.3[s] ±4.1
400	95.6 ±4.3	74.8[s] ±4.4	104.5 ±8.7	75.7[s] ±5.2	57.6[s] ±3.9
1600	59.4[s] ±6.2	47.1[s] ±4.9	88.3 ±9.8	44.1[s] ±4.8	29.4[s] ±3.1

*The retention data for experimental animals presented as mean S.E. percentages of the corresponding control values (n=10).

[s]Values significantly different from the corresponding control (P<0.05;.

Acknowledgement   This work was supported by the Scientific Research Council of S.R. Croatia. The author thanks Mrs M. Buben for her valuable technical assistance and Mrs M. Horvat for typing the manuscript.

4 REFERENCES

1. N. Gruden, In "Nutritional Bioavailability of Manganese", ACS, Washington, 1987, Chapter 7, 67.
2. N. Gruden, *Nutr. Rep. Int.* 1988, 37, 57.
3. B. Momčilović and I. Rabar, *Period. Biol.* 1979, 81, 27.
4. N. Gruden, *Nutr. Rep. Int.* 1982, 25, 849.

EFFECT OF POLYPHENOLS ON IRON BIOAVAILABILITY IN RATS

R. Brown, A. Klein and R.F. Hurrell

Nestec Ltd., Nestlé Research Centre,
Vers-chez-les-Blanc,
CH-1000 Lausanne 26, Switzerland

1 INTRODUCTION

The absorption of iron from a meal has been reported to
be reduced in man by the simultaneous consumption of
polyphenolic-containing beverages such as black tea[1]
and coffee[2]. Other beverages such as cocoa and bush teas
also contain polyphenolic compounds. In bush teas the
polyphenolics are mainly monomeric flavonoids and polyphenolic acids. Roasted coffee beans contain about 4.5%
dry weight chlorogenic acid and 2% other phenolic compounds including caffeic acid[3]. The fermentation steps
in the production of black tea and cocoa cause the
original monomeric flavonoids and polyphenolic acids to
polymerize into condensed and hydrolyzable tannins. We
have investigated the influence of different polyphenolic-
containing beverages and polyphenolic compounds on iron
absorption in rats.

2 MATERIALS AND METHODS

Whole body retention of ^{59}Fe in rats was used to study
the bioavailability of iron. Polyphenolic beverages
(coffee, black tea, cocoa and bush teas) or polyphenolic
compounds (epicatechin, a flavonoid; chlorogenic, gallic
and caffeic acids, polyphenolic acids; and tannic acid,
a hydrolyzable tannin) were administered to 24-hour fasted
rats either by oesophageal cannula as a single aqueous
dose or added to a single meal and were compared to a
water control. Rats were given three hours to consume the
meal and food was withheld from the animals for four hours
following the removal of the test meal. In order to better
investigate the mechanism of action of different poly-

phenols on iron bioavailability, the ratio of polyphenols to iron in the experimental meal was standardized at 4.0mg of polyphenol (as determined by the Folin-Denis method[4]) to 12.5µg of iron in all studies. Whole body radioactivity was determined following the meal and at 2, 6 and 8 days. The percent retained iron was used as a measure of iron bioavailability.

The bush teas tested in this study (Jack-in-the-Bush, Pepper Elder, Basil and Sour Sop) were supplied by Dr. W.K. Simmons of the Caribbean Food and Nutrition Institute, Kingston, Jamaica. They are widely consumed in Jamaica.

3 RESULTS AND DISCUSSION

The results in Table 1 show that compared to the water control, the beverages tested reduced the bioavailability of iron by 31 to 45% when administered by oesophageal cannula. The individual polyphenolic compounds were less inhibitory to iron absorption than the beverages and reduced iron bioavailability from 2 to 30%. Caffeic acid and tannic acid were the most inhibitory. When the polyphenolic containing beverages were added to a meal, the inhibition of iron absorption was less pronounced ranging from no effect with Sour Sop to 25% inhibition with black tea and 31% inhibition with basil. The standard compounds were also less inhibitory to iron absorption when added to a meal resulting in a 9 to 25% reduction.

From these results it would appear that both monomeric and polymerized polyphenolic compounds are able to bind iron *in vivo* and reduce iron bioavailability. However, in relation to human nutrition, the polyphenolic concentration of the bush teas as consumed (3-30mg total polyphenols/100 ml) is far lower than that found in black teas (136mg/100ml), coffee (89mg/100ml) and cocoa (80mg/100ml) and bush teas would be less likely to have a significant impact on iron absorption.

REFERENCES

1. P.B. Disler, S.R. Lynch, R.W. Charlton, J.D. Torrance, T.H. Bothwell, R.B. Walker and F. Mayet, *Gut*, 1975, *16*, 193.

2. T.A. Morck, S.R. Lynch and J.D. Cook, <u>Am.J.Clin.Nutr.</u>, 1983, <u>37</u>, 416.
3. M. Sivetz and N.W. Desrosier, "Coffee Technology", Avi, Westport, Conn, 1959.
4. T. Swain and W.E. Hillis, <u>J.Sci.Fd.Agric.</u>, 1959, <u>10</u>, 63.

<u>Table 1</u>   The Effect of Polyphenolic-Containing Beverages or Polyphenolic Compounds on Iron Absorption in the Rat

Treatment	Absorption of Iron mean% $\pm$ SD	
	By Stomach Tube[1]	With Meal[2]
Jack-in-the-Bush	61.9 $\pm$ 15.2*	---
Pepper Elder	49.9 $\pm$ 10.2*	---
Basil	---	44.7 $\pm$ 2.7*
Sour Sop	---	65.7 $\pm$ 3.4
Coffee	51.5 $\pm$ 10.6*	52.1 $\pm$ 7.1*
Cocoa	62.2 $\pm$ 13.3*	56.5 $\pm$ 9.3*
Assam Tea	49.6 $\pm$ 9.7*	49.0 $\pm$ 6.1*
Control (Water)	89.5 $\pm$ 6.6	65.1 $\pm$ 4.7
Epicatechin	80.2 $\pm$ 15.5	64.4 $\pm$ 8.4
Chlorogenic Acid	76.8 $\pm$ 17.0	58.9 $\pm$ 3.9*
Gallic Acid	74.5 $\pm$ 7.2	52.9 $\pm$ 5.7*
Tannic Acid	63.9 $\pm$ 8.8*	53.0 $\pm$ 3.4*
Caffeic Acid	57.2 $\pm$ 16.0*	61.9 $\pm$ 5.7*
Control (Water)	82.0 $\pm$ 8.0	70.9 $\pm$ 8.8

1. One ml of each sample containing 4.0mg of polyphenol was mixed with 0.5ml of distilled water containing 12.5µg of iron as $FeSO_4$ labelled with 2.0µCi ^{59}Fe.

2. For the meal studies, a sample containing 20mg of polyphenol was mixed with 5g of a meal (80% wheat flour & 20% oil) containing 12.5µg of iron/g of meal labelled with 2.0µCi ^{59}Fe. The control for both studies was distilled water.

* $P < 0.05$

THE EFFECT OF SAPONINS ON IRON AND ZINC AVAILABILITY

K.R. Price, S. Southon and G.R. Fenwick

Institute of Food Research, Norwich Laboratory
Colney Lane, Norwich, NR4 7UA

1   INTRODUCTION

It has been suggested that increased consumption of
saponins might be beneficial because of their ability to
lower serum cholesterol[1]. Some saponins, however, are
able to form insoluble complexes with Fe and Zn in vitro[2]
and so may reduce the amount of mineral available for
absorption in vivo. The present study, comprising three
experiments, was undertaken to determine the effect of
saponins in the diet on mineral utilization in the rat.

2   METHODS

Experiment 1. Male Wistar rats (100 g) were divided into
3 groups and given diets containing 38 mg Fe and 55 mg Zn
(Basal), 38 mg Fe and 5 mg Zn (Low Zn) or 12 mg Fe and 55
mg Zn (Low Fe). Groups were further divided so that half
the rats received diets with 12g/Kg Gypsophila saponin
(GS). Food intakes were equalised between groups. After
3 weeks Fe and Zn status was assessed.

Experiment 2. Male Wistar rats (80 g) were given basal
diet ad lib. for 7d, meal-fed for 2d, fasted overnight and
given 3g starch: sucrose paste containing $120\mu g$ Fe or
$139\mu g$ Zn labelled with ^{59}Fe or ^{65}Zn, and varying amounts
of GS. Estimates of absorption were obtained by whole-
body counting techniques.

Experiment 3. Male Wistar rats (200 g) were given basal
diet ad lib. for 7d followed by an ^{59}Fe labelled test
meal, as described for Expt. 2. Meals contained GS,
soyasaponin I or lucerne (Medicago sativa) saponins to
give a saponin:Fe molar ratio of approximately 8. Iron

absorption from the meal was estimated by whole-body counting.

3   RESULTS

<u>Expt. 1</u>   Fe and Zn status of rats fed diets containing 12g/Kg Gypsophila saponin.

Dietary treatment	Body wt. gain (g)		Hb (g/100ml)		PCV (%)		Liver Fe (g)		Femur Zn (µg/g dry wt.)	
	Mean	SE	Mean	SE	Mean	SE	Mean	SE	Mean	SE
Basal	134	2	12.5	0.3	40	1	849	55	220	10
Basal + saponin	131	2	11.9*	0.3	36*	1	672*	55	211	5
Low Fe	133	2	7.6	0.2	26	1	344	14	228	7
Low Fe + saponin	131	2	7.0	0.3	25	1	303*	10	242	10
Low Zn	134	3	12.7	0.2	40	1	825	48	155	6
Low Zn + saponin	126*	1	12.2	0.2	39	1	753	56	158	9

* Mean values significantly different ($P<0.05$) from those for rats given a similar diet without saponin.

<u>Expt. 2</u>.   Percentage ^{59}Fe absorption relative to rats given a saponin-free test meal.

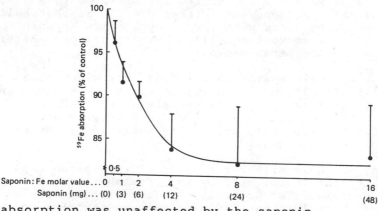

Zn absorption was unaffected by the saponin.

Expt. 3.   [59]Fe absorption from a test meal containing 16mg soyasaponin I, lucerne saponins or Gypsophila saponin (saponin:Fe ratio approx. 8).

Type of saponin in test meal	[59]Fe absorption (% of dose)		
	n	mean	se
Control (no added saponin)	15	64.0	1.5
Soyasaponin I	14	59.1	2.5
Lucerne	11	53.4*	1.7
Gypsophila	12	49.5*	2.3

* Mean value significantly different from Control ($P < 0.01$)

4   CONCLUSIONS

The results from Expt. 1. indicated that Gypsophila saponin (a non-food saponin) had an adverse effect on Fe status in the rat. Expt. 2. demonstrated that increasing amounts of this saponin given in a single meal progressively reduced the amount of Fe available for absorption. The effect reached a plateau at a saponin:Fe molar ratio of 4. Zn status and absorption appeared to be unaffected. Lucerne saponin, present in some herbal remedies, also significantly reduced Fe absorption at a saponin:Fe ratio of 8. Soyasaponin I, the main saponin found in legume seeds, had a lower, marginal effect. Recent data[3] show daily intakes of saponins to be in excess of 100 mg for some vegetarians, a level which may adversely influence Fe absorption and status in man.

5   REFERENCES

1.   D.G. Oakenfull, Food Technol. Aust., 1981, 33, 432.
2.   L.G. West, J.L. Greger, A. White and B.J. Nonnamaker, J. Food Sci., 1978, 43, 1342.
3.   C.L. Ridout, S.G. Wharf, K.R. Price, I.T. Johnson and G.R. Fenwick, Hum. Nut. Fd. Sci. & Nut., 1988, in press.

IN VITRO STUDIES OF INOSITOL TRI-, TETRA-, PENTA- AND HEXAPHOSPHATES AS POTENTIAL IRON ABSORPTION INHIBITORS

A.-S. Sandberg, N.-G. Carlsson and U. Svanberg

Department of Food Science
Chalmers University of Technology
Gothenburg

1 INTRODUCTION

Several studies in animals and humans indicate that under certain conditions phytate (inositol hexaphosphate) in the diet may decrease the absorption of dietary minerals such as zinc, calcium, magnesium and iron (1-4). Conventionally, "phytate" has been analyzed by precipitation or by ion-exchange methods including except the inositol hexaphosphate at least the penta-, tetra-, and triphosphates of inositol. In raw, unprocessed food the inositol hexaphosphate is the predominant form. Food preparation/processing e.g. germination, fermentation, extrusion cooking or digestion in the human gut, can, however, result in formation of inositol phosphates with a lower degree of phosphorylation (5-9). Consequently, a relevant question will be whether the effects of various inositol phosphates are similar, or not. We have, therefore, investigated the effects of inositol tri-, tetra-, penta-, and hexaphosphates on iron availability using an in vitro model. This model measures the iron solubility of a diet and has shown a high correlation with human studies of iron absorption (Svanberg et al, submitted for publ.).

2 METHODS

Inositol tri-, tetra-, and pentaphosphates were prepared by hydrolysis of sodium phytate in 0.5 M HCl for 7 h. The inositol phosphates formed were separated by ion-exchange chromatography with a linear gradient of 0.05-0.5 M HCl (Sandberg et al, submitted for publ.). The inositol phosphates were identified and quantified with HPLC ion-pair chromatography (10).

Pure inositol phosphates (0.125-10 μmol) were added to 1 g freeze-dried wheat roll and digestion performed in vitro simulating physiological conditions. The digestion was performed step-wise using a three enzyme system and the amount of solubilized iron at pH 6.0 was determined (Svanberg et al, submitted for publ.) and used as an index of bioavailability.

158

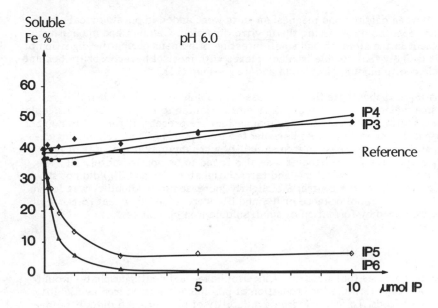

In vitro iron availability (% soluble Fe after digestion) when inositol tri-, tetra-, penta- and hexaphosphates (IP_3, IP_4, IP_5 and IP_6) were added to 1 g of wheat roll. Pure wheat roll was used as a reference. (Mean values of duplicate determinations.)

3 RESULTS

Figure 1 shows that addition of inositol penta- and hexaphosphates reduced the iron solubility. When 2.5 μmol of inositol penta- and hexaphosphates were added, only 5 % and 1 % respectively of total iron was soluble, while in the reference sample (pure wheat roll) 39 % was soluble. Addition of 0.125-2.5 μmol of inositol tri- and tetraphosphates did not influence the iron solubility, whereas higher amounts slightly increased the solubility. The solubility of iron was not affected by the pH in the interval 6.0 to 7.0 when inositol penta- or hexaphosphate was added. When inositol tri- and tetraphosphates were added under the same conditions the solubility of iron decreased when pH was increased from 6.0 to 7.0.

4 DISCUSSION

The highest amount of inositol hexaphosphate (10 μmol) added to 1 g wheat roll corresponds approximately to the amount found in wholemeal flour. The findings that inositol hexaphosphate (IP_6) has a negative effect on iron solubility, even when added in small amounts, is consistent with results obtained in human absorption studies using radionuclide technique (4). This effect was, however, only obtained when calcium and magnesium salts were added in physiological amounts with the pepsin solution during the in vitro digestion. Calcium and magnesium are present in the stomach and small intestine of humans during the digestion of food. It is likely that soluble iron complexes with inositol hexaphosphate become insoluble due to binding of calcium and magnesium (10).

Inositol hexaphosphate (IP_5) decreased the solubility of iron when IP_5 was added in a molar ratio to iron of 1:2 or more. Similar to IP_6, IP_5 forms insoluble complexes with iron if calcium and magnesium are present. If related to number of phosphate groups, IP_5 would be expected to have 5/6 of the iron binding capacity of IP_6. The decrease in iron solubility when equimolar amounts of IP_5 and IP_6 respectively were studied was also found to be approximately 5:6. The phosphate groups of inositol tri- and tetraphosphates (IP_3 and IP_4) did not show a similar effect. On the contrary, a slightly increased iron solubility was found at pH 6.0 when $5\,\mu$mol or more of IP_3 and IP_4 were added to wheat rolls, which may be explained by formation of small soluble iron complexes.

5 CONCLUSIONS

This study indicates that the sum of inositol hexa- and pentaphosphates would be accurate to determine for prediction of possible effects on iron availability in processed foods. To increase iron availability of phytate-rich diets it seems adequate to degrade inositol hexa- and pentaphosphates to lower inositol phosphates. To investigate the effects of different inositol phosphates on iron absorption further studies in humans should be performed.

REFERENCES

1. R.A. McCance and E.M. Widdowson, Journal of Physiology, 1942a, 101, 44.
2. R.A. McCance and E.M. Widdowson, Journal of Physiology, 1942b, 101, 304.
3. B. Nävert, B. Sandström and Å. Cederblad, Br. J. Nutr., 1985, 53, 47.
4. L. Hallberg, L. Rossander, A.B. Skånberg, Am. J. Clin. Nutr., 1987, 45, 988.
5. N.R. Nayini, P. Markakis, J. Food Sci., 1983, 48, 262,
6. A.-S. Sandberg, H. Andersson, N.-G. Carlsson and B. Sandström, J. Nutr., 1987, 117, 2061.
7. A.-S. Sandberg and H. Andersson, J. Nutr., 1988, 118, 469.
8. U. Svanberg and A.-S. Sandberg, 'In Proceedings on "Household level food - technologies for improving young child feeding in Eastern and Southern Africa"', Nairobi, Act., 1987 (in press 1988).
9. B.A. Phillippy, M.R. Johnston, S.-H. Tao and M.R.S. Fox, J. Food Sci., 1988, 53, 496.
10. A.-S. Sandberg and R. Ahderinne, J. Food Sci., 1986, 51, 547.
11. K. Rao Subba and B.S. Rao Narasinga, Nutr. Rep. Int., 1983, 28, 771.
12. D.J. Cosgrove, Biochem. J., 1963, 89, 172.
13. B.Q. Phillippy, K.D. White, M.R. Johnston, S.-H. Tao and M.R.S. Fox, Anal. Biochem., 1987, 162, 115.

PHYTIC ACID LEVEL OF WHITE AND WHOLEMEAL BREAD DOUGHS VARIATION WITH DIFFERENT FACTORS

P. Le François, A. Verel and Y. Audidier

BSN Branche Biscuits
Centre de Recherche
6 rue E. Vaillant
91201 Athis-Mons
France

Phytic acid is important because it binds to divalent cations and forms stable complexes with poor mineral bio-availability. The aim of this research was to assess the effect of different factors on the hydrolysis of phytic acid in doughs to improve nutritional quality of bread.

1 METHODS

Bread doughs were kneaded in standardized experimental conditions in a Brabender farinograph at 20°C and fermented in a steam oven with controlled temperature and moisture. Phytic acid was analyzed by a thiocyanate method (1) on aliquots of dough homogenized in HNO3 0.5 M.

Different assays were made to assess the effect of the following factors on the hydrolysis of phytic acid in white and wholemeal bread doughs:
- amount of bakers'yeast (1.5-6 % flour basis)
- time (45-240 mn), temperature of fermentation (32, 38°C)
- water content (90-120 % of the optimal amount)
- addition of rye flour (0, 10 % flour basis), dried skim-med milk (0-20 % flour basis), calcium carbonate (0-0.66 % flour basis), phytase (0-9 U % flour basis), lactic or acetic acid (0-0.9 % flour basis).

2 RESULTS AND DISCUSSION

The average results (mean ± S.D.) of phytic acid deter-mination for the same dough made 4 times in different batches is 0.037 ± 0.005 % for white bread, 0.468 ± 0.011 % for wholemeal bread.

<u>Table 1</u>   Residual percentage of phytic acid according to
the conditions of the assays

		F e r m e n t a t i o n		
Assay	Yeast	Time	Temperature	Phytic acid %
	YE	TI	TE	PA
1	-1	-1	-1	91
2	1	-1	-1	92
3	-1	1	-1	77
4	1	1	-1	74
5	-1	-1	1	87
6	1	-1	1	87
7	-1	1	1	70
8	1	1	1	67

Yeast: -1 = 1.5 % flour basis , 1 = 6 % flour basis
Time :   -1 = 45 mn , 1 = 120 mn
Temperature : -1 = 32°C , 1 = 38°C

<u>Predictive equation for the model</u>

$$PA = 80.625 - 8.625\ TI - 2.875\ TE - 0.625\ YE$$
$$- 0.875\ YE * TI - 0.625\ TI * TE$$

$$R\ 2 = 0.9996 \qquad F = 0.0009$$

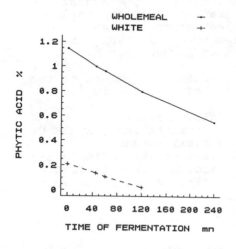

<u>Figure 1</u> Phytic acid content of
bread doughs during fermentation

<u>Figure 2</u> Phytic acid as a function
of pH and milk in wholemeal doughs

White bread

Phytic acid content is low and further decreased by hydrolysis during fermentation. The predominant factors for the hydrolysis are time of fermentation (Figure 1; r = -0.999), water content of the dough and the temperature of fermentation. The addition of dried skimmed milk inhibits the hydrolysis of phytic acid (2) which is 4 % instead of 47 % in the control.

Wholemeal bread

The effects of the amount of yeast, time and temperature of fermentation have been assessed simultaneously by a full factorial experimental design with the following assays summarized in table 1.

The effect of the time (Figure 1) and of the temperature of fermentation are the most important as they explain respectively 88 and 10 % of the total variation of the previous equation. The water content of the dough increases the hydrolysis of phytic acid, while rye flour has no significant effect.

The increasing addition of dried skimmed milk also produces a linear augmentation of pH and a reduction of the hydrolysis of phytic acid (Figure 2 ; r = - 0.999). The addition of calcium carbonate has less influence on the hydrolysis of phytic acid, perhaps because this calcium salt is not very soluble (3) and does not induce precipitation of phytic acid.

The acidification of the dough by lactic or acetic acid associated with a long fermentation time enhances the hydrolysis of phytic acid as it has been observed in sourdough fermentation (3-5). In these conditions the pH of dough is closer to the optimum pH of phytase.

REFERENCES

1. N.T. Davies and H. Reid, Brit. J. Nutr., 1979,41, 579.
2. M. Bartnik, T. Jakubczyk and M. Zarnecka, J. Cereal Sc., 1987, 5, 29.
3. W.J.S. Pringle and T. Moran, J. Soc. Chem. Ind., 1942, 61, 108.
4. F. Meuser and U. Meissner, Ernährung, 1987, 11, 2, 102.
5. H.J. Van Lonkhuysen, Getreide Mehl Brot, 1984, 38, 12, 372.

NUTRITIONAL EVALUATION OF INFANT FORMULAS FOR TRACE ELEMENTS BIOAVAILABILITY

Sunita Kakker and A. C. Kapoor

Department of Foods and Nutrition
Haryana Agricultural University
Hisar, Haryana - 125004, India

1   INTRODUCTION

A child's entire life is determined to a great extent by the quality of food provided in its first five years. Breast milk, if available in sufficient quantities, is adequate as the sole source of food during the first four to six months of age[1]. Under some circumstances where breast feeding is not possible, artificial feeding is done. In recent years, a large number of commercially available infant foods have been developed. Since trace elements play an important role in human nutrition, therefore, determination of the bioavailability of trace elements from such formulas is very important from infant nutrition point of view.

2. MATERIALS AND METHODS

Bioavailability of iron, copper and zinc was assessed in three commercial infant foods available in Haryana, namely; Sapan, Infanto and Amulspray and a synthetic diet similar in composition to those of infant formulas. Four groups of young male Wistar rats were fed with infant formulas and a synthetic diet for 28 days. During the last five days of the experiment, metabolic study was conducted. All the diets were analysed for proximate composition[2]. Trace elements in urine, faeces and diet samples were determined by Atomic Absorption Spectrophotometer[3]. Different infant formulas were also estimated for in vitro iron bioavailability[4].

3   RESULTS AND DISCUSSION

The results of proximate composition of infant foods and synthetic diet are presented in Table 1.

Table 1   Chemical composition of different diets
                (per 100g of dried powder)

Food Component		Dietary Group			
		Sapan	Infanto	Amulspray	Synthetic diet
Moisture	(g)	3.35	1.69	1.72	6.11
Protein	(g)	21.66	21.32	22.33	21.43
Fat	(g)	18.61	18.24	18.28	18.00
Ash	(g)	5.94	5.55	4.86	4.95
Energy	(kcal)	455	455	450	466
Iron	(mg)	4.20	4.19	4.07	4.30
Copper	(mg)	0.350	0.350	0.550	0.530
Zinc	(mg)	4.77	4.55	2.90	1.45

Table 2   Iron, copper and zinc intake of rats fed on
           different infant foods and synthetic diet for
           five days.

Dietary group	Iron intake (mg)	Copper intake (μg)	Zinc intake (mg)
Sapan	2.01	111.5	2.291
Infanto	1.97	109.6	2.149
Amulspray	1.95	263.3	1.388
Synthetic diet	2.75	397.7	0.928
C.D. at 5%	0.21	33.88	0.204

Table 2 revealed that iron and copper intake in the synthetic diet group was significantly higher as compared with infant formulas. Zinc intake in the synthetic diet group was the lowest in synthetic diet and highest in Sapan. Differences in trace elements intake of various groups were due to variations in dietary trace elements concentration and dissimilarity in food intake of different groups. All the groups were on positive iron, copper and zinc balance.

Apparent absorption of iron in Infanto group was the highest and differed significantly from other groups except Sapan (Table 3). Apparent retention of iron was minimum in synthetic diet group which differed non-significantly from Amulspray group and significantly from Sapan and Infanto groups. Lower apparent absorption and retention of iron in Amulspray and synthetic diet than those of other foods may be due to higher levels of copper present in Amulspray and synthetic diet. Similarly, it was observed that dietary copper affected the apparent absorption and retention of iron adversely.[5]

Table 3   Apparent absorption and retention of iron, copper
          and zinc in rats fed on different infant foods and
          synthetic diet for 5 days (average of six rats)

Dietary group	Apparent absorption (%)			Apparent retention (%)		
	Iron	Copper	Zinc	Iron	Copper	Zinc
Sapan	16.91	35.6	21.7	12.23	15.9	16.9
Infanto	17.76	36.5	21.2	12.84	16.1	16.8
Amulspray	14.87	37.7	17.5	10.11	23.1	12.9
Synthetic diet	11.63	14.2	23.8	9.35	8.9	12.2
C.D. at 5%	1.57	1.38	2.8	1.07	1.16	2.1

Copper absorption in synthetic diet group was significantly lower than those of infant formulas which indicated
that high copper intake resulted in decrease in apparent
absorption. Among infant formulas apparent absorption of
copper was lower in Sapan and Infanto formulas having lower
dietary copper levels as compared with Amulspray indicating
a decrease in apparent absorption of copper by lowering the
dietary copper levels.[5] Apparent retention of copper in
Sapan was lower as compared to Amulspray group having low
zinc concentration indicating that higher retention of
copper in Amulspray group may be due to high dietary copper
and low levels of zinc in diet.

The absorption and retention of zinc in Sapan group
was maximum and differed significantly from Amulspray and
synthetic diet group. Apparent absorption of zinc in Sapan
and Infanto group was more because of their lower copper
concentration as compared with Amulspray showing that at
lower level of copper intake, the apparent absorption of
zinc was more.

Results of bioavailability of iron in infant foods
estimated by in vitro procedure shows that Sapan, Infanto
and Amulspray contain 13.57, 14.43 and 10.36% of dialysable
iron, respectively. Correlation analysis indicated a
positive and significant ($P < 0.05$) agreement between in vitro
and human in vivo methods ($r = +0.578$).

REFERENCES

1. C.W.Weber, L.A.Vaughan and W.A.Stini, 'Nutritional Bioavailability
   of Iron', C.Kies (ed.), ACS Symposium Series 203. American Chemical
   Society, Washington, D.C. 1982 P.173.
2. D.Osis, K.Royston, K.Samachisen and H.Spencer, Develop.Spectroscopy,
   1969, 7A,227.
3. A.O.A.C., Official Methods of Analysis of the Association of
   Official Agricultural Chemists,Washington,D.C., 1980,13th edn.
4. D.D.Miller, B.R.Schricker, B.S.Rasmussen and D.V.Campen,
   Am.J.Clin.Nutr., 1981, 34, 2248.
5. B,Chaudhary, MSc Thesis, Haryana Agricultural University,India,1985.

FERRIC GLYCINATE IRON BIOAVAILABILITY IN INFANT FORMULAS DETERMINED BY EXTRINSIC RADIOISOTOPIC LABELLING

Langini,S.;Carbone,N.;Galdi,M.;Barrio Rendo,M.E.,Portela, M.L. and Valencia,M.E.

Department of Food Science and Experimental Nutrition
University of Buenos Aires
Junin 956 - 1113 - Buenos Aires, Argentina

1 INTRODUCTION

Infant formulas must provide bioavailable iron in order to cope with rapid growth and poor iron stores at birth. Ferrous sulphate is the major iron source used for fortification. However, this compound shows prooxidant properties which impair nutritional and organoleptic product quality[1] Accordingly, ferric glycinate was developed as an alternative iron source for infant formula fortification, in an attempt to reduce deterioration during storage[2]. Its catalytic activity proved lower than that of ferrous sulphate in an experimental milk-based formula[3]. This study was undertaken to evaluate ferric glycinate iron bioavailability vs ferrous sulphate in the above formula.

2 MATERIALS AND METHODS

Experimental Formula

A milk-based formula was designed as described previously[3] in order to resemble a commercially available product . Iron (100 ppm) was added either as $FeSO_4$ (FS) or ferric glycinate (FG), the latter prepared according to Galdi et al [3].

Radioiron Labelled Formulas. Aliquots of 1 mL of recently prepared FS and FG solutions (4 mg/mL) were labelled with 0.3 mL $^{59}FeCl_3$ (100 µCi/mL). Isotopic exchange was allowed for 24 h, then 0.7 mL aliquots of each milk based formula resuspended in distilled water (10g/100mL) were added. After a second 24 h exchange period, roughly 100 µL of each test formula, equivalent to

1 μCi per rat, was administered by gastric tube.

Experimental design

Twenty male Wistar weanling rats (29±1 days old) were
used in this study. Hemoglobin (Hb)[4] and Free Erythrocyte
Porphyrins (FEP)[5] were assessed and animals assigned to
one of two groups with equal average Hb value (12.7 ±
1.9 g/dL), FEP/Hb ratio (1.5 ± 0.5 μg/g) and body weight
63 ± 8 g). Rats were fasted for 4 h before radioiron
administration. Experimental formulas were fed 24 h pre and
post radioiron administration. Thereafter, rats were fed
20 % protein basal diet according to Harper[6] . Animals were
counted 2 h after radioiron dose and then daily for 2 weeks
under constant geometry. Individual whole body counts on
day 0 was taken as 100 % dose. Daily counts were corrected
for background radiation and radioactive decay. On day 14,
animals were killed and body weight recorded. One mL blood
was drawn by cardiac puncture and counted in a gamma well
counter. Blood radioactivity was referred to corrected
individual whole-body measurements. Total radioiron blood
count was calculated taking Total Blood Volume (TBV) equal
to 0.067 mL/g body weight.

Statistical analysis. Mean retention data of each time
period, for each experimental formula, were compared by
Student's t test [7]   .

3   RESULTS AND DISCUSSION

The time course of ^{59}Fe for both iron sources closely
fitted a   biphasic equation of the form:

$$\% \text{ dose retained (R)} = A\,e^{-at} + B\,e^{-at}$$

as described by Van Campen and House[8] for Zn retention.
The first component of the curve probably reflects iron
clearance from the gastrointestinal tract; the terminal
component primarily reflects endogenous iron losses.
Coefficient B , obtained by extrapolating the terminal
portion of the curve to time zero, provides an indicator of
the percentage of absorbed dose . Table 1 lists the coefficients and exponents of the retention equations. Apparent
iron absorption and iron retention were calculated as
percentages of ^{59}Fe dose. Values from rats fed FG fortified
formula were significantly higher than those for FS formula
(p<0.05). For both iron sources, whole radioiron content on
day 14 of experiment was approximately 85 % of retained
tracer.

Table 1. Mean radioiron apparent absorption, retention and percentage in blood.

Iron Source	Equation exponents(i) a	b	Apparent absorption % dose(ii)	Iron retention % dose(iii)	Percentage in blood % dose (iv)
FS	0.023	0.0018	15.8	8.9	7.5
FG	0.015	0.0008	30.9	23.3	21.8

(i) Percentage of administered ^{59}Fe retained at time t, $R = A\, e^{-at} + B\, e^{-at}$;(ii) ^{59}Fe absorption estimated from B intercept ; (iii) percentage of ^{59}Fe dose retained on day 14 of experiment and (iv) total blood percentage of adminstered ^{59}Fe on day 14 of experiment.

In the light of our present results, which demonstrate the relatively higher iron bioavailability of ferric glycinate, current iron fortification levels might be considerably reduced if FG were used. However, studies in humans are required before applying our findings to infant formula iron fortification.

REFERENCES

1. WHO Technical Report Series, N 580. Report of an IAEA, USAID, WHO Joint Meeting. Ginebra, 1975.
2. M.Galdi, PhD Thesis, University of Buenos Aires, 1987.
3. M.Galdi,N.Carbone and M.E. Valencia, J.Food Sci., 1988. Submitted for publication.
4. A. Hainline," Standard Methods of Clinical Chemistry" Academic Press,New York.1958, Vol 2, p 49.
5. S. Piomelli, J.Lab. Clin.Med.,1973, 81, 932.
6. A.E.Harper, J.Nutr.,1959, 68,605.
7. R.Sokal and J. Rohlf,"Biometry", W.H. Freeman, San Fco, USA. 1969, p. 222.
8. D.Van Campen and W.House, J.Nutr. 1973, 74, 84.

INTRINSIC LABELLING OF IRON IN MILK

J Gislason*, B Jones**, B Lönnerdal*** & L Hambraeus*

*Department of Nutrition, University of Uppsala, Sweden,
**Department of Clinical Chemistry, Swedish University
of Agricultural Sciences, Uppsala, Sweden and ***
Department of Nutrition, University of California,
Davis, USA

INTRODUCTION

Despite its high affinity to iron, lactoferrin (LF)
is only saturated to 2-4% of its iron-binding capacity
(Fransson and Lönnerdal, 1980) and LF-bound iron
constitutes 25-30% of the total iron content in human
milk. It has been shown that when an iron isotope is
added to a milk sample in vitro more than 80% occurs
bound to lactoferrin. The reported high bioavailability
of extrinsically labelled iron in human milk (Saarinen
et al., 1977), may therefore essentially be valid only
for the lactoferrin-bound iron. The bioavailability of
the other iron complexes in human milk is thus still
unknown.
    The purpose of this study was to 1) analyze the
possibility to label the various iron complexes in milk
intrinsically; 2) study the effect of iron status of the
lactating animal (mother) on the recovery of an
intravenously administered iron isotope.

MATERIALS AND METHODS

The recovery of an intravenously administered iron
isotope (^{59}Fe) was studied in five adult apparently
healthy lactating goats. The animals were studied in two
experiments under anaemic conditions during which they
were bled and in one experiment after iron supplementation. At the end of each period of treatment (bleeding
or supplementation), blood samples were collected for
haematologic analysis, the mammary glands were emptied
and the background radioactivity in the milk was
measured. Subsequently, a dose of 3.7 MBq ^{59}Fe-citrate
was injected intravenously. Milk samples were

170

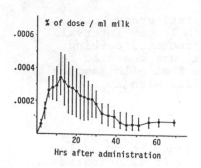

Figure 1. Distribution of ^{59}Fe excreted in milk after intravenous injection of the isotope. The dotted curve represents the mean of the three experiments and the vertical lines the range.

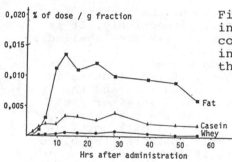

Figure 2. Distribution of ^{59}Fe in the various iron compartments in milk after intravenous administration of the isotope.

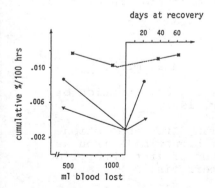

Figure 3. Correlation between iron status and recovery of iron isotope in milk in three goats (nos. 1, 2 and 3). The amount of blood loss and the duration of supplementation (number of days after the period of bleeding) is plotted against the cumulative percent recovery of injected dose in 1 ml milk portions during 100 hrs.
● Goat no. 1
▼ Goat no. 2
■ Goat no. 3

collected the following 5 days, at first, every hour
until 8 hrs after injection, then with longer intervals.
Some samples were fractionated by ultracentrifugation
(140,000g, 1hr and 4°C). Radioactivity was measured in
fat, casein and whey fractions and in 5 ml milk samples
in a gamma counter (Nuclear Chicago 1186 with a
well-type NaI detector).

RESULT AND DISCUSSION

Isotope recovery in 1 ml of milk was found to be as low
as 0.0001-0.0007% of the injected dose. As illustrated
in Figure 1 the process of iron excretion is slow, with
the maximum concentration of ^{59}Fe being reached 10 to 15
hours after intravenous injection, and then declining
slowly to a constant minimum 40 to 70 hrs after
injection.

Figure 2 shows the distribution of the isotope in
the fat, whey and casein fractions, respectively. It is
evident that all iron compartments in milk are labelled
by the intrinsic labelling technique.

Figure 3 shows the correlation between iron status
of the lactating animal and recovery of iron isotope in
milk. In three goats the amount of blood loss and the
duration of supplementation (number of days after the
period of bleeding) is plotted against the cumulative
percent recovery of injected dose in 1 ml milk portions
during 100 hrs. It is evident that with increasing blood
loss, recovery of isotope in milk is decreased.

Goat no. 1 shows the most rapid return to higher
isotope recovery although she was not supplemented with
iron after the period of bleeding. As she was one of two
goats that lost most blood in the two first experiments
the findings indicate that the iron excretion in milk is
highly prioritized during anaemia.

REFERENCES

G-B Fransson and B Lönnerdal, Iron in human milk, J
Pediatr, 1980, 96, 380-384.
B Lönnerdal, Biochemistry and physiological function of
human milk proteins. Am J Clin Nutr, 1985, 42, 1299-
1317.
UM Saarinen, MA Siimes and PR Dallman, Iron absorption
in infants: high bioavailability of breast milk iron as
indicated by the extrinsic tag method of iron absorption
and by the concentration of serum ferritin. J Pediatr,
1977, 91, 36-39.

INFLUENCE OF HEAT TREATMENT OF MILK ON AVAILABILITY OF COPPER, IRON AND ZINC - A STUDY IN MINIPIGS

Scholtissek, Johanne; Barth, C.A.

Institut für Physiologie und Biochemie der Ernährung
Bundesanstalt für Milchforschung,
Hermann-Weigmann-Str. 1, D-2300 Kiel

1 INTRODUCTION

Recent studies suggest that heat treatment modifies the functional properties of binding proteins of the whey fraction in milk which may play an important physiological role in intestinal absorption of trace elements and vitamins (Gregory, 1982). The present study was designed to compare the influence of raw-, pasteurized and UHT-milk on the serum and urine concentrations of copper, iron and zinc.

2 METHODS

Adult Göttingen minipigs weighing 30.0 ± 2.6 kg were maintained exclusively on one of three milks for a period of 3 weeks or on a balanced semisynthetic casein based diet (Barth et al., 1986) for a period of 2 weeks between the milk periods. They were provided with 0.44 MJ ME x $(kg^{0.75}$ x day)$^{-1}$ corresponding to the maintenance requirement of 262 g dry matter of milk or 350 g dry matter of the casein based diet. The animals were housed individually in experimental metabolic cages which had plastic feeders and walls and slotted tenderfoot floors to minimize intake of non dietary trace elements. Pasteurized milk was heated directly for 30" at 72°C and UHT-milk indirectly for 5" at 141°C. Table 1 shows the mineral content of the diets used.

Table 1 Copper, iron and zinc concentration of the
        diets

Diet	Cu	Fe	Zn
	μmol/kg dry matter		
raw cow's milk	83.1 ± 1.1	54.1 ± 3.6	472.9 ± 18.5
past. " milk	91.4 ± 13.3	80.0 ± 3.5	534.6 ± 14.6
UHT- " milk	80.7 ± 1.2	60.5 ± 4.1	524.6 ± 4.6
casein	283.0 ± 60.0	8024.0 ± 410.0	2364.0 ± 150.0

$\bar{x}$ ± SEM;

Fasting venous blood samples were obtained weekly
during the whole experiment. Urine and faeces were
collected in 1 week pools and analyzed in order to
calculate balances.

Serum and urine samples were introduced directly into
the atomic absorption spectrophotometer for quantification of Cu, Fe and Zn. Milk samples and casein were
wet-ashed with nitric- and perchloric acid concentrated
by evaporation and diluted with distilled deionised
water.

Non-fat-powdered milk from the National Bureau of
Standards Gaithersburg MD, USA was used as reference
material.

       3 RESULTS

In Table 2 the serum copper, iron and zinc concentrations are presented.

Table 2   Serum copper, iron and zinc

Diet	Fe	Cu	Zn
	μmol/l		
raw cow's milk	18.8 ± 3.4	39.3 ± 1.5	13.6 ± 0.4
past. " milk	18.8 ± 0.9	37.7 ± 1.7	12.8 ± 0.7
UHT- " milk	22.0 ± 4.0	31.4 ± 1.5	13.6 ± 0.9
casein	25.9 ± 2.4	33.7 ± 2.3	14.8 ± 0.1

$\bar{x}$ ± SEM; n = 3 animals; no significant differences.

The results indicate that there were no significant
differences (P> 0.05) in serum concentration (Table 2)
and in the daily urinary excretion of copper, iron and
zinc (Table 3) due to the treatment of milk.

Table 3 Urinary excretion of copper, iron and zinc

Diet	Cu	Fe	Zn
		μmol/24 h	
raw cow's milk	1.89 ± 0.15	2.88 ± 0.20	18.05 ± 1.84
past. " milk	2.39 ± 0.19	2.45 ± 0.27	23.25 ± 3.21
UHT- " milk	1.90 ± 0.16	2.84 ± 0.26	18.97 ± 1.68
casein	2.49 ± 0.32	3.10 ± 0.26	23.63 ± 2.59

$\bar{x}$ ± SEM; n = 3 animals

The studies have shown no significant differences in the availability of copper, iron and zinc in milk due to the treatment when the availability was studied by measuring urinary excretion or serum concentration. These findings will be extended by absorption and balance studies.

4 REFERENCES

1. J.F. Gregory, J.Nutr., 1982, 112, 1329.

2. C.A. Barth, M. Frigg and H. Hagemeister, J.Anim. Physiol.Anim.Nutr., 1986, 55, 128.

THE EFFECT OF YOGURT UPON IRON METABOLISM IN YOUNG RATS

N. Gruden and S. Mataušić

Institute for Medical Research
and Occupational Health
University of Zagreb
41001 Zagreb, Yugoslavia

1 INTRODUCTION

Yogurt is a popular dairy product whose consumption is
increasing and whose beneficial effect on human health
seems to be scientifically proved[1-3]. It was shown in a
recent study that yogurt diet exhibited a decreasing
effect upon radiostrontium absorption in neonatal and
weanling rats, especially when receiving a four day treatment[4]. Considering the great demand for iron at an early
age the aim of this study was to find out whether, and
to what extent, yogurt influences iron metabolism in
young rats.

2 ANIMALS AND METHODS

Experimental animals were ten- and twenty-one-day-old
albino rats. They received by the artificial feeding
procedure[5], for one or four days, either cow's milk or
yogurt marked with iron-59. Three days later the radioactivity was determined in animals' whole bodies, car-
casses, liver and spleen.

3 RESULTS AND DISCUSSION

The results for radioiron retention were calculated as
percentages of the dose received (Table 1). Yogurt -
compared to milk diet - decreased iron absorption slightly
(by 4 - 19 per cent) but statistically significant in
all experimental groups. Its inhibitory effect was most
pronounced in three-week-old rats that had been receiving yogurt for four days. Since the similar effect of
yogurt (though quantitatively more intense) was observed

176

upon the strontium metabolism[4] it might be assumed that
the longer yogurt consumption lasts, the more pronounced
its effect will be. Further studies should try to prove
this and to explain how this mechanism works. Although
not spectacular these results indicate that irons' metabolism can be influenced by a common food product, such
as yogurt.

Table 1   The effect of yogurt upon iron-59 absorption
          in young rats*

Animals' age (d)	Diet	Whole body	Carcass	Liver	Spleen
10	Cow's milk	100.98 $\pm$0.72	90.48 $\pm$1.85	13.25 $\pm$1.30	0.89 $\pm$0.09
	Yogurt	93.70^S $\pm$2.45	87.00 $\pm$2.35	12.96 $\pm$1.01	0.83 $\pm$0.06
21	Cow's milk	100.12 $\pm$1.80	88.83 $\pm$1.73	12.99 $\pm$0.65	0.91 $\pm$0.06
	Yogurt	95.73^S $\pm$0.97	82.20^S $\pm$1.38	13.52 $\pm$0.65	1.10^S $\pm$0.09
21**	Cow's milk	99.73 $\pm$1.26	85.60 $\pm$1.18	18.86 $\pm$0.82	1.18 $\pm$0.07
	Yogurt	80.91^S $\pm$4.43	68.41^S $\pm$4.26	14.40^S $\pm$1.09	1.04 $\pm$0.08

* The data presented as mean $\pm$ S.E. percentages of the
dose received (n=15).

** four days treated animals

^{S}Values are significantly different from the corresponding control.

Acknowledgement   This work was supported by the Scientific Research Council of S.R. Croatia. The authors
thank to Mrs B. Ferčec and D. Vasiljević for their care
and handling of animals and to Mrs. M. Horvat for
typing the manuscript.

4. REFERENCES

1.   T.L. Bazzare, S. Wu Lin and J.A. Yuhas, Nutr. Rep. Int., 1983, 28, 1225.

2.   E.I. Garvie, C.B. Cole, R. Fuller and D. Hewitt, J. Appl. Bacteriol., 1984, 56, 237.

3.   F.E. McDonough, N.P. Wong, P. Wells, A.D. Hitchins and C.E. Bodwel, Nutr. Rep. Int., 1985, 31, 1237.

4.   N. Gruden and S. Mataušić, Proceed. XIVth Regional Congress of IRPA, Kupari 1987, Vol. 1, 33.

5.   B. Momčilović and I. Rabar, Period. Biol., 1979, 81, 27.

IMPROVED IRON AVAILABILITY IN WEANING FOODS USING GERMINATION AND FERMENTATION

U. Svanberg and A.-S. Sandberg

Department of Food Science
Chalmers University of Technology
P.O. Box 5401, S-402 29 Gothenburg, Sweden

1 INTRODUCTION

Weaning foods in developing countries are normally prepared into thick or soft porridges based on the local staple, usually a cereal. The iron content of such staples, from endogenous origin and contamination from soil particles, is generally high (1, 2) but has a low bioavailability (3, 4). This partly explains the high prevalence of iron deficiency anaemia in developing countries.

The low bioavailability of iron from cereal diets is explained by the presence of inhibitors, out of which the fibre components, phytates and tannins (polyphenols) are of major importance (5). In developing countries, traditional household level food technologies such as dehulling, soaking, germination and fermentation could be utilized to reduce the amount of these inhibitors. The aim of this study is to investigate how such techniques could be applied on sorghum in order to reduce the phytate content and to measure the effect on the iron availability.

Conventionally, analysis of the phytate content (inositol hexaphosphate) also will include lower inositol phosphates. However, only inositol hexa- and pentaphosphates seem to inhibit the iron availability in foods (Sandberg et al., conferencepaper) and the amount of these two inositolphosphates is therefore related to the iron availability using an in vitro model. This model measures the iron solubility of a diet and has shown a high correlation with studies of iron absorption in humans.

2 METHODS

Sample Preparation

Grains from a white (non-tannin) sorghum variety (Lugugu) was cleaned and washed in distilled water. Three types of flour were prepared.

179

Processing of grains. (1) whole flour, (2) 85% extraction rate flour using a mortar and pestle and (3) whole flour of germinated (72 hrs) and dried grains.

Processing of flours. (1) soaking in water for 12 hrs and (2) lactic acid fermentation in water for 96 hrs. All samples were prepared as porridges before analysis.

Determination of Inositol Phosphates

The amount of hexa- and pentaphosphates (IP_6 + IP_5) in the porridges was measured with HPLC ion-pair chromatography (6).

Determination of Iron Solubility at Physiological Conditions

The digestion of the weaning food samples (porridges) was performed step-wise using a three-enzyme system and the amount of solubilized iron at pH 6.0 was determined by AAS (Svanberg et al., submitted for publ.) and used as an index of bioavailability.

3 RESULTS

Figure 1 shows the percentage soluble iron of differently processed sorghum porridges in relation to the amount of IP_6 + IP_5.

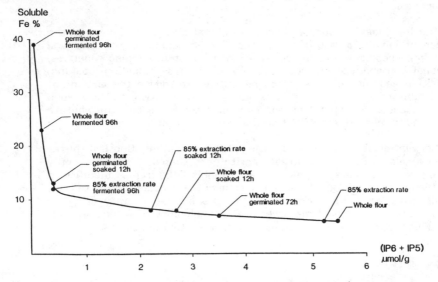

Figure 1. In vitro availability (% soluble iron after digestion) related to the amount of IP_6 + IP_5 in processed sorghum porridges.

Dehulling to 85% extraction rate removed a minor part of the phytate and germination caused a 35% decrease of the IP_6 + IP_5 content due to activated phytase degrading the inositolphosphates, however, no effect was observed on the iron solubility. Soaking the flours in water at pH = 5 in 12 hrs caused a further degradation of IP_6 + IP_5, over 90% in the flour of germinated grains which also resulted in an improved iron solubility, doubled compared to the untreated whole flour.

In the fermented samples the pH in the slurry was reduced from an initial value of pH = 6 to about pH = 4 due to the produced lactic acid. The amount of IP_6 + IP_5 was reduced by more than 90% in all samples and the fermented flour of germinated grains had no detectable amounts of IP_6 + IP_5. The lactic acid fermentation increased the amount of soluble iron with a factor 2 to 6 times, the highest value for the fermented flour of germinated grains. Obviously the combination of germination and fermentation gives the highest increase in soluble iron, and the explanation to this seems to be that the germination process activates or synthezises phytase which during the fermentation process are active under optimal pH conditions, e.g. pH = 5, due to bacterial production of organic acids, mainly lactic acid.

4 CONCLUSIONS

Traditional household level food methods such as soaking, germination and fermentation has been shown under laboratory conditions to significantly reduce the content of inositol hexa- and pentaphosphate, in white sorghum. The iron solubility and thus the iron availability increased depending on treatment with a factor two to six times. In quantitative terms this means that a diet of "low bioavailability" has changed into an "intermediate to high bioavailability" diet, which otherwise only could be achieved by including generous quantities of meat or foods containing high amounts of ascorbic acid.

REFERENCES

1. A. Besrat, A. Admasu and M. Ogbai, Ethiopian Medical Journal, 1980, 18, 45.
2. T.H. Bothwell, R.W. Charlton, J.D. Cook and C.A. Finch, 'Iron Metabolism in Man'. Blackwell Scientific Publications, Oxford, 1979.
3. L. Hallberg, Ann. Rev. Nutr., 1981, 1, 123.
4. M. Gilloly, T.H. Bothwell, J.D. Torrance, A.P. MacPhail, D.P. Derman, W.R. Bezwoda, W. Mills and R.W. Charlton, Br. J. Nutr., 1983, 49, 331.
5. G.O. Latunde-Dada and R.J. Neale, J. Food Techn., 1986, 21, 255.
6. A.-S. Sandberg and R. Ahderinne, J. Food Sci., 1986, 51, 547.

EFFECT OF PREPARATION METHODS ON THE IN VITRO BIOAVAILABILITY OF IRON FROM A LOCAL CEREAL-BASED WEANING FOOD

Carl M. F. Mbofung

Department of Food Science and Nutrition,
Ensiaac Ngaoundere University Centre,
Ngaoundere-Cameroon.

1 INTRODUCTION

In several parts of Africa and in particular, in Northern Cameroon,
maize gruel is used as a weaning food and breakfast cereal.
Occasionally, the gruels are prepared with the addition of peanut
(extracted into water) and/or lemon juice. The aim of this study
was to determine to what extent these different ways of preparing
maize gruel affect iron content and its bioavailability.

2 MATERIALS AND METHODS

Maize flour obtained via a local process of milling (using pestle
and mortar) and sieved through a .25mm mesh size was used as the base
for the preparation of the gruels in distilled water: MGP0–plain
maize flour gruel; MGP20– maize + peanut gruel in the ratio of
1:0.2.   In like manner, MGP40 (1:0.4); MGP50 (1:0.5); MGP60 (1:0.60);
MGP80 (1:0.80) and MGP100 (1:1). Another set of MGP0, MGP50 & MGP100
gruels was similarly prepared adding to each 25ml of fresh lemon juice.
The gruel samples were dried to a constant weight and subsequently
pulverised into a fine powder.   Aliquots were then used for in vitro
determination of iron availability while others were analysed for
total iron, total proteins, phytate and neutral detergent fibre (NDF).

Relative iron availability was estimated using, with slight
modifications, the in vitro method of Kane and Miller[1]. The method
involves a two-stage digestion at 37°C and continuous shaking
(pepsin at pH2 for 2 hours and pancreatin-bile at pH7.5 for 2 hours)
of a 100g sample of each gruel (made into a slurry with 0.1M HCl)
followed by the dialysis of subsamples of the digest. The dialysate
was analysed for bathophenanthroline disulphate reactive iron which
was considered as the amount of available iron in the gruel. Blank
digest were run with each batch of samples and the results used for
correcting for possible contamination arising during the procedure.

Table 1   Total and Available Iron (μg/100g) Total Protein (g%) Phytate (mg/100g) and Neutral Detergent Fibre–NDF (g%) content of Gruels.

Gruels	Total Iron	Avail.Iron	Total Protein	Phytate	NDF
MGP0	1850	50	8.10	230	16.0
MGP20	2540	102	10.90	250	23.0
MGP40	3010	112	13.10	280	28.1
MGP50	3250	125	13.80	290	32.0
MGP60	3420	126	14.50	320	30.2
MGP80	3780	135	15.30	290	31.0
MGP100	4100	140	16.80	350	27.0

Table 2   Correlation Coefficient (r) between % Available Iron and Other Components in Gruels containing Peanut Extract.

Component	r	P value
Total Iron	−0.87	0.02
Total Proteins	−0.87	0.02
Phytate	−0.82	0.05
NDF	−0.15	0.8

Table 3   Effect of Addition of Lemon Juice (LJ) on the Availability of Iron (μg/100g) from Gruels

Gruel	Total Iron	Available Iron		% Increase in Av. Iron
		No LJ	With LJ	
MGP0	1850	50	90	80
MGP50	3250	125	164	31.1
MGP100	4110	140	201	43.6

To avoid sample contamination, only distilled water was used in all cases.   All glassware was washed thoroughly with liquid detergent, rinsed several times with distilled water, soaked for 12 hours in 1M HCl and rinsed thrice with glass distilled water.   All reagents used were of pure grade (Sigma Chemical Co.).

Chemical analysis: The total iron in each gruel was analysed by atomic absorption spectrophotometry, total protein content by Kjedahl method[2],   phytate by the method of Mohammed et al[3],   and neutral detergent fibre (NDF) by the method of Van Soest as modified by Reinhold et al[4].

3   RESULTS AND COMMENTS

The addition of peanut extract led to an increase in the total iron content of the gruel.   The changes in the iron content of the

gruels with increase in the amount of peanut extract added was
highly correlated with changes in protein content. The percent
available iron in the gruels containing peanut extract was inversely
related to the amount of phytate (r = -0.82; P<0.05) and NDF
(r = -0.150; P>0.05) as well as the amounts of total iron and protein.
(Table 2).   The addition of varying levels of peanut to maize flour
in the preparation of the gruels led to increases in the relative
availability of iron ranging from 3.4 to 3.9% with an overall mean
of 3.7%.   The relative increase was higher in gruels MGP20, MGP40
and MGP50 than those with a higher peanut extract content.   In
absolute terms however, the amount of iron available from the gruels
increased with the total iron and peanut component of the gruel.
Gruels prepared with peanut extract in the ratio of 1:1 showed an
increase of 180% in iron availability compared to plain maize gruel
(50 µg *vs* 140µ g).

Iron in the gruels prepared with fresh lemon juice was more
available than in gruels without lemon juice (Table 3).   The
increased effect on relative iron availability was higher in plain
maize gruel (MGP0, 80%) than in gruels containing peanut extract
(MGP50, 31%; MGP100, 43%).   However the absolute amount of iron
available was much higher from MGP100 than from MGP0.   Generally
the effect of lemon juice on the relative availability of iron
decreased with increase in the iron content of the gruels.   Lemon
juice is a rich source of vitamin C and might have been responsible
for the increased dialysable iron[5].

In conclusion, some of the methods of preparing maize gruels
seem to have beneficial effects on their nutritive value.

4   REFERENCES

1. A.P.Kane and D.D. Miller, 1984, Am J. Clin. Nutr. 39, 393-401
2. AOAC (Association of Official Analytical Chemicsts), 1975,
    Washington, DC.
3. A.I. Mohammed, P.J. Perera and Y.S. Hafez, 1986, Cereal Chem.
    63, 475-478.
4. J.G.Reinhold and J.S.Garcia, 1979, Amer. J. Clin. Nutr. 32,
    1326-1329.
5. H. Brise and L. Hallberg, 1962. Acta Med. Scand. 171 Suppl.
    376, 51.

INFLUENCE OF PROTEINS ON IRON ABSORPTION IN MAN

R.F. Hurrell[a], M. A. Juillerat[a], S.R. Lynch[b] and
J.D. Cook[b]

a Nestlé Research Centre   b University of Kansas
  Nestec Ltd   Medical Center,
  Vers-chez-les-Blanc   Kansas City
  CH-1000 Lausanne 26   Kansas / USA
  Switzerland

1 INTRODUCTION

Iron bioavailability from vegetable sources is generally
low due to the presence of inhibitors of iron absorption
such as phytate, dietary fibre and polyphenols. Animal
tissue on the other hand has the property of enhancing
non-heme iron absorption from inhibitory meals. This has
been attributed to the effect of peptide-digestion products derived from tissue proteins[1]. In this study, we
have compared the influence of different protein sources
on iron absorption in man.

2 MATERIALS AND METHODS

The protein sources (Table 1) and the hydrolysed soy
proteins (Table 2) were purchased commercially. The phy-
tate-reduced soy isolates and the high and low phytate
7S and 11S soy proteins (Table 2) were prepared in a
pilot plant by isoelectric precipitation and thorough
washing. Phytate was measured by a modified method derived
from Makover et al[2]. Iron absorption measurements were
made in human volunteers using the extrinsic tag technique
with radioiron[3]. Each test contained 6-10 subjects and 4
separate iron absorption measurements were made on each
subject who consumed 4 different meals. One meal in each
test was the standard liquid formula meal of Cook and
Monsen[4] consisting of 35g egg white, 35g corn oil, 67g
hydrolysed maize starch, 12ml vanillin extract and 200ml
deionized distilled water. The test proteins were substituted for egg white isonitrogenously. The extrinsic tag
contained sufficient iron to bring the iron content of
each meal to 4.1mg.

Table 1   Relative effect of different protein sources
          on non-heme iron absorption from a liquid
          formula meal (from Refs 1, 4 and 5)

| Substitute | Percentage Mean Iron Absorption | | Relative Absorption ((A/B)x100) |
	Substitute (A)	Egg White Control (B)	
No Protein	10.6	3.0	353
Beef muscle	5.1	1.7	300
Bovine serum albumin	5.7	3.0	190
Wheat gluten	2.1	6.7	31
Casein	3.7	6.7	55
Whey protein	1.0	2.5	40
Soy protein isolate	0.5	2.5	20

Table 2   Influence of phytate-removal and enzyme hydro-
          lysis on iron absorption from soy isolate and
          soy proteins

| Substitute | %Phytate | Percentage Mean Iron Absorption | | Relative Absorption ((A/B)x100) |
		Substitute (A)	Egg White Control (B)	
Soy Isolate A	1.70	0.28	3.10	9
B	0.84	0.72	4.42	16
C	0.15	1.79	5.84	30
Hydrolysed soy proteins				
24% hydrolysis	0.23	1.86	3.10	60
52% hydrolysis	<0.05	5.33	3.10	172
Soy proteins 7S	2.52	1.87	5.84	32
7S	0.04	2.59	5.84	44
11S	0.65	0.97	4.42	22
11S	0.06	5.48	4.42	124

3 RESULTS AND DISCUSSION

Compared to the protein-free meal (Table 1), all substitute proteins were inhibitory. It is suggested that binding of iron in the duodenum to the peptide-digestion products of some food proteins can inhibit iron absorption, although the influence of non-protein factors such as Ca, P and phytate was not controlled in these studies. Lowering phytate in soy isolate from 1.7% to 0.15% increased relative iron absorption 3 fold (Table 2), although the isolate was still very inhibitory. Lowering phytate in the 7S protein from 2.52% to 0.04% increased absorption only slightly. Theoretically the 4.1mg of iron in each meal could be bound by 12.4mg phytate (assuming unreastically that no phytate is bound to other minerals or protein). This would correspond to a phytate content in the protein fraction of about 0.04%. Lowering phytate in the 11S protein from 0.65% to 0.06% increased iron absorption substantially as did prior extensive hydrolysis of soy proteins. It is concluded that the iron-binding properties of the peptide digestion products from the 7S protein are mainly responsible for the inhibitory effect of soy isolate on iron absorption. Phytate contributes to this inhibition , particularly when in presence of the 11S protein, and it is probable that iron is jointly bound between phytate and the peptide digestion products.

REFERENCES

1. R.F. Hurrell, S.R. Lynch, T.P. Trinidad, S.A. Dassenko and J.D. Cook, Am.J.Clin.Nutr., 1988, 47, 102.
2. R.U. Makower, Cereal Chemistry, 1970, 47, 288.
3. T.H. Bothwell, R.W. Charlton, J.D. Cook and C.A. Finch, "Iron Metabolism in Man", Blackwell Scientific, Oxford, 1979.
4. J.D. Cook and E.R. Monsen, Am.J.Clin.Nutr., 1975, 28, 1289.
5. R.F. Hurrell, S.R. Lynch, T.P. Trinidad, S.A. Dassenko and J.D. Cook, Am.J.Clin.Nutr., 1988, in press.

IN VITRO IRON AND PROTEIN AVAILABILITY FROM MEALS

E Carnovale, G. Lombardi-Boccia, G. Di Lullo, M. Cappelloni

Istituto Nazionale della Nutrizione
Roma, Via Ardeatina n. 546

INTRODUCTION

Availability of both protein and iron is affected by food processing. Moreover , because protein digestion products are involved in the nonheme iron absorption, the study of the availability of these nutrients is strictly connected.

In the present study in vitro iron and protein availability from meals, composed of 50% of meat and 50% of vegetables, steamed and dried in three different processes, were determined. In addition, the same meals were studied after fortification with electrolytic iron powder (3mg/100g).

Protein availability

In vitro protein digestibility (1) available lysine (2) and available methionine (3) of the meals other than aminoacids composition, were determined. Results are shown in table 1. In vitro protein digestibility, which had a high correlation with in vivo estimation (r=0,98), showed a decrease, although not significant, depending on cooking and drying treatments; the most pronounced effect was shown by the drum-dried meal. The total lysine content showed a reduction from raw to processed meals of about 20%, whilst the available lysine showed a smaller reduction, lower than 10%. Also the total content of methionine was affected by processing, the reduction ranging from 9.7 to 17.8%; its availability was affected to a less extent. However, since the sulphur-containing aminoacids were limiting, the decrease in methionine content induced a reduction of protein quality, evaluated as chemical score. Protein and aminoacid availability was affected to a greater extent in the drum-dried meals.

TABLE 1 - Protein and aminoacid availability.

	Raw meal	Freeze dried meal	Drum dried meal	Spray dried meal
In vitro protein digestibility %	82.78	82.22	80.53	81.43
Total lysine *	8.20	6.58	6.22	6.50
Avail. lysine *	7.88	6.18	5.59	6.17
Total methionine *	1.96	1.69	1.61	1.77
Avail.methionine *	1.79	1.57	1.58	1.60

* Expressed as g/16gN

Iron availability

The iron availability of the meals was evaluated by the in vitro method of Miller (4) and the results are shown in table 2. The raw meal showed an availability of 9.36% and a remarkable reduction (about 23%) occurred in processed meals. The meals had a very similar composition, also as regards the presence of those factors influencing iron availability, such as phytic acid, dietary fiber and ascorbic acid; so the observed reduction in availability can be attributed to the effect of cooking and drying processes. In order to balance losses due to processing, the meals were fortified with electrolytic iron powder (3mg for 100g of meal). Fortification induced an improvement in iron dialyzability in cooked meals, the average percentage of reduction from raw to processed meals being 8%. The addition of electrolytic iron powder masked the effect of treatments on native iron; the differences between raw and processed meals in fact were not significant contrary to what occurs in unfortified meals. The improvement in availability could be explained by a better solubilization of added iron, compared to native iron, due to processing.

TABLE 2 - Iron availability from meals

	Total Fe mg/100g	Available Fe %	Reduction %
Unfortified meals			
raw	6.1	9.36	
freeze-dried	5.8	7.00	25.2
drum-dried	6.0	7.40	21.0
Fortified meals			
raw	14.6	8.58	
freeze-dried	13.4	8.00	6.4
drum-dried	13.3	7.89	8.0
spray-dried	13.7	1.05	8.8

In conclusion, considering the effects of processing on bioavailability of nutrients, the effect on nonheme iron appears particularly interesting and deserves further study in relation to protein modifications.

Research work supported by CNR, Italy-Special Grant IPRA, subproject 3, paper n. 1803.

REFERENCES

1) Satterlee, L.D., Marshall, H.F., Tennyson, J.M. J. Am. Oil Chem. Soc. 1979;56,103
2) AOAC. Official Methods of Analyses. 1984;14th ed.
3) Ford, J.E. Br. J. Nutr. 1964;18,449
4) Miller, D.D., Schricker, B.R., Rasmussen, R.R., Van Campen, D. Am. J. Clin. Nutr. 1981;34,2248

BIOLOGICAL EVALUATION OF IRON AVAILABILITY OF MIXED MEAT AND VEGETABLE MEALS

Corcos Benedetti P., Tagliamonte B., Ciarapica D.,
Turrini A.

Istituto Nazionale della Nutrizione - Roma - Italy

1 INTRODUCTION

Technological treatments may affect the bioavaila
bility of many nutrients in foods (aminoacids,oligoe-
lements).In previous research (no published results) we
showed that protein value of a mixed meat and vegetable
meal,steam heated and then drum dried,was significantly
decreased compared with a freeze-dried sample.

Since meat is the major dietary source of iron,we
investigated the Fe availability of the same mixed meat
and vegetable meals knowing that meat proteins enhance
the absorption of ·non haem Fe (1) while thermal
processing may change its oxidative state (2).

Fe availability was tested using the official AOAC
repletion method (3); all the diets were isonitrogenous
and isocaloric.Haemoglobin Fe gain was used as response
parameter in dose response bioassay .

2 RESULTS

As shown in table 1 only the rats fed diet with raw
meat showed an increased weight gain in relation to the
Fe level. Haemoglobin Fe gain in all groups,was gradually
increased as the Fe level of the diet rose:the maximum
value was obtained with the test diets at the highest
Fe level and it was approximately equal to that of the
second Fe level in the standard diet. Moreover no differences were detectable among the three test diets at any
level studied.

This study was supported by CNR,Italy, Special Grant
IPRA, subproject 3 paper N.1862

Tab. 1 Feed intake, weight gain, and haemoglobin iron
       gain* at the end of repletion period

Fe in diets mg	Food intake g/14 days	weight gain g	Iron intake mg	Hb g/100ml	Hb Fe gain mg
FeSO4					
1.27	270	76	3.42^{a1}	8.3	3.19
1.39	267	84	3.83^{a2b2}	9.8	4.45^{a2}
1.63	341	94	5.14^{a2b2}	10.2	5.80^{a2}
A**					
1.44	240	73^{a1}	3.45^{a2}	8.0	2.60^{a1}
1.72	260	92^{a2}	4.45^{a3b3}	7.6	3.17^{a3b2}
2.28	274	107^{a2}	6.24^{a3b3}	8.8	4.65^{a3b2}
B**					
1.43	257	75	3.45^{a1}	8.2	2.71^{a1}
1.69	283	91	4.79^{a1}	8.0	3.49^{a1}
2.23	212	85	4.72^{a2}	8.0	3.39^{a1}
C**					
1.44	269	82	3.91^{a1}	7.8	2.75^{a1}
1.71	262	75	4.49^{a3b2}	7.8	3.27^{a1}
2.27	244	91	6.23^{a3b2}	8.0	4.45^{a3b1}

*Difference between total haemoglobin iron in blood,at
end and beginning of repletion period ,was calculated
assuming blood to be 7% of body weight and haemoglobin
to contain 0.34% iron.Average weight and haemoglobin
concentration at the beginning of the repletion period
were in the range of 236-271 g and 4.71-5.75 g/100 ml
respectively.
**A:raw meal,B steam-heated and freeze-dried, C steam-
heated and drum dried.Iron content of the three products
was mg 6% .
a) significant v. the first iron level in the diet
b)   "   between second and third iron level
1- P<0.05   2- P<0.01   3- P<0.001.

        Fig. 1 shows RBV (relative biological value) for Fe
availability with their 95% confidence limits. The values
of each test diet v.the standard one, were lower and
statistically different because the fiducial limits do
not include the 100%. These results are confirmed by the
analysis of variance for parallelism (4), which shows a
significant difference (P<0.05) for all test diets
v.reference standard but no significant difference among
themselves.
        In Fig.2 we can see that Total Iron Binding Capacity
(TIBC) is very similar in all experimental diets;serum Fe
with the third Fe level of reference diet is very high

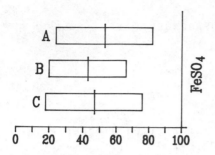

Fig.1 Vertical lines=RBV
v.FeSO4 diets Horizontal
bars= 95% fiducial limits

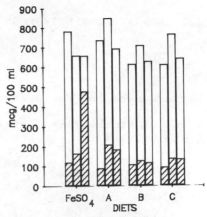

Fig.2 Serum Fe
and LIBC

and thus the Latent Iron Binding Capacity (LIBC) is reduced .No significant differences are noted in the other three diets.

Perhaps the release of Fe v. red cell precursors for haemoglobin regeneration is facilitated when the transferrin contains more bound iron.

From data to hand we can conclude that steam-heating treatment did not induce changes in Fe availability of the mixed meat and vegetable meals examined,this is evidenced by the not statistically significant changes in RBV values of B and C samples v.A; serum Fe and TIBC values also account for this hypothesis.These results agree with those of other authors who observed that none of the major cooking methods reduced the bioavailability of meat Fe (5). Neither do the different drying treatments induce any change.

REFERENCES

1. J.D. Cook and E.R. Monsen,Am.J.Clin.Nutr.,1976,29,859
2. B.R. Shricker, D.D. Miller, J. Food Sci., 1982, 47,740
3. A.O.A.C. Official Methods of Analysis,1984, n.43,268
4. P.Gyorgy and W.N.Pearson, The vitamins, Ac. Press. New York 1967, cap.2, vol.6, pag.50
5. O.Jansuittivechakul, A.W. Mahoney, D.P. Conforth, D.C. Hendricks and K.Kangsadalampay, J.Food Sci.,1985, 50, 405

IN VITRO IRON AVAILABILITY FROM SOYABEANS

G.O. Latunde-Dada and *R. J. Neale

Department of Biochemistry   *Dept. of Applied Biochemistry
Ogun State University   & Food Science
Ago-Iwoye   School of Agriculture
Nigeria   University of Nottingham
                               Sutton Bonington LE12 5RD

1 INTRODUCTION

The in vitro estimation of chemically available iron from
foods has proved to be very useful in situations requiring
the screening of a large number of samples.   The technique
has however been subjected to different modifications viz
(i) neutralization with NaOH or $NaHCO_3$ (ii) the use of
digestive enzymes and surfactants such as gastric juice
and bile extracts, (iii) the use of different response
parameters such as percentage soluble iron, iron profiling,
and (iv) the employment of different peptic and pancreatic
digestion time courses.

In this paper, three response parameters were employed
in studying the chemical availability of extrinsically -
labelled ^{59}Fe from soyabean products (Defatted Flour(DF);
Soya Concentrate (SC), and Soya Isolate (SI).   The effect
of pancreatic pH on the solubility of ^{59}Fe in these soya
products was also investigated.   The soya products were
subjected to simulated gastro-intestinal digestion using
peptic and pancreatic enzymes with subsequent measurement
of the soluble and dialyzable ^{59}Fe.

2 RESULT AND DISCUSSION

Data for the total soluble ^{59}Fe (%) obtained from the various soyabean products at different stages of pepsin - pancreatic digestion are given in Table 1.   The solubility of
^{59}Fe was highest in SI (P<0.05).   Secondly, when dialysed
exhaustively for 72 hours, the proportion of dialyzable
low-molecular weight ^{59}Fe increased generally with digestion time.   It was, however, significantly higher (P<0.01)

Table 1   Soluble ^{59}Fe (%) from Soya Products During
In vitro Simulated Digestion

Digestion Conditions	Soya Products DF	SC	SI
Pepsin, pH 1.5, 1½ hrs.	32.5 ± 1.08	24.2 ± 0.89	26.6 ± 2.03
Neutralization (NaHCO$_3$)	34.3 ± 2.4	25.8 ± 0.45	47.2 ± 0.65
Pancreatin, pH 7.0,			
1 hour	34.2 ± 1.9	32.3 ± 2.2	52.7 ± 0.86
2 hours	36.1 ± 0.2	32.6 ± 0.91	54.8 ± 0.71
4 hours	41.0 ± 1.9	33.8 ± 1.32	58.0 ± 0.2

in SI than those of other products (Table 2). This low
molecular weight ^{59}Fe was also expressed as a percentage
of the total food iron. Finally, a digestion technique
that estimates available iron as percentage of the total
food iron[2] dialyzed during the digestion process was
employed.   In this method, a maximum dialysis time of
4 hours was allowed. Values of dialyzable ^{59}Fe obtained,
though lower than in method 2 above, followed the same
trend for the soyabean products (Table 3). Similar low
values of percentage dialyzable iron have been reported
for soya products in meals when this method was employed.[3]

   The soluble iron was found to vary with pancreatic
pH. The values at pH 5, 6 and 7 were respectively 72.1%
54.1% and 36.1% for DF and 48.1%, 43% and 32.6% for SC.
For SI, however, solubility increased with pH (15.8%,
35.7% and 58% at pH 5, 6 and 7 respectively). The observation for DF agrees with those of other workers.[4]

Table 2   Total Low-Molecular Weight ^{59}Fe (%) from Soya
Products after 72 hours Dialysis

Digestion Conditions	Soya Products DF	SC	SI
Pepsin, pH 1.5, 1½ hrs.	7.92 ± 0.30	5.85 ± 0.23	9.09 ± 0.14
Neutralization (NaHCO$_3$)	8.81 ± 0.49	6.77 ± 0.4	12.5 ± 0.33
Pancreatin, pH 7.0 Digestion Conditions			
1 hour	8.96 ± 0.49	7.72 ± 0.78	15.1 ± 0.79
2 hours	9.29 ± 0.58	7.73 ± 0.08	15.0 ± 1.58
4 hours	11.1 ± 0.56	8.83 ± 0.23	16.7 ± 0.54

Table 3   Dialyzable ^{59}Fe(%) during digestion and
            simultaneous dialysis of Soya Products

Pancreatic digestion and dialysis time	Soya	Products	
	DF	SC	SI
30 minutes	1.04$\pm$0.04	1.53$\pm$0.05	1.07$\pm$0.08
1 hour	1.87$\pm$0.23	1.95$\pm$0.05	2.11$\pm$0.07
2 hours	2.17$\pm$0.05	2.11$\pm$0.06	2.51$\pm$0.19
4 hours	2.17$\pm$0.05	2.28$\pm$0.06	3.2 $\pm$0.03

Peptic digestion prior to pancreatic digestion was at pH 1.5
for 1½ hours.

Values in Tables are means of three samples $\pm$ SE.

The primary aim of an in vitro digestion technique
is to simulate in vivo conditions in such a way that a
good correlation is obtained between the two assays.
Although the dialyzable ^{59}Fe during in vitro digestion
(Table 3) measures only a fraction of the total low molecular weight ^{59}Fe (Table 2), it is now widely accepted
since it compares well with human absorption values for
some food items.   Nevertheless, it is probably an under-
estimation of the available iron particularly from foods
that stay longer than 2 hours in the gut.   Furthermore
iron absorption continues beyond the duodenum.[5]   The
total low-molecular weight ^{59}Fe (Table 2) was also found
to correlate well (r = 0.97) with the values obtained for
rats fed intragastrically the same soya products.[6]   It is
therefore important to standardize with an iron salt in a
semi-synthetic diet the different in vitro techniques.
Relative iron availability of the test diet could therefore be estimated.   Thus the composition of foods, digestion pH, response parameters are important considerations
in in vitro solubility studies.

REFERENCES

1.   T. Hazell, D.A. Ledward and R.J. Neale, Br. J. Nutr., 1978,
     39, 631.
2.   D.D. Miller, B.R. Schricker, R.R. Rasmussen & D. Van Campen,
     Am. J. Clin. Nutr., 1981, 34, 2248.
3.   B.R. Schricker, D.D. Miller & D. Van Campen, J. Nutr., 1982,
     112, 1696.
4.   F. M. Clydesdale and A.L Camire, J. Fd. Sci., 1983, 48, 1272.
5.   M.S. Wheby, Scand. J. Haematol, 1970, 7, 56.
6.   G.O. Latunde-Dada and R.J. Neale, J.Fd. Tech., 1986, 21, 255.

THE IRON BIOAVAILABILITY OF Leucaena leucocephala TEMPEH

Mary Astuti, Retno Indrati and Yotti Atmajaya

Faculty of Agricultural Technology
Gadjah Mada University
Yogyakarta, Indonesia.

1   INTRODUCTION

Leucaena leucocephala, a leguminous plant of the mimosa family, is found throughout the tropics[2]. It can produce nutritious forage, fire wood and organic fertiliser but is not recommended for extensive use for food because of the presence of the toxic water-soluble amino acid, mimosine in large amounts in leaf and seed. It has produced one or more of the following syndromes: loss of hair, abortion, infertility, low milk secretion and other abnormalities[4].

In Indonesia Leucaena leucocephala is used for food. Young pods are eaten raw, mature seeds are cooked or fermented. Fermentation by mold of the Rhizopus sp. reduces the phytic acid content[6] and mimosine content[3]. The purpose of the present study is to investigate the effect of tempeh production on the iron bioavailability of anaemic rats.

2   MATERIALS AND METHODS

Preparation of Tempeh

Tempeh was prepared according to Indonesian traditional ways, as follows: Whole dried seed of Leucaena leucocephala were soaked for 24 h in water at room temperature, the soaking water was discarded and the seeds boiled in excess water for about 3 h. The cooking water was discarded. The seeds were dehulled by hand and washed. The cleaned seeds were cooked in steam for 20 min and were spread onto a perforated bamboo tray to drain off the excess water then air dried for 15 min. The seeds were inoculated with a traditional inoculum (usar). Usar is the traditional inoculum for tempeh fermentation in Indonesia and usually contains one or usually more Rhizopus sp. together with some yeasts and a range of aerobic bacteria. The well-mixed inoculated seeds were wrapped in

banana leaves, incubated for 48 h in room temperature.   Fresh tempeh
was steamed for 10 min, dried and pounded.

Diets

Table 1   Diet formulation (g/kg)

Item	DS	DT	DW	DD
Skim milk	294	–	–	294
Tempeh	–	384	–	–
Whole seed	–	–	287	–
Corn oil	77	63	63	77
Sucrose	119	110	127	553
Corn starch	434	385	467	–
Mineral mixture	12*	36*	34*	12*
Vitamin mixture	22	22	22	22
Cellulose	42	–	–	42

DS :   skim milk as protein source
DT :   tempeh as protein source
DW :   whole seed of <u>Leucaena leucocephala</u> as protein source
DD :   skim milk as protein source, not added with iron
Mineral Mix :   AOAC, 1970
Vitamin Mix :   AOAC, 1970
* iron excluded: all of the diet is protein and calories.

Animal experiment

30 male and female weanling Wistar rats were individually housed in
plastic cages.   Housing was in a temperature controlled room with
a 12 h day and night lighting circle.   The rats were made anaemic
by feeding with a diet deficient in iron (DD diet, 3.5 ppm iron) for
7 weeks by which time their Hb level dropped to about 5 mg/dl.   Diet
and deionized water were given <u>ad libitum</u>.   The anaemic rats were
divided into 4 groups according to their hemoglobin level.   DS group
was fed with skim milk diet;   DT group was fed with tempeh diet;
DW group was fed with whole seed <u>Leucaena</u> diet and DD group was fed
with iron deficient diet.   During 2 weeks repletion period, weight
gain and food intake records were kept, faeces were collected.   At
the end of the experiment the rats were decapitated and autopsied for
liver and heart analysis.

Analytical methods

Hemoglobin was determined on tail blood by the cyano methemo-
globin method[1].   Iron in the diet and faeces were determined

following dry ashing, by colorimetric method[1], protein by Kjeldahl nitrogen, proximate analysis by AOAC, phytic acid by Makower method[11] and mimosine was determined by colorimetric method[8].

3   RESULTS AND DISCUSSION

The mimosine content of tempeh and whole seed Leucaena is compared in Table 2, which shows that the level of mimosine decreased about 99% during tempeh production.   Mimosine is soluble in water and destroyed by heating to more than 70°C.   According to Komari (personal communication) soaking, boiling and dehulling removed more than 95% of the mimosine content in the seed.   Reduction by fermentation is only small.   All of the treatments during tempeh production resulted in a decrease of phytic acid content by about one third from 1.25% in whole seeds to 0.85% in tempeh.   The reduction of phytic acid content can be accounted for by the activity of phytase elaborated by the mold responsible for the fermentation[6,7].

The iron absorption in rats fed with tempeh diet was greater in all four groups with absorption rates 23 to 87% and the difference was statistically significant (P 0.05).   The reduction of phytic acid and mimosine content during tempeh production caused the iron to be more available.   Derman et al[10] showed that the fall in pH during fermentation increases the soluble Fe content.   In DS diet Ca in skimmed milk competes with the iron.   Our results of iron absorption are similar to the previous study by Schriker et al[5].   They reported that the iron status did not influence the bioavailability of iron. Table 3 shows the iron intake and iron absorption.

Table 2   The composition of tempeh and whole seed Leucaena

Item	Whole seed (%)	Tempeh (%)
Crude protein	34.88	26.06
Crude fat	5.73	4.41
Ash	5.40	3.65
Carbohydrate	36.39	48.99
Moisture	8.55	15.94
Mimosine	7.89	0.103
Phytic acid	1.25	0.85

Table 3   Iron intake, iron in faeces and iron absorption

Item	Iron intake mg	Iron in faeces mg	Apparent absorption mg
DS group			
male (n=4)	1.98 ± 0.09	0.66 ± 0.21	66.72 ± 13.47
female (n=4)	1.71 ± 0.14	1.92 ± 0.10	45.92 ± 9.16
DT group			
male (n=4)	10.85 ± 0.75	1.36 ± 0.22	87.38 ± 5.94
female (n=4)	9.12 ± 0.34	1.25 ± 0.13	86.26 ± 13.29
DW group			
male (n=4)	2.52 ± 0.86	1.62 ± 0.18	35.87 ± 11.75
female (n=4)	2.95 ± 0.67	1.86 ± 0.43	37.02 ± 15.55
DD group			
male (n=5)	0.43 ± 0.25	0.32 ± 0.21	23.76 ± 13.35

DS group = skimmed milk diet, 14.99ppm Fe
DT group = tempeh diet, 65.73 ppm Fe
DW group = whole seed diet, 72.10 ppm Fe
DD group = iron deficient diet, 3.5 ppm Fe

Table 4   Hemoglobin level and iron in the organ

Item	Hb level mg/dl	Liver organ weight g/100 g b.w.	Liver iron mg/100g b.w.	Heart organ weight g/100g b.w.	Heart iron mg/100g b.w.
DS group					
male (n=4)	6.73	4.43	1.79	0.45	0.37
female (n=4)	6.49	4.38	1.98	0.44	0.48
DT group					
male (n=4)	9.63	3.67	1.65	0.40	0.37
female (n=4)	9.09	3.41	2.06	0.38	0.68
DW group					
male (n=4)	5.12	3.42	2.28	0.58	2.08
female (n=4)	4.92	3.65	2.59	0.51	1.03
DD group					
male (n=5)	4.54	4.18	1.43	0.47	0.43

Among the 4 groups of rats, the Hb level after 2 weeks repletion period in DT group was significantly (P 0.05) higher than with the other groups. The iron intake for DT and the other diet was significantly different (P 0.05), this suggests that the amount of iron in the diet influences the iron bioavailability. The low iron intake in DW group is caused by the low food intake of the rats. Although the iron absorption in DW group was very low the iron storage in the organs was greater than the other groups. Table 4 shows that the weight of the heart in DW group is greater than in normal Wistar rats of the same age. It is suggested that the higher mimosine content in whole seed of Leucaena has a toxic effect on that organ.

In conclusion, tempeh production has a good effect on the reduction of toxic substance mimosine and iron inhibitor, phytic acid. Tempeh is a fermentation product and good iron source.

REFERENCES

1. AOAC, Official method of analysis, Association of Official Analytical Chemists, Washington DC, 1970.
2. Anonymous. Leucaena, promising forage and tree crop for the tropics, NAS, Washington DC, 1977.
3. Ganjar I. Report on fermentation of Leucaena leucocephala seed, Nutrition Research Center, Indonesia, 1979.
4. Hamilton R.I., Donalson L.E. and Lamborne, L.J. Leucaena leucocephala as a feed on the calf for dairy cows. Aust. J. Res. 22: 681–692, 1971.
5. Schricker, B.R., Miller, D.D. and van Campen, D. Effects of iron status and soy protein on iron absorption by rats. J.Nutr. 113: 996–1001, 1983.
6. Sudarmadji S. and Markakis, P. The phytate and phytase of soybean tempeh. J.Sci. Food Agric. 28, 381–383, 1977.
7. Sutardi and Buckle, K.A. Reduction in phytic acid during tempeh production, storage and frying. J. Food Sci. 50: 260–263, 1985.
8. Matsumoto and Sherman G.D. A Rapid colorimetric method for the determination of Mimosine, Arch. Biochem. Biophys. 33, 195–200, 1951.
9. Astuti, M., Uehara M. and Suzuki K. Effects of soy tempeh powder on iron, copper and zinc bioavailability. J. Agric. Sci. Tokyo Univ. of Agric. 32: 106–114, 1987.
10. Derman D.P. et al, Br. J. Nutr. 43: 271–279, 1980.
11. Makower, R.U. Cereal Chem. 47: 288, 1970.

DETERMINATION OF BIOAVAILABLE IRON IN TYPICAL PAKISTANI FOODS

S. Arif Kazmi, Shireen Ghani, Kishwer Sabih, S.E.M. Shawoo and Samina Siddiqui.

Department of Chemistry, University of Karachi, Karachi, Pakistan

1. INTRODUCTION

It is now well established that like most other nutrients, iron bioavailability is also variable and depends both on the nature of the food intake as well as on the factors inherent to the subject itself. In prevention of the nutritional deficiency anaemia, both the increase in dietary iron and an increase in the availability of this iron should be simultaneously considered. The availability of dietary iron varies markedly in different types of food. We report here the results of our estimation of bioavailable iron in different types of typical Pakistani foods as a function of other ingredients and of the method of preparation of these foods.

For our studies we have chosen an in vitro assay as opposed to an animal bioassay such as rat haemoglobin regeneration test or a human bioassay involving administration of labelled iron. In vivo assays in addition to being cumbersome and demanding extensively elaborate protocols, suffer from disadvantages of intersubject variability and interspecies variability in iron absorption so that comparative evaluation of different types of foods for their efficacy in alleviating nutritional anaemia would be obscured. Consequently we have chosen an in vitro procedure. This method simulates the digestive process of stomach (2hr pepsin digestion at pH2) and that of small intestine (2hr pancreatin and bile salts, pH5-7). Finally absorption through mucosa is simulated by passage through a dialysis bag which allows iron which is unpolymerized, soluble, free ionic or bound to small molecules to pass. This iron in dilysate is then estimated spectrophotometrically.

2. EXPERIMENTAL

The cooked food was homogenized. 50g aliquot was adjusted to pH2 with HCl and incubated with 10mg Pepsin/g Protein at 37° for 2hrs. One 20ml aliquot of this digest was titrated against standard KOH to determine titrable acidity. An equivalent amount of $NaHCO_3$ in 25ml H_2O was taken in a dialysis bag which in turn was placed in a second 20ml aliquot of the pepsin digest. This as well as a third 20ml aliquot were placed on a water bath at 37°C. After 30 minutes, 10ml of pancreatin and bile salt mixture were added and incubation continued for 2hr. The dialysis bag was taken out, rinsed and its contents analysed for Fe after precipitation of protein by TCA. The procedure for Fe analysis was based on the absorbance of the Fe(II) complex with o-phenanthroline at 510nm. Hydroxylamine HCl or ascorbate were used as reducing agents to ensure all iron is in form of Fe(II) and the medium was acetate buffer of pH4.5. Total iron was similarly determined in the whole pancreatin digest. The % bioavailable iron is the ratio of the dialysable iron to total iron times 100.

Table 1

Food	Main Ingredients	% Bioavail. Fe
Beef Curry	M,375g+A	35.7
Mutton Curry	M,375g+A	12.5
Chicken Curry	M,375g+A	15.4
Beef Curry w/yogurt	M,375g+A+Yogurt,150g	8.4
Beef Curry w/tomato	M,375g+A+Tomato,150g	18.3
Beef Curry + Bread	Equal Wts of Curry & Bread	2.12
Beef Curry + Bread	Curry:Bread = 10:4	7.4
Beef Liver	Liver,370g+B	19.95
Chicken Liver	Liver,370g+B	36.6
Mutton Liver	Liver,370g+B	25.8
Beets	Veg,500g+C	16.3
Spinach	Veg,500g+C	59.5
Guar (Legume)	Veg,500g+C	13.9
Dal Mash (P.Mungo)	Dal,50g+D	5.8
Dal Mung (P.Aureus)	Dal,50g+D	12.1
Dal Masoor (C.Erietinum)	Dal,50g+D	10.1

Ingredients; A=Onions,250g+Oil,30g+Water,0.5L; M=Boneless Meat; B=Shortening,20g+Water0.5L; C=Oil,30g+Water,0.5L.

3. RESULTS AND DISCUSSION

Results of our determination of percent bioavailable iron (PBI) are shown in Table 1. The trends in meat curries

is that beef has higher PBI than does chicken which in turn
has a slightly higher value than mutton. Furthermore, our
values for beef curry are higher than those of the test
meals of Miller and Shricker containing ground beef[2,3].
Their test meal additionally contained bread and milk.
Ingredients of both these products have been implicated in
lowering of iron absorption. Our curries had a high proportion of onions which is rich in ascorbate - a factor known
to enhance iron absorption. In fact, when milk was replaced
by orange juice in the test meal based on ground beef, the
percent iron absorption jumped from 4.8 to 24[1] - a value
much closer to our results. Similarly when we mixed our
beef curry with bread the PBI dropped drastically to levels
closer to that of ref. 1. Our results show greater PBI when
ratio of curry to bread was increased. If one was to assume
that phytate alone is responsible for decrease in
bioavailability of iron caused by bread, then these results
would be surprising. It has been showed that iron forms 3
complexes with phytate, i.e., monoferric, diferric and
tetraferric phytates. Among these, monoferric is soluble
and absorbable while the other two are not[7]. Thus when the
iron:phytate (or curry:bread) ratio is high the equilibrium
should shift towards di and tetraferric complexes and the
PBI should be low; conversely, when this ratio is low,
equilibrium should remain towards the monoferric species and
results should indicate a higher PBI. The results are
opposite. We therefore suggest that dietary fibre, in
addition to phytate in bread, inhibits iron absorption. We
notice that curry when cooked in yogurt and to a lesser
extent in tomato gives a smaller value of PBI. Yogurt may
retain some of the factors in milk which complex iron and
reduce its PBI value. Also, the process of making yogurt
involves growth of bacteria which release powerful iron
chelators (siderophores), the presence of which might reduce
PBI. The result of curry cooked with tomato is more
surprising since tomatoes are rich in vitamin C. It may be
that pigments or chelators bind Fe to lower the PBI.

4. REFERENCES

1. D.D. Miller and B.R. Schricker in 'Nutritional Bioavailability of
    Iron', Am.Chem.Soc.Symp., Ser.No. 203, 1982, pp.11-26, C. Keis ed.
2. D.D. Miller et al., Am.J.Clin.Nutr., 1981, 34, 2248-56.
3. B.R. Schricker et al., Am.J.Clin.Nutr., 1981, 34, 2257-63.
4. M.A. Eastwood and R.M. Kay, Am.J.Clin.Nutr., 1979, 32, 364.
5. Y.M. Feuillen, Acta Ped., 1954, 43, 181.
6. S.R. Lynch and J.D. Cook, Ann.NY Acad.Sci., 1980, 355, 32-44.
7. U.R. Morris and R. Ellis, 'Nutritional Bioavailability of Iron',
    Am.Chem.Soc.Symp., Ser.No. 203, 1982, pp.121-41, C. Keis, ed.

BIOAVAILABILITY OF IRON IN FERRIC ORTHOPHOSPHATE, FERROUS GLUCONATE AND CARBONYL IRON TO RATS.

T. Kosonen and M. Mutanen.

Department of Nutrition
University of Helsinki
00710 Helsinki, Finland.

In Finland the enrichment of flour with iron as ferrum reductum has been allowed since 1974. The bioavailability of this iron source in flour or in bread baked with this flour is not known. The present study was conducted to determine the relative biological availability (RBV, $FeSO_4$ = 100 %) to rats of the carbonyl iron, ferric orthophosphate and ferrous gluconate in flour and the carbonyl iron and ferric orthophosphate in bread.

Weanling male rats were fed on a Fe-deficient (3.3 mg/kg) casein based diet for 28 days followed by either continued depletion or repletion for 16 days with additional 6, 12 or 24 mg Fe/kg as ferrous sulphate or three test sources of iron. The hemoglobin iron was used as the criterion of body iron status. The bioavailability was estimated with the slope-ratio method as the gain in the hemoglobin iron (mg) <u>versus</u> the intake of iron (mg). The carbonyl iron in flour was omitted because the statistical validity of the slope-ratio method was not fullfilled with this iron source. The RBV's for ferric orthophosphate and ferrous gluconate in flour were 45 and 76 %, respectively and ferric orthophosphate and carbonyl iron in bread 36 and 35 %, respectively. Except for ferrous gluconate other iron sources tested differed significantly from the standard ($p < 0.05$).

EFFECT OF PROTEIN QUALITY AND DIETARY LEVELS OF IRON, ZINC AND COPPER ON APPARENT ABSORPTION AND TISSUE TRACE ELEMENTS CONCENTRATION IN THE RATS

A. Brzozowska, A. Sicińska, J. Witkowska and W. Roszkowski

Institute of Human Nutrition
Warsaw Agricultural University SGGW-AR
02-766 Warsaw, Poland

1 INTRODUCTION

Dietary deficiences or excesses of some elements create disorders in absorption and utilization of others. It is interesting that if the quantities of iron, zinc and copper are increased in proportion to their normal requirements, the adverse interactions are much less apparent, if they occur at all[1]. So, the aim of this study was to determine the effect of protein quality on iron, zinc and copper concentration in rat tissues at different level but constant ratios of these elements in the diets.

2 MATERIALS AND METHODS

The experiment was performed on male Wistar rats with initial weight 102 g. The animals were housed individually in plastic cages with free access to semipurified diet and redistilled water. The experimental diets contained 20% of protein. Casein (C), wheat gluten (G) or mixture (1:1) of both (CG) were used as a source of protein. Iron citrate, zinc acetate and copper carbonate were used to obtain the minerals levels as follows:

    LM - low level of Fe, Zn and Cu simultaneously
        (60% of recommendation),
    SM - standard level, recommended for rats i.e.
        Fe 35 mg, Zn 12 mg, Cu 5 mg per kg of the diet[2],
    HM - high level (300% of recommendation).

During experiment faeces collection was done in three 4-days periods. After 6 weeks iron, zinc and copper were determined in tissues, diets and faeces after dry ashing using AAS method.

3 RESULTS

The apparent absorption of examined trace elements was significantly influenced by the source of protein in the diets (Table 1). This effect was marked stronger for zinc and copper than for iron. For rats eating G and CG diets the average apparent absorption of zinc were less effective than those on C diets, while the average absorption of copper was significantly lower on G diets than on C and CG diets.

Under conditions of this experiment rats absorbed iron (av. 39.6%) less efficiently than copper (av. 48.8%) and zinc (av. 51.2%). Apparent absorption of these metals was inversely related to their dietary levels. The highest difference between LM and HM diets was observed for copper from C and CG diets. One potential reason for this is that the levels of copper in the CLM and CGLM diets were somewhat lower than assumed 60% of recommendation i.e. 1.33 and 1.99 mg/kg diet, respectively.

Tissue concentration of zinc, iron and copper was also influenced by protein source. The growth of rats on G diets was slower than on C or CG but they absorbed more minerals per g of weight gain. Thus among rats on G diets the highest concentration of examined minerals in most tissues was observed. As dietary level of minerals was higher the iron concentration in liver, spleen, kidney and testes increased, the same relation for zinc in kidney,

Table 1 Apparent absorption in % (mean ± S.E.)

Diet	Iron	Zinc	Copper
CLM	49.5 ± 4.3	68.6 ± 3.1	75.5 ± 1.7
CSM	45.2 ± 1.8	60.4 ± 3.0	48.1 ± 1.8
CHM	40.1 ± 4.2	49.9 ± 4.0	42.0 ± 5.2
GLM	43.1 ± 3.7	52.3 ± 2.1	45.5 ± 1.4
GSM	37.6 ± 4.6	46.8 ± 1.6	42.3 ± 4.0
GHM	26.4 ± 3.0	37.8 ± 2.4	33.7 ± 3.5
CGLM	45.9 ± 6.7	57.4 ± 2.5	68.4 ± 1.8
CGSM	41.4 ± 3.0	47.7 ± 2.7	44.2 ± 1.3
CGHM	27.3 ± 3.6	40.3 ± 2.0	39.5 ± 2.2

	Analysis of variance (P-values)		
Protein	0.0137	0.0001	0.0001
Minerals	0.0001	0.0001	0.0001
PxM	NS*	NS	0.0002

* Not significant, i.e. $P > 0.05$

<u>Table 2</u> Ratios in the rat livers (mean ± S.E.)

Diet	Fe:Zn	Fe:Cu	Zn:Cu
CLM	2.58 ± 0.32	17.3 ± 1.8	7.28 ± 0.69
CSM	2.51 ± 0.11	12.6 ± 0.7	5.51 ± 0.57
CHM	4.17 ± 0.38	29.4 ± 2.4	7.34 ± 0.61
GLM	2.78 ± 0.45	16.5 ± 1.4	5.96 ± 0.57
GSM	3.33 ± 0.14	21.0 ± 1.3	6.19 ± 0.40
GHM	4.83 ± 0.23	30.5 ± 2.0	6.26 ± 0.49
CGLM	1.60 ± 0.08	10.9 ± 0.8	6.77 ± 0.49
CGSM	2.20 ± 0.10	12.7 ± 0.5	5.92 ± 0.16
CGHM	3.21 ± 0.17	22.2 ± 1.5	6.70 ± 0.45

	Analysis of variance (P-values)		
Protein	0.0001	0.0001	NS*
Minerals	0.0001	0.0001	0.0152
PxM	NS	NS	NS

* Not significant, i.e. $P > 0.05$.

femur, hair and for copper in liver, kidney and femur was
observed.
Moreover the ratio of iron to other metals in liver
(Table 2), spleen, testes and femur was higher on G diets
than on C or CG diets. As the diets contained more
minerals the liver, spleen and testes Fe:Zn and Fe:Cu
ratio also increased. On the contrary to the above, the
ratio of Zn:Cu in spleen, kidney and femur was the lowest
on G diets as well as this ratio in spleen and kidney
decreased as dietary minerals were higher. In hair the
metals ratios were relatively constant.
The absorption and tissue distribution of iron, zinc
and copper were influenced by both their dietary level and
source of protein. Though the proportions of these
elements in the diets were constant the adverse
interactions occured, which changed metal ratios in some
tissues.

REFERENCES

1. G.K. Davies, <u>Ann.N.Y.Ac.Sc.</u>, 1980, <u>355</u>, 130.
2. 'The Laboratory Rat', H.J. Baker, J.R. Lindsey and
   S.H. Weisbroth, Academic Press, New York, 1979,
   Vol. I, Chapter 6, p. 128.

This work was supported by CPB-R Grant no. 10-16/67.

NEUTRON ACTIVATION FOR ^{59}FE-LABELING OF ORAL IRON PREPARATIONS FOR BIOAVAILABILITY MEASUREMENTS IN MAN

H. C. Heinrich, R. Fischer and E. E. Gabbe

Division of Medical Biochemistry, University-Hospital-Eppendorf,
University of Hamburg
2000 Hamburg 20, Martinistrasse 52, Fed. Rep. Germany.

The reliable quantitative and direct estimation of the bioavailability of iron in commercial oral iron preparations requires their ^{59}Fe-labeling so that the ^{59}Fe-absorption can be calculated from the measured whole body retention (WBR) of absorbed ^{59}Fe. The necessary ^{59}Fe-labeling can be done either by the manufacturers using the same procedure as for their commercial products, or by neutron activation (NA) of commercial iron preparation in the thermal flux of a nuclear reactor.

1. Neutron Activation ^{59}Fe-Labeling of Commercial Oral Iron Preparations

The 10 MW nuclear research reactor FRJ-1 (MERLIN) at the Kernforschungsanlage Jülich/Fed. Rep. Germany was used for the NA of several oral Fe(II) and Fe(III) containing oral iron preparations. Individual solid samples (tablets, capsules, dragees etc.) of the iron preparations (80-105 mg Fe) were vacuum sealed in polyethylene foils and liquid samples filled into polypropylene vials and then exposed behind a thermal column to a thermal neutron (10^{-4} - 10^0 eV) flux of $10^{11} \cdot cm^{-1} \cdot sec^{-1}$ (fast to thermal neutron flux ratio 0.01; γ-dose rate 10^4 rad/h) for 3-14 days at + 30°C. The natural 0.33% ^{58}Fe-content was sufficient for obtaining a specific radioactivity of 1 µCi(=37 kBq) ^{59}Fe/100 mg Fe by the $^{58}_{26}$Fe(n/γ) $^{59}_{26}$Fe NA-reaction. The radiochemical purity of all neutron activated iron preparations was investigated after 2 weeks with a high purity germanium detector. Trace contaminations of the commercial iron preparations with stable ^{50}Cr and ^{59}Co were converted by NA to traces of 1 - 6% ^{51}Cr and 1 - 4% ^{60}Co. The ^{51}Cr- γ -photons of 320 keV were discriminated from the ^{59}Fe energy window (500 - 1700 keV) of the used 4π-geometry whole body radio-activity detector (= WBRD) with liquid organic scintillator whereas the small amount of ^{60}Co was corrected by considering its activity as measured in the sum peak (2,500 keV) area of its spectrum.   The commercial oral iron preparations were controlled for quality before and after NA-^{59}Fe-labeling.   No measurable differences were observed and espec. the "in vitro" release of iron in artificial gastric and duodenal juice at pH 1.2 and 6.8 respect. was identical.   The bioavailability of ^{59}Fe from a NA-^{59}Fe-labeled commercial Fe(II) capsule (Eryfer) was shown by intra-individual comparison in 9 subjects to be identical with the ^{59}Fe-bioavailability from an aqueous ^{59}Fe(II)-ascorbate solution (reference for relative bioavailability RBA = 100%) because of a 15-days ^{59}Fe whole body retention (=WBR) ratio of 0.96 $\pm$ 13% and did also agree with earlier results when the same preparation was labeled during production in the company.

2.   Quantification of ^{59}Fe Absorption by Measurement of ^{59}Fe-Whole Body Retention

^{59}Fe-labeled commercial iron preparations (80-105 mg Fe) were orally administered to male volunteers with normal or depleted iron stores.   The subjects were starved for between 10 hours before and 2 hours after oral iron uptake in order to avoid iron absorption promoting or inhibiting effects of food constituents.   Up to 5 different oral iron preparations were studied at 2 week intervals in each individual by comparison with an aqueous solution of ^{59}Fe(II) -ascorbate (= 100 mg ^{59}Fe) as the reference standard for RBA = 100%. The ^{59}Fe-absorption was calculated from the WBR of absorbed ^{59}Fe as measured within the 4π geometry of the WBRD always 14 days after each uptake.   The additional radiation absorbed dose for a NA-^{59}Fe -labeled preparation (1 μCi ^{59}Fe oral dose and 8.2% absorption) was calculated to be 4.8 mrem (= 48 μSv) or 1.6% of the natural radiation burden of man (~300 mrem/year) and therefore without radiobiological relevance.

3.   Bioavailability of Iron in Commercial Oral Fe(II) and Fe(III) -Preparations

3.1   Administration of an Oral Iron Preparation on an Empty Stomach is Imperative for not Decreasing the Characteristic Bioavailabilities of Each Commercial Preparation

The bioavailabilities of even the well absorbable oral Fe(II) preparations (RBA = 70 - 100%) can be severely inhibited by a great number of natural iron chelating compounds as contained particularly in vegetable foods and drinks as tea, coffee, milk etc. to such an extent that the oral iron can be rendered ineffective.   A 2 rolls with butter and cheese and 300 ml tea (extract of 4.2 Ceylon tea) including standard breakfast reduced the absorption of ^{59}Fe from an aqueous ^{59}Fe(II) ascorbate solution (100 mg Fe) from $\bar{X}A \pm SEM =$ = 10.2 $\pm$ 0.54% to only 1.27 $\pm$ 0.16% in subjects with normal iron stores and to a similar degree from 18% to 3% with depleted iron

stores. The bioavailability of ^{59}Fe in a commercial oral ^{59}Fe
-(II)-glycine-sulphate preparation (ferro sanol duodenal) with quick
and complete Fe(II) release in the duodenum was decreased from 7.09
$\pm$ 0.65% to 3.49 $\pm$ 0.46% (RBA = 51%) in 9 subjects with normal iron
stores by a standard breakfast containing 40g crisp bread, 25g butter
and 300 ml Ceylon tea.

3.2 <u>Full RBA (90-100%) of Iron in Aqueous Solutions and Solid Fe(II)-
Preparations with Quick and Complete Release of Fe(II) in the
Stomach</u>

From an aqueous ^{59}Fe(II)ascorbate solution (100mg Fe) subjects
with normal Fe stores absorbed an average of between 7.7 and 8.5% of
mg Fe whereas depleted Fe-stores caused an increased average absorption between 15 and 18% in different groups of volunteers. This Fe
-absorption was set equivalent to a RBA = 100%. Healthy male volun-
teers with normal Fe-stores were shown to absorb $\overline{X}A \pm$ SEM = 7.70 $\pm$ 0.50
(Eryfer) and 7.63 $\pm$ 0.53 (Ascofer) equivalent to RBA-values of 97 and
96% respect. from Fe(II)ascorbate containing gelatine capsules with
quick and complete Fe(II) release already in the stomach. The ^{59}Fe-
absorption was increased to 16.2 $\pm$ 1.8% (Eryfer, RBA = 100%) and
15.1 $\pm$ 1.7% (Ascofer, RBA = 100%) in persons with depleted iron stores.
From ^{59}Fe(II)-diaspartate (Spartocine) containing gelatine capsules
7.02 $\pm$ 0.56% (RBA = 88%) were absorbed with normal Fe-stores and 14.0
$\pm$ 1.75% (RBA = 96%) with depleted iron stores. It was demonstrated
in earlier studies that patients with mild (9-12 g Hb/dl) and severe
(5-9 g Hb/dl) iron deficiency anaemia do absorb $\overline{X}A \pm SD_9 = 28 \pm 9.4\%$
(RBA = 100%) and 25 - 5.4% (RBA=100%) respect. from a ^{59}Fe(II)ascor-
bate quick releasing capsule (Eryfer). The bioavailability of ^{59}Fe
from a ^{59}Fe(II)-gluconate plus citric acid and tartaric acid in addition to ascorbic acid containing sparkling tablet (Losferron) was
reduced to 3.11 $\pm$ 0.27% (RBA = 39%) with normal iron stores and to
8.24 $\pm$ 1.18% (RBA = 51%) with depleted iron stores possibly due to an
iron absorption inhibiting effect of the other organic acids.

3.3 <u>High RBA (70 - 90%) of Iron in Fe(II)-Preparations with Quick
and Complete Release of Fe(II) in the Duodenum</u>

The bioavailability of ^{59}Fe from an oral (Fe(II)-preparation
with "delayed" rapid Fe(II)-release in the duodenum at pH = 5.5 - 6.8
(ferro sanol duodenal, containing ferrousglycinesulphate in many small
gastric juice resistant coated pellets within a gastric juice soluble
gelatine capsule) was slightly reduced to 6.55 $\pm$ 0.39% (RBA = 83%) in
subjects with normal iron stores and to 14.5 $\pm$ 1.6% (RBA = 90%) with
depleted iron stores.

3.4 <u>Reduced RBA (40 - 70%) of Iron in Fe(II)-Preparations with Slow
and Complete/Incomplete release of Fe(II) in the Jejunum and
Colon</u>

The ^{59}Fe-bioavailability from a sustained or controlled released

filmtablet with a delayed but finally complete iron release(Kendural
C = Fero-Grad 500 in USA contains 105mg Fe(II) and 500mg ascorbic acid
within a plastic matrix with an "in vitro" release of only 38% after
1 hour at pH 1.2 plus 1 hour at pH 6.8 at + 37°C) was reduced to 4.52
$\pm$ 0.42% (RBA = 57%) in persons with normal iron stores and to 9.89 $\pm$
1.21% (RBA = 61%) with depleted iron stores.   The ^{59}Fe-absorption
from a mucoproteose containing ^{59}Fe(II)-SO$_4$-dragee (Tardyferon) with
a slow and incomplete "in vitro" iron release (only 60% after 1 hour
at pH 1.2 and 5 hours at pH 6.8) was diminished to 3.37 $\pm$ 0.23%
(RBA = 43%) with normal iron stores and to 10.7 $\pm$ 1.00% (RBA = 66%).

3.5 Low RBA (10 - 20%) of Iron in Trivalent Iron Containing Fe(III)-
     Citrate and Fe(III)-Hydroxide Dextrin or Polymaltose Complexes.

     The ^{59}Fe-bioavailability from a trivalent iron containing ^{59}Fe(III)
-citrate complex in solution (Ferrlecit drops) was considerably decreased to 1.58 $\pm$ 0.12% (RBA = 18.5%) in volunteers with normal iron
stores.   Earlier studies had demonstrated also a very low ^{59}Fe-ab-
sorption of 2.30 $\pm$ 0.60% (RBA = 13%) from a polymeric ^{59}Fe(III)-
citrate complex in subjects with depleted iron stores.   The lowest
^{59}Fe-bioavailability ever described was observed with a Fe(III)-
hydroxide-polymaltose complex (Ferrum Hausmann drops and juice).
By intraindividual comparison with an aqueous ^{59}Fe(II)-ascorbate
solution (RBA = 100%) a ^{59}Fe-absorption of only 0.81 $\pm$ 0.06% (RBA =
9.5%) was measured in subjects with normal iron stores.   Earlier
studies with an exchange labeled Fe(III)hydroxide polymaltose complex
had already demonstrated very poor bioavailabilities of 0.49 $\pm$ 0.12%
(RBA = 6.2%) in persons with normal iron stores and only 1.34 $\pm$ 0.23%
(RBA = 9.2%) with depleted iron stores.   This particular Fe(III)-
preparation was then shown to be therapeutically ineffective at a
daily dose level of 100 and 200 mg Fe(III) in patients with mild and
severe iron deficiency anaemia.   A similar or identical oral Fe(III)
-preparation is also on the USA market (Niferex).

     An iron-chelate-tablet (Albion Laboratories, USA) was claimed to
contain only ferrous iron chelated to soya-bean proteins and protein
hydrolysate and to be 3.8 times better available than the Fe(II) in
Fe(II)-sulphate.   This preparation did, however, contain 80% of its
total iron as trivalent iron and its bioavailability was decreased
from 8.72 $\pm$ 0.92% (^{59}Fe(II)SO$_4$ reference solution, RBA = 100%) to
4.01 $\pm$ 1.01% (RBA = 46%) in 12 subjects with normal iron stores and
from 18% ^{59}Fe(II)-ascorbate-solution) to 10.1 $\pm$ 1.68% (RBA = 56%)
in 8 blood donors with depleted iron stores.   The reduced bioavailability of the iron-chelate-complex was either due to the poor
absorbability of the trivalent iron and/or an iron absorption
inhibiting effect of the soya-bean protein hydrolysate.

THE HOMEOSTATIC REGULATION OF ZINC ABSORPTION AND SECRETION IN ZINC DEPLETED MAN

C.M. Bosworth, J. Bacon (1), I. Bremner and P.J. Aggett
Biochemistry Division, Rowett Research Institute, Greenburn Road,
Bucksburn, Aberdeen.   AB2 9SB
(1) Macaulay Land Use Research Institute, Craigiebuckler,
Aberdeen.   AB9 2QJ

1. INTRODUCTION

Zinc homeostasis in animals is maintained by regulation of intestinal zinc absorption and excretion[1] but little is known of these control mechanisms in man. In some investigations, the percentage of true zinc absorption was found to be inversely related to dietary zinc intake[2,3]. In another study, involving only one male volunteer, the intestinal secretion of zinc varied in response to changes in zinc supply[4]. However no information is available on the mechanisms involved in the maintenance of zinc homeostatis when dietary zinc intakes are very low. A metabolic study has therefore been carrried out in which zinc absorption and secretion were measured, using zinc-70 as marker, in male subjects fed a formula diet with a low zinc content.

2. METHODS

Three healthy men, aged 37-40 years and of normal weight (BMI 19.1-21.8) took part in a 55 day metabolic study in which they received a formula diet according to their energy requirements. The basal diet, which was fed from days 16-40, provided only 12.2-13.2 µmoles zinc per day. During the initial and final stages of the trial (days 1-15 and 41-55) the diet was supplemented with zinc sulphate to provide a total of 84.8-85.8 µmoles zinc/day. On days 6, 31 and 46, the subjects were given 3.5 µmoles zinc-70 in their diet. Serial 5-day metabolic balance studies were conducted throughout the trial.

The abundance of stable isotopes of zinc in dry ashed faecal samples was determined by thermal ionisation mass spectrometry after separation of the zinc by ion exchange chromatography. The mass of zinc-70 in the samples was calculated[5]. Total zinc concentrations were determined by atomic absorption spectrometry.

213

The luminal disappearance or apparent absorption of zinc-70 was calculated from the difference between the amount fed and that recovered in the faecal pool. The absorption of the stable isotope of zinc was assumed to represent that of total luminal zinc. The intestinal loss of endogenous zinc was calculated by subtracting the amount of unabsorbed exogenous zinc from the total zinc in the faecal pool.

3. RESULTS AND DISCUSSION

During the intial period (days 1-15), the absorption of zinc-70 was 32% (Table 1). The subjects went into negative zinc balance of -23.8 to -49.3 µmol/day when given the zinc-deficient diet. The size of the zinc deficit became less as the trial proceeded and after 25 days on the low zinc diet it was only -10.5 to -14.5 µmol/day, and there was a decline of 55% in faecal zinc and 42% in urinary zinc output.

Table 1 Changes in the absorption of zinc in three subjects fed a low zinc diet

	Zinc absorption % (µmol/day)		
	Baseline	Depletion	Repletion
Subject			
1	31.0 (26.4)	91.8 (12.6)	39.9 (34.2)
2	33.6 (28.6)	97.5 (13.4)	82.8 (71.0)
3	30.9 (26.2)	92.0 (12.0)	83.8 (71.1)

The efficiency of zinc-70 absorption increased substantially when the subjects received the low-zinc diet and had a mean of 94% after 15 days of zinc depletion. Conversely, the efficiency of zinc-70 absorption decreased to 69% after 5 days of zinc repletion. This was accompanied by a restoration of a positive zinc balance (mean value 45.2 µmol/day).

There were also changes in the loss or secretion of endogenous zinc during the trial (Table 2). This was equivalent to about 30 µmol/day during the initial and final periods, when the zinc-supplemented diet was fed, but decreased to 11 µmol/day during zinc depletion. Urinary zinc losses during the initial, depletion and repletion phases were 14.5 to 21.9, 8.3 to 12.3 and 7.8 - 19.3 µmol/day respectively.

Table 2 Intestinal loss of endogenous zinc in three subjects fed a low zinc diet

	Intestinal zinc loss (μmol)		
	Baseline	Depletion	Repletion
Subject			
1	44.6	9.7	26.4
2	22.8	13.0	25.8
3	15.6	18.0	54.0

This experiment has demonstrated that humans have a considerable ability to adapt to a severely restricted zinc intake. The efficiency of intestinal zinc absorption increased to over 90% after a brief period of zinc deprivation and there were also substantial reductions in loss of endogenous zinc *via* the intestinal and urinary tracts. These adaptive changes were not sufficient to allow the subjects to attain positive zinc balance but they did lead to a reduction in the severity of the negative balance.

Direct comparison of these results with other studies in which stable isotopes have been used is difficult because of differences in the quantities and route of administration of the isotope. However, there is a general agreement insofar as the efficiency of absorption has increased as zinc supply has decreased[2-4]. Moreover the fact that zinc secretion, but not zinc absorption, returned to normal during the brief zinc repletion period supports the suggestion that zinc secretion responds more rapidly to changes in dietary zinc supply[4].

REFERENCES

1. E. Wiegand and M. Kirchgessner, Nutr. Metabl., 1978, 22, 101.
2. N.W. Istfan, M. Janghorbani and V.R. Young, Am. J. Clin. Nutr., 1983, 38, 187.
3. L. Wada, J.R. Turnlund and J.C. King, J. Nutr., 1985, 115, 1345.
4. M.J. Jackson, D.A. Jones, R.H.T. Edwards, I.G. Swainback and M.L. Coleman, Br. J. Nutr., 51, 199.
5. J.R. Turnlund, J.C. King, W.R. Keyes, B. Gong and M.C. Mithel, Am. J. Clin. Nutr., 1984, 40, 1071.

ACKNOWLEDGEMENTS

We thank the Medical Research Council, Rank Prize Funds and Scottish Education Department for financial support.

EXERCISE BIOCHEMISTRY - AN OXYGEN RADICAL APPROACH

O.I. Aruoma and B. Halliwell

Department of Biochemistry
University of London King's College
Strand, London WC2R 2LS UK

Oxygen free radicals are increasingly implicated in molecular and tissue damage arising in normal metabolic process accompanying aging and in particular in increased oxidative metabolism associated with strenuous exercise.

Exercise causes an increased oxygen consumption in vivo and a small part of this oxygen uptake leads to the formation of reactive tissue damaging oxygen radicals. Hydroxyl radicals $\cdot OH$ produced by the Fenton-type reaction

$$Fe^{3+} + O_2^- \longrightarrow Fe^{2+} + O_2$$
$$Fe^{2+} + H_2O_2 \longrightarrow Fe^{3+} + \cdot OH + OH^-$$

$$Net\ H_2O_2 + O_2^- \underset{catalyst}{\overline{\quad Iron\ complex \quad}} \longrightarrow \cdot OH + OH^- + O_2$$

in biological systems can cause damage to DNA, lipids, proteins and carbohydrates.

Generation of the highly reactive oxygen species requires catalytic metal complexes especially those of iron. However, proving that oxidative damage in biological systems is due to $\cdot OH$ radical is extremely difficult. This highly reactive radical once generated will combine very quickly with adjacent molecules and so is almost impossible to scavenge.

In normal cells, (erythrocytes for example) antioxidant defence are afforded by the enzymes superoxide dismutase, catalase and glutathione peroxidase and its substrate glutathione (GSH). When these cells are damaged (as may be the case in foot-strike haemolysis), the

216

antioxidants of the cells are diluted. Haem may also be degraded releasing iron which is a pro-oxidant. Hence biological systems must sequester iron to prevent it from circulating around in free form. In vivo, iron is normally bound to transport and storage proteins, transferrin, lactoferrin, ferritin and haemosiderin. Indeed, at pH 7.4, apotransferrin and apolactoferrin are able to bind iron ion and protect against ·OH radical generation promoted by iron added as $FeCl_3$ or by iron released from ferritin in the presence of ascorbate or a superoxide radical generating system, hence supporting the proposal that under normal conditions, iron binding proteins function as antioxidants in vivo.

One of the methods for the measurement of free radical reaction in vivo, aromatic hydroxylation, involves the use of a non toxic aromatic compound (aspirin for example) with a high rate constant for reaction with ·OH. The end products of ·OH attack must be stable in vivo and not identical with those produced in vivo via normal enzyme mechanisms. Another method in use involves the measurement of the levels of uric acid and its oxidation product allantoin. (Uric acid is a product from the degradation of purines). This would serve as a potential index of free radical attack in vivo. However, compared with the salicylate method, the measurement of allantoin is favoured although a rather complex derivatisation is involved (see Grootveld and Halliwell 1986, 1987).

It has been observed that human sweat contains catalytic iron (Fe) and copper (Cu) capable of catalysing ·OH reactions. This may be irrelevant (with respect to ·OH radical reaction) since sweat is an excretory product. However, there exist suggestions that iron loss during exercise is associated with sports anaemia. Hard training athletes and indeed endurance performers have greatly accelerated sweat loss and sometimes, especially for women, develop iron deficiency anaemia. By comparing the plasma levels of zinc, iron and copper before and after a period of controlled exercise with losses of the metals in sweat together with changes in plasma volume and haematocrit, it may be possible to gain an insight into the significance of metal metabolism in exercise (see Aruoma et al 1988).

The increased ratio of uric acid to allantoin levels following exercise (Table 1) is significant. However, the apparent increase in uric acid levels may be accounted for by observed changes in plasma volume, and increased purine breakdown. Allantoin, the product of uric acid oxidation may itself be oxidized hence resulting in

Table 1   Uric Acid and Allantoin Analysis

Subject	Uric Acid μM	Uric Acid / Allantoin	Uric Acid μM	Uric Acid / Allantoin
	(Before exercise)		(After exercise)	
A	300	10.8	359.5	16.8
B	309.5	24.4	342.9	31.5
C	243	13.6	345.2	20.9
D	359	10.1	304.2	24.0
E	442.9	18.2	504.8	26.3
Mean±SD	330.9±75	15.4±5.9	371.3±77.4	23.9±5.5

Table 2   Sweat metal content as a function of body site. (Number of samples analysed by atomic absorption spectroscopy are given in parenthesis).

Site studied	μmol/l (mean±SD) of:		
	Fe	Cu	Zn
Abdomen	8.8±7.0(14)	14.0±9.9(8)	12.7±13.0(10)
Arm	5.0±2.5(10)	8.2±7.5(4)	6.8±7.3(6)
Chest	8.9±10.8(15)	11.5±11.6(8)	6.4±7.9(11)
Back	3.6±3.2(19)	8.8±6.8(14)	7.3±8.8(20)

increased uric acid:allantoin ratio following a period of exercise on cycle ergometer over 50 minutes with a work load of 210 watts at standard laboratory conditions. In addition to antioxidant enzymes the body has non-enzymic antioxidants derived from diets, for example, vitamins E, C, selenium (an important component of glutathione peroxidase) and beta carotene from which vitamin A is derived. The antioxidant status of the training athletes or exercising subjects is indeed important, in view of the possible oxygen radical damage. Do antioxidants develop during exercise? Perhaps dietary supplementation may be significant as a preventative measure should the answer be no. Clearly more work is required on this aspect.

Typical data (Table 2) show that appreciable amounts of iron are lost during exercise and that this varies between sites. Appreciable amounts of copper and zinc are also lost <u>via</u> the sweat route. Given the relatively lower pool of zinc and copper <u>in vivo</u> compared with iron, these losses are biologically significant. There was a tendency for losses of copper and zinc in sweat from all sites to be greater than losses of iron although there was considerable variation between subjects (see Aruoma <u>et al</u> 1988).

The variability, even between male subjects of similar age and body mass in such parameters as sweat rate, plasma volume changes and changes in the metal contents of plasma (see Aruoma <u>et al</u> 1988) suggests that real sports anaemia or indeed significant deficiencies in the zinc content of the body, may be features only of certain individuals. The nutritional implication of the work would centre on the recommendation for dietary supplementation with not only iron but copper and zinc.

We thank the Sports Council for support.

SUGGESTED READING

B. Halliwell and J.M.C. Gutteridge, 'Free Radicals in Biology & Medicine', Clarendon Press, Oxford, 1985.
G. Benzi, L. Packer and N. Siliprandi (editors) 'Biochemical Aspects of Physical Exercise',Elsevier Science Publishers, Amsterdam, 1986.
M. Grootveld and B. Halliwell, <u>Biochem. J.</u>, 1986, <u>237</u>, 499.
M. Grootveld and B. Halliwell, <u>Biochem. J.</u>, 1987, <u>243</u>, 803.
B. Halliwell and M. Grootveld, <u>FEBS Lett.</u>, 1987, <u>213</u>, 9.
O.I. Aruoma and B. Halliwell, <u>Biochem. J.</u>, 1987, <u>241</u>, 273.
L.A. Fredrickson, J.L. Puhl and W.S. Runyan, <u>Med. Sci. Sports Exerc.</u>, 1983, <u>15</u>, 271.
O.I. Aruoma, T. Reilly, D. MacLaren and B. Halliwell, <u>Clin. Chim. Acta</u>, 1988, (Accepted for publication).

MATERNAL ZINC AND FETAL GROWTH DURING ORAL IRON SUPPLEMENTATION IN PREGNANCY. A PRELIMINARY STUDY.

N.R. Williams, D.L. Bloxam, Y. Morarji and P.M. Pattinson-Green

Royal Postgraduate Medical School Institute of Obstetrics and Gynaecology
Queen Charlotte's Maternity Hospital
Goldhawk Road
London   W6 OXG

1. INTRODUCTION

The practice of giving iron to women during pregnancy is widespread, in spite of a lack of information regarding its effects on the mother and fetus. While it is accepted that an unsupplemented woman faces a risk of anaemia in late pregnancy or post-partum, there is no evidence that non-anaemic pregnant women positively benefit from oral iron. On the other hand, many investigations have shown that altering the intake of essential metals can affect the bioavailability of others.[1] This has been shown in animals and humans, and the possibility that excessive oral iron can reduce zinc status has been raised.[2]

This is important because zinc is required for many metabolic processes (including DNA and protein synthesis), and there is an extra demand for zinc during pregnancy for fetal growth. Some studies have found associations between low maternal plasma or leucocyte zinc concentrations with congenital malformations, fetal growth retardation and a variety of complications of parturition.[3]

In order to test the hypothesis that oral iron supplementation during pregnancy may reduce maternal zinc status and so possibly affect fetal growth, we carried out a small double-blind trial in which two matched groups of women were given either a commercial iron preparation or an iron-free placebo in their second and third trimesters. Serial blood samples and ultrasound scans of the fetal femur and biparietal diameter (head size) were obtained, and the maternal zinc status and fetal growth of the groups compared.

220

2. SUBJECTS AND METHODS

Twenty pregnant non-vegetarian Caucasian women remained in
this study from forty who were originally recruited when
attending an antenatal clinic at about 16 weeks' gestation.
Each was assigned to either an iron supplemented group
(two Fefol-Vit Spansule capsules per day, each containing
multivitamins and 47 mg elemental iron as ferrous sulphate)
or placebo group (multivitamins only). The groups were
matched for parity, weight, smoking and maternal age. Data
were excluded from mothers who did not comply with the
instructions, whose haemoglobin fell below 10.4 g/dl or
who developed a significant medical condition. Two non-
Caucasians were removed because of the known effects of
race on birthweight. This left 13 supplemented and 7
placebo group women. There were no significant differences
in the matching factors mentioned above between the two
groups. Fuller details of the study design have been
published.[4] Blood was collected and ultrasound scans
given at 16 weeks' gestation (zero time of the study) and
periodically thereafter. Zinc was measured in diluted
plasma by atomic absorption spectrophotometry.

Results are expressed as means$\pm$SEM, and differences
analysed by Student's t-test or 2-way analysis of variance
as appropriate.

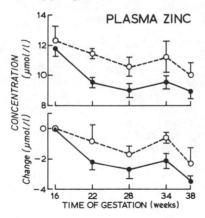

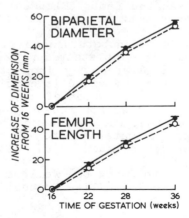

Figure 1. Effect of iron
supplementation on plasma
zinc concentration.
Supplemented •——•;
placebo o— — —o.

Figure 2. Effect of iron
supplementation on fetal
head and femur growth.
Supplemented •——•;
placebo o— — —o.

3. RESULTS

Indices of iron status of the two groups of women (blood haemoglobin, serum ferritin and plasma transferrin saturation) were not different at the start of the study. After 12 to 18 weeks of the trial they became significantly greater in the supplemented group compared to the placebo group. As shown in Figure 1, there was a significant fall in plasma zinc by the sixth week of the trial ($P=0.0002$), which was not due to a change in the concentration of albumin (the major plasma zinc-binding protein) as this was increased in the supplemented mothers. At the same time the biparietal diameters and femur lengths of the fetuses increased more in the supplemented than the placebo group (Figure 2; $P=0.047$, 0.011, respectively). The birthweights of the babies of the supplemented mothers tended to be greater than those of the placebo group, but the difference was not statistically significant (supplemented: 3.69 ± 0.11 kg; placebo: 3.38 ± 0.11 kg; $P=0.076$).

4. DISCUSSION

The results from this study indicate that oral iron supplementation during pregnancy reduces the plasma zinc concentration, and appears to enhance, not reduce, the growth of fetal head and femur (Figures 1 and 2). Thus zinc availability was not limiting to fetal growth in our subjects.

The effects on both plasma zinc and fetal growth occurred almost completely during the first six weeks of the study, long before the iron status was affected. This rapid fall of plasma zinc is consistent with inhibition of the intestinal absorption of zinc by the inorganic iron as has been documented for non-pregnant subjects. The results also suggest that the enhancement of fetal growth was not due to improved maternal iron status, but to an earlier change, perhaps related to the altered zinc availability.

We wish to thank the Wellcome Trust, Smith, Kline and French and the SmithKline Foundation for financial support.

5. REFERENCES

1. C.F. Mills, *Ann. Rev. Nutr.*, 1985, 5, 173.
2. N.W. Solomons, *J. Nutr.*, 1986, 116, 927.
3. J. Apgar, *Ann. Rev. Nutr.*, 1985, 5, 43.
4. D.L. Bloxam, N.R. Williams, R.J.D. Waskett, P.M. Pattinson-Green, Y. Morarji and S.G. Stewart, *Clin. Sci.*, (in press).

EFFECTORS OF SMALL INTESTINAL ZINC ABSORPTION
-studies with an in vitro perfusion technique
and on brush border membrane vesicles

H. Daniel, M. Auge and G. Rehner

Institute of Nutritional Sciences
Justus-Liebig-University
D-6300 Giessen, F.R.G.

INTRODUCTION

Transport of zinc across the brush border membrane of mucosal cells
of the small intestine occurs by a series of steps. It has been suggested that a low molecular weight ligand complexing zinc acts as a
carrier in transmembrane transport. However, the identity of this ligand has been controversial (1,2,3). Therefore we studied the effect of
picolinic acid (PA), citrate (CA), histidine (HIS) and cysteine (CYS) on
transmural transport (TT) and tissue accumulation (TA) of $^{65}ZnCl_2$
using an in vitro perfusion technique with isolated segments of rat
small intestine. Additionally influx and binding of ^{65}Zn in brush
border membrane vesicles (BBMV) was investigated.

Transmural transport and tissue accumulation

METHODS
To study TT and TA segments (5cm) of either duodenum, jejunum or
ileum of rats (220-250g;WISTAR) were removed and incubated for up
to 60 min. in isotonic HEPES/MES based media of pH 6.0, 7.4 or 8.0
containing no complexing agents. The serosal side was continuously
perfused with a medium pH 7.4 at a rate of 0.3ml/min. Ligands were
only added to the mucosal solution.

RESULTS
When the ligands CA, HIS and CYS (1mM) were added the time dependent TT of Zn (1μM) showed saturation kinetics. With PA however Zn
uptake increased linearly to time up to 60 min.
TA exceeded TT 100-300 times. All ligands increased TT but reduced
TA compared to the control. No statistical differences were found between the different regions of the small intestine at pH ≥7.4. A low
mucosal buffer pH (6.0) however increased TT and TA of free Zn in
the duodenum 2 to 3 times compared to the jejunum and ileum.

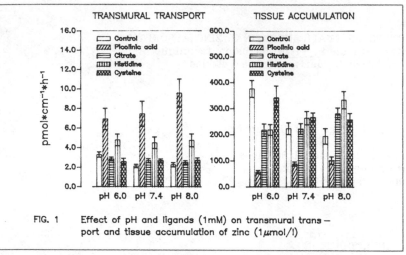

FIG. 1   Effect of pH and ligands (1mM) on transmural trans –
          port and tissue accumulation of zinc (1μmol/l)

As seen in fig. 1 at a Zn:ligand ratio of 1:1000 only PA increased TT
and reduced TA significantly whereas the other ligands showed only
moderate effects. TT as a function of HIS and CYS concentration (at
1μM Zn) increased dose dependently but TA decreased parallel to it.
From these experiments it may be concluded that TA represents binding to the tissue rather than uptake into the cells. Half maximal
stimulation of TT was observed at a Zn:ligand ratio of 1:2500.

Studies with BBMV

METHODS

BBMV were prepared with the Ca–precipitation technique according to
Kessler (4) and incubated in Na–free media containing 300mM
mannitol, 20mM HEPES/TRIS (pH >7.0) or MES/TRIS (pH 6.0), and 1mM
MgSO$_4$. Uptake studies were carried out according to Berner (5).

RESULTS

Uptake of ^{3}H–D–Glucose (30μM) into BBMV in the presence of a 100mM
NaCl gradient showed an overshoot of 14 times the equilibrium values
at 10 sec of incubation. This indicates highly efficient transporting
vesicles. Addition of ZnCl$_2$ decreased initial glucose uptake dose dependently (50% inhibition at 4μM Zn).
Time dependent uptake of 1μM ^{65}Zn (ZnCl$_2$) into BBMV of duodenum,
jejunum and ileum showed similar kinetics. The equilibrium values
exceeded the theoretical value 200 times as calculated from the glucose space (1,5μl/mg protein). This indicates that almost all the zinc
was bound to the membrane; only 2% of the total Zn was transported
into the intravesicular space. Uptake sudies on vesicles shrunk by
adding mannitol to the incubation medium revealed no detectable
uptake into osmotic reactive space either at 10 sec or at 60 min of

incubation. Binding to the membrane increased linearly to the Zn concentration with a slope of 267 ± 33 pmol·mg^{-1}·µM^{-1}. Low pH (6.0) reduced the binding capacity of the membrane by 50–70% compared to pH 7.4 or 8.0. Addition of the ligands (1mM) to the incubation medium abolished the initial glucose uptake in the presence of Na$^+$ indicating a Na$^+$–cotransport system for these ligands. Binding kinetics of Zn to the BBMV as a function of ligand concentration are given in fig. 2.

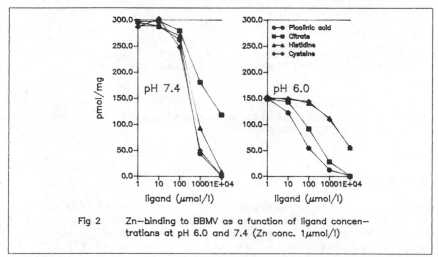

Fig 2   Zn–binding to BBMV as a function of ligand concentrations at pH 6.0 and 7.4 (Zn conc. 1µmol/l)

Addition of ligands led to a pH and dose dependent reduction of binding capacity with a concomitant increase of Zn transport into the intravesicular space.

DISCUSSION

From the experiments it may be stated that non–proteinogenic and proteinogenic low molecular weight ligands increase Zn transport in the small intestine by chelating Zn. This occurs via solubilization of zinc which is trapped at the brush border membrane and by increased transmural transport probably as a complex. Additionally in the duodenum a special transport system for free zinc operating at low pH may be involved in overall Zn absorption. Under physiological conditions especially the amino acids HIS and CYS may act as the Zn carrier.

REFERENCES
1.G.W. Evans; P.E. Johnson, *Pediatric Research* 1980, 14, 876–880
2.L.S. Hurley et al, *Proc. Nat. Acad. Sci.* 1977, 74 3547–3549
3.R.A. Wapnier et al, *J. Nutrition,* 1983, 113, 1346–1354
4.M. Kessler et al, *Biochim. Biophys. Acta,* 1978, 509, 348–359
5.W. Berner et al, *Biochem. J.,* 1976, 160, 467–474

EFFECTS OF PHARMACOLOGIC DOSES OF FOLATE ON ZINC ABSORPTION AND ZINC STATUS

N.F. Krebs, K.M. Hambidge, R.J. Hagerman, P.L. Peirce, K.M. Johnson, J.L. English, L.L. Miller and P.V. Fennessey

Department of Pediatrics
University of Colorado Health Sciences Center
Denver, Colorado, USA 80262

1   INTRODUCTION

Recent reports have suggested that increasing the oral intake of folate interferes with intestinal absorption of zinc,[1,2] although the specific mechanism of the interaction has not been established. Pharmacologic doses of folate are frequently used in the management of the Fragile X Syndrome, the most common familial form of mental retardation. The objectives of this study were to assess the zinc status of patients with the Fragile X Syndrome who were being treated with pharmacologic quantities of folate, and to determine the effects of similar quantities of folate on zinc absorption in normal adults.

2   METHODS

The study design involved two separate components. In the first, zinc status was evaluated in 8 subjects (7 males) with the Fragile X Syndrome. Mean age was 24 ± 11 years ($X \pm S.D.$), and all had been receiving 10-20 mg/day of folate for at least 1 year. Fasting morning blood levels of plasma zinc, alkaline phosphatase, albumin, and delta-amino-levulinic acid (DALAD) were determined by routine methods as indices of zinc status.

In the second component of this study, intestinal absorption of a stable isotope of zinc(^{70}Zn) was measured in normal adults with and without the simultaneous administration of folate. Preliminary data presented are on 3 subjects (2 females) with ages ranging from 23-35 years. Each subject received 2 doses of an accurately weighed quantity of ^{70}Zn at intervals of 2-3 weeks, administered in a gelatin capsule after an overnight fast. Subjects remained in a fasting state for an additional 4 hours after the dose of isotope. On one of the two occasions, 30 mg of folate was given orally 5 minutes prior to the ^{70}Zn. One subject received the folate with the first dose of isotope, and 2 subjects received it with the second dose of ^{70}Zn. The quantity of ^{70}Zn administered in the enriched preparation ranged from 0.81 to 1.83 mg; the quantity for the 2 doses for each individual subject differed by <0.25 mg.

All faeces for $\geq$10 consecutive specimens after administration of isotope were collected in plastic bags and stored at -20°C. The samples were subsequently weighed to the nearest 0.1 g, dried to constant weight under infra-red lamps, and ground into a fine powder in a plastic food processor. Weighed aliquots of the dried sample were dry ashed at 450°C and the ash was then dissolved in 6 N HCl. An aliquot of the dissolved ash was used for total zinc determination by flame atomic absorption spectrophotometry.

Zinc was separated from other inorganic components of the dissolved ash by ion exchange column chromatography (AG-1 ion exchange resin). Zinc stable isotope enrichment was determined by fast atom bombardment mass spectrometry using VG7070 mass spectrometer equipped with a fast atom gun[3].

3 RESULTS AND DISCUSSION

The mean plasma zinc concentration for the subjects with Fragile X Syndrome was 84.4 + 6.0 µg/dl, which was not significantly different from the control mean of 87.1 ± 12.2 µg/dl. Levels of alkaline phosphatase, albumin, and DALAD were also within normal limits for all of these subjects.

Cumulative faecal excretion of ^{70}Zn as a percentage of the administered isotope dose was adjusted for calculated excretion of resecreted ^{70}Zn to give a final figure for the excretion of non-absorbed ^{70}Zn. Thus, by subtraction, percentage true absorption was calculated Results for the 3 subjects are given below in the table.

Table 1   Calculated True Absorption of ^{70}Zn

Subject	Without folate	With folate	Δ
1	68.3%	65.2%	-3.1%
2	67.4%	62.1%	-5.3%
3	57.5%	52.6%	-4.9%

These data demonstrate a consistent pattern of slightly lower absorption of ^{70}Zn when administered with folate (mean decrease 4.4 ± 1.1%).

Although a mutually inhibitory interaction between zinc and folate at the intestinal mucosa has been suggested by studies in rats[2], studies of such effects on absorption in humans is more limited. Milne et al[1] noted increased faecal excretion of zinc with supplementation of modest quantities of folate. The preliminary data on 3 subjects in the present study suggest that a pharmacologic dose of folate slightly decreases zinc absorption in the fasting state. The data for the subjects with Fragile X Syndrome indicated apparently normal zinc status despite long term pharmacologic folate therapy. These results are similar to those reported for a group of women with cervical dysplasia who were being treated with similar quantities of folate[4]. The results of the present study suggest that the effect of folate on zinc absorption is relatively minor and is not clinically signficant.

Acknowledgements

Supported in part by a grant from the National Institutes of Health, NIADDKD, 5 R22 AM12432, and grant RR-69 from the National Institutes of Health, General Clinical Research Center, and grant RR 01152 from the National Institutes of Health, Clinical Mass Spectrometry Resource.

4   REFERENCES

1.   D.B. Milne, W.K. Canfield, J.R. Mahalko, H.H. Sandstead, Am J Clin Nutr, 1984, 39, 535.
2.   F.K. Ghishan, H.M. Said, P.C. Wilson, J.E. Murrell, H.L. Greene, Am J Clin Nutr, 1986, 43, 258.
3.   P.L. Peirce, K.M. Hambidge, C.H. Goss, L.V. Miller, P.V. Fennessey, Anal Chem, 1987, 59, 2034.
4.   C.E. Butterworth, K. Hatch, P. Cole, H. Sauberlich, T. Tamura, P.E. Cornell, S. Soong, Am J Clin Nutr, 1988, 47, 484.

THE EFFECT OF MAILLARD REACTION PRODUCTS ON ZINC BIOAVAILABILITY

S.J. Fairweather-Tait and L.L. Symss

AFRC Institute of Food Research
Colney Lane
Norwich NR4 7UA
England

1.   INTRODUCTION

Maillard reaction products (MRP) are formed during various processing procedures, such as in the heating and toasting of maize to produce cornflakes. Several reports in the literature suggest that MRP have an adverse effect on zinc nutrition, either by reducing zinc absorption[1] or by increasing urinary excretion[2]. The present study was designed to investigate the effects of MRP formed from a heated mixture of monosodium glutamate (MSG) and glucose on zinc absorption and excretion in rats.

2.   MATERIALS AND METHODS

Monosodium glutamate and glucose (1:1 molar ratio) were heated to 100 °C in water for 3 hours to produce MRP and the resultant mixture freeze-dried.

Zinc absorption experiment

Thirty male Wistar rats (Mean wt. 178g, SEM 3g) fed control semi-synthetic diet containing 45µg Zn/g were fasted overnight. The following morning each rat was given 3g wholewheat flour plus 0.3g freeze-dried MRP's (n=15) or 0.145g MSG and 0.155g glucose (n=15). Each meal was made into a paste with distilled water and the zinc (60µg) labelled extrinsically with 37kBq ^{65}Zn (ZnCl$_2$, Amersham International, Bucks). After consuming the meal, the rats were counted individually in a small animal whole body counter (WBC, NE8112, Nuclear

Enterprises, Edinburgh, Scotland) to determine the
amount of ^{65}Zn-labelled food consumed; food pots
containing control diet were returned 3 hours later.
The animals were counted again on days 7-14 post-dosing
and the % ^{65}Zn retention calculated. The $\log_{10}$ of the %
whole body retention was plotted against time, and true
zinc absorption estimated from regression analysis by
correcting for endogenous losses of absorbed ^{65}Zn.

Zinc excretion experiment

Thirty male Wistar rats (mean wt. 332g, SEM 4g)
were fasted overnight and given 3g wholewheat flour
labelled with ^{65}Zn. Three hours later, after counting
in the WBC, they were provided with low zinc semi-
synthetic diet (11μg Zn/g) <u>ad lib</u>; half the animals
received diet containing 2% w/w MRP and half 2% w/w
unreacted MSG plus glucose (1:1 molar ratio). Each rat
was counted daily in the WBC for 14 days and the daily
rate of loss of ^{65}Zn calculated from regression analysis
of log % ^{65}Zn retention between days 6-14 post-dosing.

3.   RESULTS AND DISCUSSION

Mean zinc absorption from wholewheat flour was 36.3%
(SEM 1.1), with a daily loss of ^{65}Zn of 2.2% (SEM 0.1),
in the presence of MRP, and 34.7% (SEM 1.7), daily loss
of ^{65}Zn of 2.3% (SEM 0.1), in the presence of unreacted
MSG and glucose. These were not statistically
different, thus it may be concluded that the MRP had no
effect on zinc absorption from the test meal.

In the zinc excretion experiment, mean zinc absorption from wholewheat flour was 50.0% (SEM 1.7) in the
group fed control diet containing 2% w/w MRP's during
the 14 days following the ^{65}Zn test meal, and 44.5 %
(SEM 2.0) in the control group. The difference between
the groups was not sigificant. The daily rate of loss
of ^{65}Zn was constant between days 6 and 14 post-dosing
and did not differ between the groups: 0.66% (SEM 0.03)
in animals fed diet containing MRP and 0.72% (SEM 0.04)
in the controls, as shown in Figure 1. The rate of loss
of zinc was only about one third of that found in the
first experiment, primarily because the rats were
responding to the low zinc diet by reducing endogenous
losses, in order to conserve body zinc.

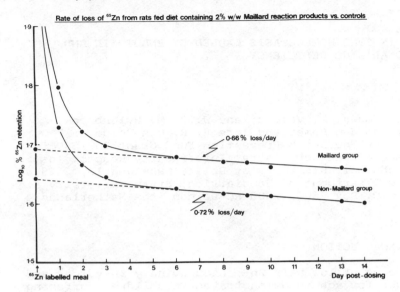

Figure 1. Rate of loss of ^{65}Zn from rats fed diet containing 2% w/w Maillard reaction products vs. controls.

4. CONCLUSIONS

The results from this study suggest that MSG-glucose Maillard reaction products do not have an adverse effect on zinc bioavailability. Even when high levels (10% w/w) were added to a food, there was no reduction in zinc absorption, nor was zinc excretion higher in animals fed a low zinc diet containing 2% w/w MRP.

ACKNOWLEDGEMENTS

This work was funded by the M.A.F.F.

REFERENCES

1.   G.I. Lykken, J. Mahalko, P.E. Johnson, D. Milne, H.H. Sandstead, W.J. Garcia, F.R. Dintzis and G.E. Inglett, J. Nutr., 1986, 116, 795-801.
2.   J.M. O'Brien, P.A. Morrisey and A. Flynn, Proc. Euro. Food Tox., II, 1986, 214-220.

CHANGES IN ZINC HOMEOSTASIS CAUSED BY ENDOTOXIN AND NUTRITIONAL ZINC DEFICIENCY

J. P. Van Wouwe, M. Veldhuizen, J. J. M. Uylenbroek,
C. J. A. Van den Hamer and late H. H. Van Gelderen
Supported by The Dutch Prevention Fund Grant 28-1549
Department of Radiochemistry, Interfaculty Reactor Insti-
tute, Technical University at Delft, Mekelweg 15, 2629 JB
Delft and Department of Paediatrics, State University at
Leiden, P.O. Box 9600, 2300 RC Leiden, the Netherlands

1 INTRODUCTION

The presence of low hair Zn-, high urinary Zn-values and
low height for age is demonstrated in children suffering
from recurrent upper respiratory tract infection (1). The
interpretation is hazardous: Zn deficiency can be both a
cause and an effect of the recurrent infection. Therefore,
a controlled metabolic study on rats is performed.

2 MATERIALS AND METHODS

Animals and Diets

Four groups of 8 weanling male Wistar rats [CPB Zeist
NL] are individually housed in macrolon cages with stainless steel lids and placed in a climate controlled environment. Body weight is monitored. The animals are pairfed
either an IRI-OB Zn Deficient diet, containing 30 micromol
Zn/kg (by analysis) or a Control diet containing 150 (2).
They are injected with Endotoxin E.coli 055:B5 [Sigma] or
Saline i.p., in the first experiment on d(ay) 4, 7, 10, 13
and 16, while dissection takes place on d 21, and in the
second experiment on d 10, 8 h before dissection.

Zn Homeostasis

Each experiment is performed on 4 animals, which are
fed the deficient resp. control diet and injected with
endotoxin (D-E resp. C-E) or saline (D-S resp. C-S).
First Experiment. Long term changes in Zn homeostasis
are studied with 5 nmol 65Zn [50 GBq/mol, Amersham U.K.]
given i.p. on d 1. During 1 week URine and FEcals are

collected to measure 65Zn activities. Whole body countings
are performed by placing a container with the animal in a
tank, filled with pseudocumene and equipped with a multi-
channel analyser. The tracer UR and FE excretions, REtention and T-b, biological half life are determined (2).

Second Experiment. Care is taken to maintain metabolic steady state while Zn homeostasis is studied in the
remaining animals on d 10, using oral 65Zn. Dissection is
performed 30 min post Dose and 65Zn activities are measured in PLasma, washed ERythrocytes, rinsed DUodenum,
LIver left lobe, PAncreas, flexor digitorum longus MUscle
and tibia BOne. Values are converted into total tissue
activities using, where appropriate, reference values for
the tissue masses (3). The sum of activities yields the
65Zn absorption during 30 min. The single values are considered part of a closed system in steady state and are
used in a modified kinetic model to calculate the transfer
rates of 65Zn activity between the various tissues (4).
The transfers to and from the tissues are used to estimate
the tissue dilution (inflow = outflow in steady state),
which is multiplied by the molar Zn inflow. This is calculated from the albumin bound PL Zn, estimated to be 70% of
the total PL Zn and supposed to be saturated with 65Zn.

Statistical Analysis is performed by analysis of
variance (ANOVA). Sensitivity and specificity is calculated by the overlap index according to Hertz (5).

3 RESULTS AND DISCUSSION

Growth

    Zn Deficiency results in anorexia and growth retar-
dation affecting the animals in D-S and D-E alike.

Zn Homeostasis

    First Experiment. In every aspect, the data in the
Table show accumulation and slow release of activity in D-
S. In C-E, endotoxin has not affected 65Zn availability
and turnover, in spite of lower UR and FE excretions, as
it has in D-E. In several tissues specific activities have
changed differently in D-E or C-E (not shown). More reliable, the estimated exchageable Zn fractions in the tissues indicate the occurrence and extent of deficiency (6).
    Second Experiment. In D-S the transfer rates are not
affected as they are in C-E and D-E, especially those to
and from LI. The sum of activities agree well with the
values for the i.p. RE d 0 (first experiment). The exchangeable Zn pools in all tissues studied are diminished

Table. Effects of Endotoxin on 65Zn Excretion, Retention, Biological Halflife, Fluxes and Exchangeable Zn Pools.

	D-E	D-S	C-S	C-E
UR %D 7 d	#*.7	*.3	1.0	#.7
FE %D 7 d	#* 40	* 25	57	# 50
RE %D d 0	# 66	* 72	55	56
SUM %D d 21	# 42	* 57	39	39
T-b in d	# 100	* 235	130	120
Total Activity and Fluxes per 30 min on d 10:				
SUM %D	#* 71	* 90	44	43
PL to ER	.001	.001	.005	.002
LI	# .118	.092	.068	#.136
PA	.0001	.0001	.002	.0001
BO	.150	.123	.111	.121
MU	.631	.683	.614	.542
ER to PL	*.030	.029	.022	.013
LI	*.031	.029	.022	.016
PA	.0001	.0001	.0001	.0001
BO	*.020	.024	.012	.009
MU	# .016	.024	.017	#.009
DU	.033	.031	.031	#.027
Estimated Exchangeable Zn on d 10, nmol per Tissue				
ER	*.004	*.004	.09	#.005
LI	.5	.5	1.9	.4
PA	*.005	.007	.012	#.001
BO	* 3	* 3	6	# 2
MU	* 32	* 43	102	# 11

*: p <0.05 and overlap <50%, compared to C-S
#: idem, compared to the corresponding diet -S

by endotoxin more than by nutritional deficiency.

  Conclusion. More than in Zn deficiency, endotoxin diminishes exchangeable Zn pools in several tissues. In concurrent Zn deficiency it also reduces Zn retention and enhances fecal and urinary Zn excretion.

REFERENCES

1.   J. P. Van Wouwe, H. H. Van Gelderen and J. H. Bos, Eur J Pediatr, 1987, 146, 293.
2.   A. A. Van Barneveld, `Trace Element Absorption and Retention Studies in Mice', Thesis, Catholic University at Nijmegen, the Netherlands, 1983, chapter 4.
3.   K. Gaertner, W. Reulecke, H. Hackbarth and F. Wollnik, Dtsch tieraerztl Wschr, 1987, 94, 52.
4.   D. M. Foster, M. E. Wastney and R. I. Henkin, Math Biosc, 1984, 72, 359.
5.   A. J. Hertz, Arch Pathol Lab Med, 1984, 108, 65.
6.   Anonymous, Nutr Rev, 1987, 45, 346.

MILK AND ZINC ABSORPTION IN POSTMENOPAUSAL WOMEN

R. J. Wood, D. A. Hanssen and J. Zheng

Nutrient Bioavailability Laboratory
USDA Human Nutrition Research Center on Aging
Tufts University
Boston, MA   02111   USA

1.   INTRODUCTION

The major food sources of calcium in the U.S. diet are milk and milk-based products. A recent National Institutes of Health consensus conference has recommended higher levels of calcium intake in women to protect against bone loss. Thus, it is reasonable to assume that the consumption of milk will increase in the female population as the awareness about calcium needs grows.

Studies in humans have suggested, however, that zinc absorption can be inhibited by milk (1-3). Since the zinc content of diets consumed by older women in the U.S. is reported to be inadequate, increased consumption of foods which lower zinc bioavailability could compromise zinc nutritional status. We have, therefore, evaluated the effect of milk on zinc absorption in postmenopausal women. We have also investigated whether the presence of other foods components modify the effect of milk on zinc absorption.

2.   METHODS

Fractional zinc absorption was determined by a dual-isotope technique utilizing 65Zn with 51Cr, as a nonabsorbable fecal marker (4). Radioactivity was measured in a large volume gamma counter in individual fecal samples and in the orally administered isotope dose. Fractional zinc absorption was calculated by the following equation:

235

Zn absorption = [(100 - %51Cr dose in sample) -
(100 - % 51Cr dose in sample)]/% 51Cr dose in sample.

Radioactive isotopes were administered in either
water or cow milk to 12 postmenopausal women after an
overnight fast. The zinc content of both test drinks
was adjusted to 92 μmol with zinc chloride. Another
group of 7 postmenopausal women fasted overnight and
consumed the radioactive tracers with or without cow
milk along with a standardized breakfast consisting
of: oatmeal (28g), brown sugar (15g), butter (5g),
wheat bread (30g), grape jelly (15g), coconut
non-dairy beverage (68g) and coffee (1g). The zinc
content of both test meals were adjusted to contain 38
μmol.

3.   RESULTS

Fractional 65Zn absorption, measured in 12
postmenopausal subjects without a meal was 55+ 4%
(mean ± S.E.M.) when 65Zn was consumed with water
alone. When 200 ml cow milk was consumed with the
65Zn fractional 65Zn absorption decreased
significantly (p < 0.01) to 24 ± 4%.

Fractional 65Zn absorption measured in
postmenopausal subjects fed a standardized breakfast
without added milk was 25+4%. Zinc absorption in these
subjects was similar, 26+7%, when 200 ml milk was
added to the breakfast.

4.   DISCUSSION

This study indicates that milk significantly
inhibits the absorption of zinc when both are fed
together without a meal. This finding would be
consistent with previous observations (1-3) showing an
inhibitory effect of milk on zinc absorption in
humans.

Our findings also suggest that the consumption of
other non-milk food components in the standardized
meal given to the women also compromised zinc
absorptive efficiency. Similar to milk alone in the
first study, zinc absorption was also low (25%) when
the breakfast alone (without milk) was ingested in the
second study. Lower absorption of 65Zn in the
presence of a "meal" has also been noted by other
investigators (reviewed in ref. 5).

It is noteworthy that even though milk can inhibit zinc absorption the addition of a physiological dose of milk to a meal had no additional negative effect on zinc absorption efficiency. This finding suggests that the practice of substituting a glass of milk for a low calcium-containing beverage in a mixed meal could do much to improve poor calcium nutriture with little risk of compromising zinc status.

Finally, from the perspective of methodological considerations in bioavailability studies, our studies illustrate the need for caution to avoid making erroneous extrapolations from simplified single food or food component absorption studies (e.g., milk alone and zinc absorption) of the nutritional importance of various nutrient-nutrient interactions in the setting of normal eating habits.

5. REFERENCES

1. A. Pecoud, P. Donzel and J.L. Schelling, <u>Clin. Pharmacol. Ther.</u>, 1975, <u>17</u>, 469.

2. F.J. Oelshlegel and G.J. Brewer, 'Zinc Metabolism: Current Aspects in Health and Disease', S. Prasad. and G.J. Brewer, Liss, New York, 1977, p. 299.

3. P.R. Flanagan, J. Cluett, M.J. Chamberlain and L.S. Valberg. <u>J. Nutr.</u>, 1985, <u>11</u>, 111.

4. K.B. Payton, PR Flanagan, E.A. Stinson <u>et al</u>, <u>Gastroenterol.</u>, 1982, <u>83</u>, 1264.

5. N.W. Solomons, <u>Am. J. Clin. Nutr.</u>, 1982, <u>35</u>, 1048.

DIALYZABLE ZINC AFTER IN VITRO DIGESTION IN COMPARISON WITH ZINC ABSORPTION MEASURED IN HUMANS

B. Sandström and A. Almgren

Research Department of Human Nutrition
The Royal Agricultural University
DK-1958 Copenhagen, Denmark and
Department of Clinical Nutrition
Gothenburg University
S-413 45 GOTHENBURG, Sweden

1 INTRODUCTION

The absorption of trace elements from a diet is influenced by low molecular weight ligands e.g. organic acids and peptides promoting or facilitating absorption as well as complexing agents like phytic acid depressing absorption. For some of the trace elements, isotope techniques are available to study the effects of these factors on human trace element absorption. However, these techniques require expensive equipment and/or are very tedious and consequently there is a need for in vitro methods to estimate available trace element content in foods. In this study we have evaluated the potential use of an in vitro digestion technique to estimate the availability of zinc from composite meals by a direct comparison with zinc absorption in humans served the same diets.

2 METHODS

Dialyzable zinc after in vitro digestion. The effect of in vitro digestion on zinc in foods and added ^{65}Zn was studied by a modification of two methods used for studies of iron availability[1,2]. Weighed amounts of freeze-dried foods (ca 3 g) were tranferred to six Erlenmeyer flasks. To two of the flasks 50 mL of saline was added and to the other four, 50 mL of "gastric juice" (0.32 g pepsin, 2 g NaCl and 10 mL HCl (25 %) ad 1000 mL). To each flask 0.02 MBq ^{65}Zn was added. Segments of dialysis tubing (MW cut off 6000-8000) containing 15 mL of saline or gastric juice without pepsin were placed in the two flasks with NaCl and in two of the flasks with gastric juice, respectively. The flasks were incubated in a 37°C shaking waterbath for 30

238

min for the samples in saline and 2 h for the other
samples. The dialysis tubes were removed and the pH was
adjusted to 8 by adding ammonium hydroxide (25 %). Trypsin
(30 mg) was added and the flasks were incubated at 37°C
for 4h with dialysis tubing containing 15 mL of gastric
juice (without pepsin) adjusted to pH 8. The content of
zinc and [65]Zn in the dialysates was determined.

Absorption measurements. The absorption of zinc was
determined by a radionuclide technique[3]. The meals were
labelled with 0.02 MBq [65]Zn by careful mixing with the
food during preparation. The meals were served to healthy
volunteers, 6-12 for each meal, after 12 h of fasting. The
retention of the radionuclide was measured in a human
whole-body counter 14 days after intake of the labelled
meal. Allowance was made for endogenous excretion of [65]Zn
in the period between intake and retention measurements to
give the estimated absorption figure.

Meals. Eighteen composite meals were studied. Ten of
the meals were based on whole-meal cereals with a range of
phytic acid content from 100 μmol to 615 μmol and with a
protein content of 12 g[4]. Eight of the meals were based on
white beans with a phytic acid content of 330-600 μmol and
varying levels of animal protein giving a total protein
content from 14 to 44 g[5]. The zinc content of the meals
varied from 24 μmol to 69 μmol.

3 RESULTS AND DISCUSSION

Dialyzable zinc after in vitro digestion. Only a small
amount of zinc, 8$\pm$7 %, was dialyzable in NaCl. In vitro
digestion at pH 1 rendered 74$\pm$13 % dialyzable and after
increasing the pH to 8 and further digestion 20$\pm$22 % was
dialyzable. [65]Zn was dialyzable to the same extent as the
native zinc.

Zinc absorption. The absorption of zinc from the
cereal based meals varied from 8 % in an oatmeal meal[4] with
a phytic acid content of 615 μmol to 27 % in a meal with a
phytic acid content of 100 μmol. From the high protein
meals the absorption varied from 19-32 % depending on the
zinc and protein content[5].

Dialyzable zinc as an estimate of zinc absorption in vivo.

A close correlation between dialyzable zinc at pH 8
and the in vivo measurement of zinc absorption in humans
was observed r = 0.94 p<0.001, Figure 1. Dialyzable zinc at
pH 1 showed no correlation to zinc absorption.

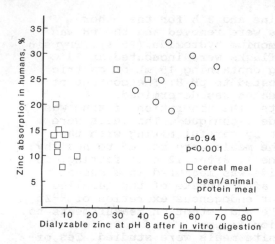

Figure 1 The relation between zinc absorption in humans and in vitro measurement of dialyzable zinc after pepsin and trypsin digestion of meals.

This direct comparison of an in vitro method and in vivo measurements in humans indicates that the amount of zinc present as "free" ions or bound to low molecular ligands at duodenal pH reflects the degree of absorption. The in vitro method confirms a low availability of zinc from cereal meals with a high phytic acid content and a higher availability from high protein meals. Although, the in vitro digestion method can never be as sensitive as radioisotope techniques used in humans, it seems to give a reasonable estimate of zinc availability.

REFERENCES

1.   L. Hallberg and E. Björn-Rasmussen, Am. J. Clin. Nutr., 1981, 34, 2808.
2.   D.D. Miller, B.R. Schricker, R.R. Rasmussen, D. Van Campen, Am. J. Clin. Nutr., 1981, 34, 2248.
3.   B. Arvidsson, Å. Cederblad, E. Björn-Rasmussen and B. Sandström, Int. J. Nucl. Med. Biol., 1978, 5, 104.
4.   B. Sandström, A. Almgren, B. Kivistö, Å. Cederblad, J. Nutr., 1987, 117, 1898.
5.   B. Sandström, A. Almgren, B. Kivistö and Å. Cederblad, Trace Elements in Human Health and Disease, 2nd Nordic Symposium, Odense 1987, Abstract C6.

ZINC INTAKE AND BIOAVAILABILITY IN A TEHRAN SUBURB WHAT IS THE MINIMUM REQUIREMENT ?

M. Kimiagar, L. Navai, M. Yassai, F. Malek and B. Samimi

Institute of Nutrition Sciences and Food Technology
Beheshti University of Medical Sciences.
P.O.BOX 19395/4741, Tehran, Iran.

1 INTRODUCTION

Zinc is an element whose bioavailability is affected by a number of factors and therefore is a controversial question. [1,2] In addition, the recommended dietary intake for this mineral has not been set on firm grounds and rather, on approximations with a wide margin of safety. The purpose of this research work was to examine the relationship between serum zinc levels and its daily intake along with some dietary factors affecting its bioavailability in a suburban area, in order to test how fitting the recommendations for zinc are with this popula - tion.

2 METHODOLOGY

Shahryar, a rural suburb 35 Km south - west of Tehran, the capital city of Iran, with 200,000 inhabitants resid - ing in 180 villages was surveyed. Food consumption was assessed in 361 families in 60 randomly selected villages. The 24 - hour - recall method was employed to evaluate zinc, calcium, iron and phytic acid intakes. The nutrients intakes were compared with those of NRC recommendations. [3] Serum zinc levels were measured in 236 subjects using an atomic absorption spectrophotometer (Varian Techtron Model 63) at 213.9 nm and slit width of 0.2 mm. Certified Atomic Absorption Standard Zinc Reference Solution 1,000 ppm (Fisher Scientific Company, Chemical Manufacturing division, Fairlawn, N.J. 07410, U.S.A) was used as standard.

241

Table 1   State of Zinc Intake in the Subjects

Percentage of RDA Consumed	Number of Families	Cumulative Percentage of Families
< 50	80	22.2
< 60	139	38.5
< 80	239	66.2

3 RESULTS

Table 1 shows the number and percentage of families un-able to consume at least 50, 60 and 80% their recommended intake, respectively.

Table 2 presents the number and percentage of families with phytate : zinc molar ratio intake of above 8.

Mean serum zinc level was 112 µg/dl and only 3 out of 236 subjects had values below 70 µg/dl. On the average 33% of zinc in the diet was derived from animal foods. Dietary iron intake was satisfactory in over 90% of the population. The requirement for calcium was met by almost half of the families, suggesting that no disproportionate consumption of major bivalent minerals existed.

4 DISCUSSION

Our results demonstrate that assuming an intake of 80% Recommended Dietary Allowance as a level below which is undesirable, almost two-thirds of the subjects will have to be presumed zinc-deficient. However, serum zinc measurements revealed a satisfactory level of this mineral in over 98% of the subjects. Even if we take 60% of the

Table 2   Molar Ratio of Phytate : Zinc in the Diet

Phytate: Zinc Molar Ratio	Number of Families	Cumulative Percentage of Families
>15	10	2.8
>12	46	12.7
>10	84	23.3
>8	137	38.0

recommended intake as the cut - off point, it is observed
that over 38% of the subjects have failed to receive this
much. Moreover, 22% of the subjects fell short of secur-
ing at least half of their recommended intake. These
observations lead one to conclude that the recommendations
for zinc are set at too high a level, at least for this
population.

Although bread of high extraction flour is the
staple food in this population, but the results presented
in Table 2 indicate that the phytate : zinc ratio was
not so high as to interfere with zinc absorption. Also,
the fact that no mineral was consumed disproportionately,
suggests that the competition among the bivalent metals
for absorption sites or carriers is not a matter of
concern in these subjects. However, making an attempt
to meet the need for zinc in these people based on the
NRC recommendations, could pose the danger of its
deleteriously competing with the other essential minerals
whose intakes are marginal. This is especially important
in areas where there is a general state of undernutrition
such as ours. Moreover, exaggerated recommendations may
hamper proper estimation of dietary adequacy and objective
identification of those at risk. In other words allowing
too wide a margin of safety while making recommendations
for the nutrients intake, poses the danger of desensitiz
- ing food consumption survey as a tool in nutritional
assessments.

We, therefore, conclude that :
I - Recommendations for zinc intake need to be re - evaluated
II - Establishing a universal figure for zinc intake seems
     to be inappropriate and each community should establish
     its own requirements based on the specific food habits
     of its people.

5 REFERENCES

1. A.S. Prasad. Proc XIII Int Cong Nutr. T.G. Taylor and
   N.K. Jenkins (eds). John Libbey, London 1985,p.516

2. N.W. Solomons Amer. J. Clin. Nutr. 1982, 35 : 1048.

3. National Research Council " Recommended Dietary
   Allowances " 9th edn. Washington D.C. National Academy
   of Sciences, 1980.

BIOAVAILABILITY TO RATS OF ZINC FROM A CAMEROONIAN PLANTAIN-BASED DIET: INFLUENCE OF ZINC AND CASEIN SUPPLEMENTATION

A. BELL, L. NEONSI, F. ABOLO, T. SIMGBA and MENUNGA

Centre for Nutrition
P.O. Box 6163, Yaounde, Cameroon.

1. INTRODUCTION

Low zinc absorption has been reported on rats fed on a diet similar to that usually consumed in rural areas of the Southern Cameroon, with plantain (Musa paradisiaca L.) as staple food.[1] This diet was low in proteins and the phytate: zinc molar ratio was high (Table 1).

In addition to phytate and cations, dietary zinc and proteins[2,3] may influence zinc absorption from a composite meal. Moreover, protein and calcium contents of the diet modulate the effect of phytate on zinc absorption: the first inhibits it;[4] the second enhances it.[5]

2. RESULTS

Zinc Supplementation of the Diet

It significantly improved zinc balance (+ 164%) and liver zinc concentration (+ 33%) but had no effect on growth and femur zinc (Table 2).

Casein Supplementation of the Diet

All parameters were significantly increased by casein supplementation alone: weight gain by 62%; zinc balance by 96%; liver, femur zinc concentrations and log of total femur zinc by 61, 10 and 10% respectively.

Further addition of zinc did not have significant effects.

244

Table 1.   Composition of the Diets

Control diet (C)		Basal diet (B)*	
Corn starch, g/kg	726	Corn starch, g/kg	112
Casein, -"-	131	Plantain flour,g/kg	588
Dl-methionine	4	Fish flour	50
Peanut óil	50	Groundnut flour	100
&-Cellulose	20	Red palm oil	45
Vitamin mix	22	Dried green leaves	95
Mineral mix	47	Kitchen salt	10
Agar agar	30	Agar agar	30
Proteins, g/100g DM	12.7	Proteins, g/100g DM	10.4
Fibre, g/100g DM	3.1	Fibre, g/100g DM	3.8
Zn, mg/100g DM	6.7	Zn, mg/100g DM	2.3
(Phytate)/(Zn) ratio	2.0	(Phytate)/(Zn) ratio	22.8
(Phytate)(Ca)/(Zn) ratio	42	(Phytate)(Ca)/(Zn) ratio	156

*In the zinc-supplemented diet (Zn), 30 ppm of zinc as zinc sulfate were added.   In the casein-supplemented diet (Cas), 45g of casein with 1.3g Dl-methionine were added at the expense of corn starch.   In the casein plus zinc-supplemented diet (Cas x Zn), both were added.

Table 2.   Weight Gain, Zinc Balance, Liver and Femur Zinc Concentrations in Rats Fed the Different Diets.

Group	B	Zn	Cas	CasxZn	C
Weight gain, g at 20 days	52.6	55.9	85.2***	85.8***	121.3***
Zn balance					
Intake, mg/10d	2.5	6.1***	3.0*	6.7***	10.1***
Feces, mg/10d	1.8	4.5***	1.8	5.6***	6.0***
Urine, mg/10d	0.11	0.10	0.10	0.15**	0.08
Balance,mg/10d	0.53	1.4***	1.0**	0.94*	4.1***
Balance, % int.	21.6	23.0	34.0*	14.0*	40.3***
Liver Zn, Ug/g WW	17.1	22.9*	27.7***	28.3***	24.5**
Femur Zn Ug/g DW	167	175	183 **	181 **	186 **
log tot femur Zn	1.54	1.60	1.67*	1.66*	1.74***

Values in the same line are significantly different from the B group; *P< 0.05; **P< 0.01; ***P< 0.001.

3. CONCLUSIONS

Improving dietary protein alone rendered the native zinc highly available and 23 ppm were then adequate while in the basal diet, zinc absorption was adversely affected by low dietary protein and probably high phytate: zinc molar ratio.

Since feeding patterns are monotonous in rural areas of the Southern Cameroon, zinc requirements are likely not to be met, especially among pregnant and lactating women, young children and low socio-economic groups whose protein intakes are more likely to be inadequate.

4. REFERENCES

1. A. BELL and B. LONNERDAL, 7th ISTRC Sympos, Gosier, 1985.
2. C. A. MAGEE and F.P. GRAINGER, Nutr Repts Int, 1979, 20, 771.
3. B. LONNERDAL, Prog. Food Nutr., 1985, 9, 35.
4. B. SANDSTROM and A. CEDERBLAD, Am. J. Clin. Nutr., 1980, 33, 1778.
5. H.J.A. LIKUSKI and R.M. FORBES, J. Nutr., 1965, 85, 235.

ZINC BIOAVAILABILITY OF THE DIET CONSUMED BY THE LOW INCOME POPULATION OF SÃO PAULO - BRAZIL (STUDY IN RATS)

R.P. Dantas, and S.M.F. Cozzolino.

Faculdade de Ciencas Farmaceuticas - Universidade de São Paulo

1. INTRODUCTION

The presence or absence of inhibiting or enhancing factors of zinc bioavailability in a diet determines the possibility of obtaining required zinc 1,2,3,4. Economic status determines food choice profile and is particularly important in developing countries. Brazilian population of low income groups have a growing tendency to consume more foods of vegetable origin, with inhibitors of zinc absorption and retention 1,5,6. In this study we determined zinc bioavailability in the diet consumed by the low income groups of São Paulo state population.

2. METHODS

The experimental diet (DRSP), based on an estimate of the main foods consumed by the low income group of São Paulo state, was prepared using normal home preparations, dried at 60°C in ventilated oven, and analysed for nutrients by AOAC methods (Table 1). Three groups were formed: Experimental (DRSP), and casein control (CA) groups fed "ad libitum", and a "pair fed" casein control group. The groups were fed for 60 days; deionized water was available "ad libitum".

At the end of the experimental period, all animals were anesthetized with ether, and killed by cardiac puncture. Feces, (collected during the experimental period) and whole carcass were analysed for zinc, by atomic absorption spectrophotometry. Analyses of variance and Tukey's test were made in order to test differences between groups.

247

Table 1   Composition of regional diet of São Paulo
state (low income group).

Foods	g/100g
Cereals and grain products	36.1
Potatoes and starchy roots	5.8
Sugar	10.7
Legumes (bean)	9.7
Green vegetables	2.0
Other vegetables	6.3
Fruits	5.2
Meat and meat products	5.7
Eggs	1.3
Milk and milk products	9.3
Fats	3.8
Miscellaneous	3.6

3.   RESULTS AND CONCLUSION

The chemical composition of the experimental and
control diets is shown in Table 2

Table 2 – Chemical composition of regional diet of São
Paulo (DRSP), and casein diet (CA), used in the study.

COMPOSITION		DRSP	CA
Energy	KCAL	379.1	389.0
Moisture	%	5.6	9.6
Protein	%	11.5	11.8
Lipids	%	5.6	8.0
Carbohydrate	%	70.7	65.5
Fiber	%	3.9	1.1
Ash	%	2.7	3.0
Zinc	%	11.1	11.6

The absorption parameters for zinc of the control and
experimental groups are shown in Table 3.

Conclusion
      Zinc bio-availability in (DRSP) was lower than
that in the (CA) control diet.   There was a positive
correlation (r=0.9023 n=14) between zinc intake and
carcass zinc.

Table 3 — Ingested Z_n ($Z_n I$), fecal Z_n ($Z_n F$), absorbed Z_n ($Z_n A$), and absorption index ($IA_{Ap}Z_n$), of animals fed with DRSP and CA, for 60 days.

Groups	Zinc (mg)			$IA_{Ap}Z_N$
	Ingested	Fecal	Absorbed	
	* a	a	a	a
DRSP	7.0	6.2	0.8	11.10
"Ad	0.4	0.5	0.5	7.31
libitum"	(6)	(6)	(6)	(6)
Control 1	a	b	b	b
"Pair	7.3	3.0	4.3	58.35
feeding"	0.0	0.3	0.4	4.28
CA	(6)	(6)	(6)	(6)
Control 2	b	a	c	b
"Ad	12.8	5.1	7.7	60.05
libitum"	1.0	1.2	1.2	7.94
CA	(6)	(6)	(6)	(6)

(Values expressed as mean $\pm$ SD)

* — Different superscripts for figures in each vertical column, indicate significant differences at $P < 0.05$.

Numbers of animals in brackets.

REFERENCES:-

1. Davies, N.T. & R. Nightingale, Br. J. Nutr. 1975, 34 243.
2. Henkin, R.I. and R.L. Aamodt. In: Nutritional bioavailability of zinc. Am. Chem. Soc., 1983, p. 82-105.
3. O Dell, B.L. Am. J. Clin. Nutr. 1969, 22, 1315.
4. Sandstron, B., & A. Cederblad. Am. J. Clin. Nutr. 1980, 33, 1778.
5. Donangelo, C.M. & C.E. Azevedo. Arch. Latinoamer 1984, 34 290.
6. Shrimpton, R. et alii. Acta Amazonica, 1983, 132 73.

The Bioavailability of Other Minerals and Toxic Metals

BIOAVAILABILITY OF CALCIUM AFFECTED BY LUMINAL AND MUCOSAL FACTORS IN THE SMALL INTESTINE

Hiroshi Naito, H.Gunshin and T.Noguchi

Department of Agricultural Chemistry
The University of Tokyo
Bunkyo-ku 113, Tokyo, Japan

1.INTRODUCTION

To elucidate the question that milk and dairy foods are highly effective in improving the bioavailability of Ca, separate studies were done with two major milk components , lactose and casein, by using absorption experiments in vitro and in vivo.
   The well known effect of lactose on Ca absorption seems to occur at a site of mucosal membrane, although only little has been evidenced. Casein gives rise to intra-intestinal formation of phosphopeptides(CPPs), a potent inhibitor against the precipitation of calcium phosphate.[1-2]

2.INTRA-LUMINAL FORMATION AND ACTION OF CPP

CPPs are macrophosphopeptides derived during the small intestinal digestion of α-sl- and ß-casein of cow's milk[1-2]. The amino acid sequence of a CPP isolated from the intestinal contents of rats fed ß-casein is following

   NH_2-Asn-Val-Pro-Gly-Glu-Ile-Val-Glu-SerP-

   -Leu-SerP-SerP-SerP-Glu-Glu-Ser-Ile-ThrOH

   The intra-luminal formation of peptide fractions exhibiting a CPP-like activity was also obtained after feeding of cheese, which was evidenced by an increased amount of the luminal soluble-Ca.
   When a preparation of CPP from whole casein with trypsin digestion was supplemented to a soya protein diet , the in situ absorption of Ca from ligated small

253

Table 1   Effect of Feeding CPP on the Net Absorption of
          Calcium from Undisturbed Ligated Loops of Rats

Addition of CPP (g/100g diet)	0	5	10
Soya Protein Isolate (g/100g diet)	20	15	10

Soluble Ca of Contents $10\overset{3}{x}$(mg Ca/mg Polyethylene glycol)

0 min.	67 ± 4*	97 ± 8	123 ± 16
60 " "	38 ± 4	58 ± 3	87 ± 7
Net Absorption	29	39	36

* Averages and SEM from five rats.

intestine, whose contents were unflushed.Correction for
luminal contents were made by simultaneous ingestion of
polyethylene glycol as an indicator.

As shown in Table 1, the supplement of CPP to a soya
protein diet increased almost proportionally the solubility
of intra-luminal Ca.

The net absorption of Ca(disappearance of the amount
of soluble Ca during 60min. of _in situ_ ligation) was also
significantly increased with CPP, but the effect seemed to
be almost saturated near 5% level.

3. MECHANISM OF ACTION OF LACTOSE ON CALCIUM UPTAKE BY SMALL INTESTINE

While the fact that lactose stimulates Ca absorption has
been generally acceptable, little of evidence is known.

We have confirmed the lactose-bearing stimulation of
Ca uptake by using brushborder membrane vesicles(BBMV)from
the small intestine of the rat.

The stimulation of ^{45}Ca uptake by lactose, as the
relative value with that obtained by an iso-osmotic concn.
of mannitol, could be seen(Table 2). This specific effect
of lactose was inhibited by the previous treatment with
cycloheximide, and markedly promoted with BBMV isolated
from vitamin D-deficient rats.

Table 2   Relative Activities of Calcium Uptake by
          Isolated Brushborder Membrane Vesicles
             (Mannitol as the Control)

Mannitol	100	Cellobiose	69
α –Lactose	128	Sucrose	88
ß–Lactose	123	Glucose	73
Lacturose	94	Galactose	84
Raffinose	78	Sorbitol	79
Maltose	102	Xylose	103

Following ingredients in mmol/l were mixed and ^{45}Ca
uptake was measured during 10min incubation after pre-
incubation with a sugar for 3hr at 0°: Sugar 100, Ca
50, NaCl 100,Hepes/Tris 10 pH7.0.

     These results may shed light on the improvement of
Ca bioavailability of many foods with less available
properties.

                    REFERENCES

1. Y.S.Lee, T.Noguchi and H.Naito, Br.J. Nutr.,1983,49,67
2. H.Naito, Proceedings XIII Intern.Congress of Nutrition,
   John Libbey,London,1986

GLUCOSE AND CALCIUM BIOAVAILABILITY IN HUMANS

R.J. Wood, J. Zheng, J. Knowles, A. Gerhardt
and I.H. Rosenberg

Nutrient Bioavailability Laboratory
USDA Human Nutrition Research Center on Aging
Tufts University
Boston, MA 02111   USA

1.   INTRODUCTION

Various studies have indicated that certain simple dietary sugars, such as lactose and glucose, can increase calcium absorption in humans. During the past several years our laboratory has been investigating the effects of glucose and more complex glucose polymers on calcium absorption in humans (1-4).

We summarize here the results from three recent studies done in our laboratory investigating the effect of glucose on calcium bioavailability in humans. Our findings indicate that the administration of an oral glucose load with calcium significantly enhances calcium absorption, but apparently does not increase net calcium retention.

2.   METHODS

Measurement of Fractional Ca Absorption

Fractional calcium absorption was measured in adult subjects in two experiments, essentially as described by Wills (5), by measuring the rise in forearm radioactivity 4 hours postdose in a large volume gamma counter following separate oral and iv doses of radioactive 47Ca on different days. The oral doses were given with 5 mmol elemental Ca as Ca chloride in 200 ml water, with or without carbohydrate. Fractional absorption was calculated from the ratio of normalized arm counts after oral and iv 47Ca. In the first study, we assessed the ability of 280 mmol of orally administered glucose to enhance fractional calcium absorption. Glucose was compared in that study (2) to an equal dose of glucose polymers, a carbohydrate source which we had previously shown to increase calcium absorption (1). In the second absorption study (3), we investigated the ability of various oral glucose loads (0, 56, 222 and 444 mmol) to stimulate calcium absorption.

Measurement of Whole Body Calcium Retention

Whole body calcium retention was measured as described by Shipp et al (6). Radioactive 47Ca was administered to fasting adult subjects in an aqueous solution (200 ml) containing 5 mmol elemental Ca with or without 222 mmol glucose. Whole body radioactivity was measured one hour postdose and again 14 days later to determine 47Ca retention. 51Cr was used as a nonabsorbable marker to verify that all the unabsorbed 47Ca had been excreted by day 14.

3. RESULTS

Effects of Glucose and Glucose Polymers on Ca Absorption

Compared with water alone, coadministration of 280 mmol of glucose or glucose polymers significantly increased fractional calcium absorption. The mean $\pm$ SEM calcium absorption with water was 43 $\pm$ 3%. Calcium absorption following the coadministration of glucose was 52$\pm$ 4% and after glucose polymers absorption was 54$\pm$3.

Effect of Various Glucose Loads on Ca Absorption

Fractional Ca absorption was increased by orally administered glucose in an apparent linear fashion up to a dose of 222 mmol of glucose. The linear regression equation relating fractional Ca absorption (Y) and oral glucose dose (X, in mmol) over this dose range was $Y = 0.08 X + 44$. The highest dose of glucose (444 mmol) coadministered with 47Ca caused no further enhancement of fractional Ca absorption above that which occurred when 222 mmol was given.

Effect of Glucose on Ca Retention

Recently, we have used a similar study design as just described, in which demonstration of positive effect of orally administered glucose on fractional Ca absorption, to investigate the effect of 222 mmol of oral glucose on 47Ca whole body retention. Glucose had no effect on 47Ca retention. The retention of 47Ca was 42+5% under control conditions with water alone and 43+5% following coadministration of carbohydrate.

4. DISCUSSION

Numerous studies have now shown that glucose can increase intestinal Ca absorption in humans. However, our study, investigating the effect of an oral dose of glucose on Ca retention in humans, suggests that glucose does not improve Ca bioavailability. This disparity between a positive effect on intestinal absorption yet no net change in retention presumably can be explained by the independent ability of sugars to increase urinary calcium losses (7).

5. REFERENCES

1. S.E. Kelly, K. Chawla-Singh, J.H. Sellin et al., Gastroenterol., 1984, 87, 596.

2. R.J. Wood, A. Gerhardt and I.H. Rosenberg, Am. J. Clin. Nutr., 1987, 46, 699.

3. J.B. Knowles, R.J. Wood and I.H. Rosenberg, Am. J. Clin. Nutr., 1988, in press.

4. L. Bei, R.J. Wood and I.H. Rosenberg, Am. J. Clin. Nutr., 1986, 44, 244.

5. M.R. Wills, E. Zisman, J. Wortsman et al, Clin. Sci., 1970, 3, 225.

6. C.C. Shipp, C.J. Maletskos and B. Dawson-Hughes, Calcif. Tissue Int., 1987, 41, 307.

7. J. Lemann, E.J. Lennon, W.R. Piering et al, J. Lab. Clin. Med., 1970, 75, 578.

BIO-AVAILABILITY (BAV) OF ZINC AND CALCIUM FROM BRAZILIAN STAPLE FOOD.

R.C. de Angelis, M.L. Ctenas, A.K. Oguido, G.A. Orozco

Nutrition Center-Dept. of Physiology and Biophysics - Institute of Biomedical Sciences-University of São Paulo Av.Prof.Lineu Prestes 1524 - 05508 São Paulo,SP,Brazil.

1 INTRODUCTION

Brazilians consume cereals and legumes as their staple food. The proposed diet for Brazilian children as the cheapest and more complete recommended diet/day (E) contained: milk, 400 ml; wheat flour, 20g; vegetables, 100g; meat, 60g; egg, 25g; rice, 50g; beans, 40g; bread, 25g; oil, butter, salt, containing: protein, 15%; lipids, 30%; carbohydrates, 55%; zinc, 30.4mg/Kg.

BAV of Zinc, in rats

Weanling rats were fed E, or, E+5mg Zinc/Kg, and compared to rats fed with isoproteic and isoenergetic diets of casein, without or, with 5mg Zinc/Kg added. In Table I the results for body weight variation (BW), Zinc in red cells (ZnR), Zinc in hair (ZnH) are correlated to the Zinc intake (ZnI), or, to Zinc absorbed (ZnA-ZnI-Zn$_{fecal}$), for Cas or E diets.

TABLE I

| y | x | REGRESSION FOR | |
		Cas diet	E diet
BW	ZnI	y=83 +22 x	y=12 +10 x
ZnR	ZnI	0.2 +1.7 x	2.2 +0.42x
ZnH	ZnI	-0.05+0.37x	-0.35+0.05x
ZnF*	ZnI	0.1 +0.6 x	-3.0 +0.71x
ZnR	ZnA	1.0 +2.75x	-5.25+0.77x

ZnF-Zinc in feces

259

The regression coefficients, as well as the y-intercepts
were lower for E diets than for Cas diets.
The exception was for ZnF/ZnI, where Zinc excretion
increased more rapidly with E diets.
The kinetic study of ZnA relative to ZnI showed an
impairment of intestinal Zinc absorption by the presence
of E diet.

Calcium BAV-Study in rats

We are developing a kinetic methodology for the study of
Ca-BAV. 2ml of solution containing Ca from different sources
(pre-digested with HCl,pH,2, and then neutralized to pH,6)
containing increasing Ca concentrations was introduced into
the lumen of a segment from the small intestine. In each
case the Km and Vmax were determined. Comparing the results
from different Ca sources with those of patterns with Ca
from $CaCl_2$, the relative BAV was calculated. The Km and
Vmax for $CaCl_2$ obtained were 220 and 400 µg of Ca,
respectively.

Study in men

Adult volunteers were fed for five days with two experimental diets "ad libitum", containing: rice, beans, milk,
meat, vegetables and fruits. In the first period the food
offered was complete. In the second all food of animal
origin was withdrawn. All food intake was controlled.
Stools and urine were collected, and the period was defined
by the appearance of an ingested marker in the feces. The
Ca and Zn balances in relation to intake are shown in
Table II, in mg/Kg/day.

TABLE II

	PERIOD I		PERIOD II	
	Intake	Balance	Intake	Balance
Calcium	17.43*	1.159	2.87	- 0.297
	(1.54)	(0.208)	(0.54)	(0.408)
Zinc	0.157	-2.019	0.042	- 0.664
	(0.081)	(0.081)	(0.018)	(0.105)

*Mean ± (SD)

The correlations between Ca and Zn Balances and the total
bean intake (BI) are shown in Table III.

TABLE III

y	x*	Regression	r
Balance of Ca	BI	1.63 - 0.31 x	0.74
Balance of Zn	BI	0.30 - 0.12 x	0.90

*BI - Beans Intake

These results suggest that the presence of beans in the food plays an important role impairing the body relation of Ca and Zn and it is disadvantageous when the energy concentration coming from beans increases in the diet (second period).

CONCLUSION

The presence of beans in the staple Brazilian diet impairs the BAV of Zinc and Calcium in the body. Therefore, the nutrient recommendation for our population must be reviewed. Meanwhile, it is important to remember that beans contain fiber which is relevant for other purposes; thus, further studies are necessary to evaluate the best equilibrium conditions: improving BAV maintaining food habits and adequate fiber consumption.

Acknowledgements:

The authors wish to acknowledge: J.H. Scialfa; I. Klemps; J.C. Bento Gonçalves for technical support. This study was partially supported by a grant from FAPESP (Fundação de Amparo à Pesquisa do Estado de São Paulo) (# 85/0212-6). We are also grateful to G.G. Giuli, R.N. Rogano, and M.G. Vecchia for the processing of human samples.

EFFECT OF DIETARY FIBRE OF COOKED VEGETABLES ON THE AVAILABILITY OF MINERALS IN RATS

Y. Saito and S. Sato

Department of Food Science and Nutrition
Koriyama Women's College
Kaisei Koriyama Fukushima Japan

1 INTRODUCTION

Several studies have indicated that components of dietary fibre are affected by cooking. It was found that boiling results in an increase in NDF, ADF and cellulose contents and a decrease in pectic materials. Frying produced a drastic decrease in NDF, ADF, cellulose and lignin contents. However, in our data, NDF, ADF and cellulose contents did not necessarily increase by boiling, and in some kinds of vegetables the fibre contents actually decreased by boiling. When vegetables were sauted, the dietary fibre content increased in most kinds of vegetables. Since each fibre component differs in its physical property and physio-logical effect cooking may change the physical property and physiological role of dietary fibre in vegetables. Indeed, McConnel et al reported that cooking did not affect the water-holding capacity, but has a varied effect on the cation capacity. The present investigation was undertaken to study the effect of dietary fibre of saute carrot on the availability of calcium and magnesium.

2 EXPERIMENTAL

Preparation of Dietary Fibre. Sliced carrot was sauted in oil until tender. Sauted and raw carrot were homogenized in acetone, and dehydrated and defatted with acetone and ether (fibre-A). The fibre-A was boiled in 85% methanol and again it was dehydrated by acetone(fibre-S). NDF was separated from fibre-A using the Van Soest procedure. Fibre-A and -B contained about 50% and 70% of dietary fibre respectively, as determined by the enzyme method.
Animal Feeding. The growing rats were fed the diets shown in Table 1 for two weeks. At the end of two weeks Ca and

Table 1   Composition of diets(g)

| | Control-1 | Fibre-A | | Control-2 | Fibre-B, | NDF |
		Raw	Saute		Raw	Saute
Starch	70	70	70	70	60	60
Casein	20	20	20	20	20	20
Oil	5	5	5	5	5	5
Salt mix	4	4	4	4	4	4
Vitamin mix	1	1	1	1	1	1
Cellulose	4	0	0	0	0	0
Fibre A, B or NDF	0	20	20	0	10	10
Total	104	120	120	100	100	100

Mg contents in the diets, feces and urine were determined for three days by atomic absorption spectrophotometry.

3   RESULTS AND DISCUSSION

Food consumption of fibre-A raw, and fibre-B raw and saute groups, was slightly lower than that of the control and other groups.   Therefore body weight gain of fibre-A raw group and fibre-B raw and saute group was about 20% and 10% less than that of control groups respectively. Fibre-A saute and NDF raw and saute did not affect food intake and body weight gain.   Mean dry fecal weight of control-1 group exhibited an increase of 50% more than that of control-2 group and the increment approximated the weight of cellulose consumed.   Dry fecal weight of fibre-A raw and saute groups increased to two, and one and a half times that of fibre-free group.   The difference between the raw and saute groups was significant.   But there was no difference between dry fecal weight of the raw and saute groups in fibre-B and NDF.   On the other hand, in fibre-A, cecum weight of the raw group was mostly equal to that of the saute group, which was about three times the fecal weight of the fibre-free group.   From this result we can think that fibre-A saute might be digested in large intestine, but raw fibre might not be so much digested and be excreted. The cecum weight of fibre-B saute group was 40% heavier than that of the raw group.   Thus fibre-B saute might be more difficult to digest than fibre-B raw. There was no difference of cecum weight of NDF raw and saute group, and cecum weight of the NDF group was equal to that of the fibre-B saute group.   These results suggest that carrot dietary fibre increases feces but part of the fibre might be digested in intestine.

    Absorption and balance of Ca in the fibre-A saute

Table 2   Absorption and balance of Ca and Mg

		Ca		Mg	
		Absorption	Balance	Absorption	Balance
Control-1		$39.0^{\pm}2.2\%$	$29.4^{\pm}1.3$mg	$51.6^{\pm}3.8\%$	$2.3^{\pm}0.8$mg
Fibre-A	raw	$26.2^{\pm}6.4$	$14.2^{\pm}6.5$	$34.0^{\pm}5.1$	$0.2^{\pm}0.4$
	saute	$40.4^{\pm}5.6$	$28.6^{\pm}3.9$	$52.2^{\pm}5.9$	$1.5^{\pm}0.9$
Control-2		$48.0^{\pm}4.9$	$39.8^{\pm}7.0$	$60.6^{\pm}2.0$	$2.4^{\pm}0.4$
Fibre-B	raw	$32.7^{\pm}4.7$	$31.2^{\pm}4.3$	$56.5^{\pm}4.6$	$2.3^{\pm}0.3$
	saute	$39.7^{\pm}2.1$	$31.4^{\pm}3.8$	$58.9^{\pm}3.7$	$3.3^{\pm}0.6$
NDF	raw	$47.1^{\pm}1.1$	$37.8^{\pm}3.1$	$59.8^{\pm}2.7$	$1.8^{\pm}0.5$
	saute	$45.9^{\pm}1.8$	$37.1^{\pm}2.8$	$57.9^{\pm}5.0$	$1.9^{\pm}0.4$

group was almost equal to that of control-1, but with raw
fibre-A both Ca absorption and Ca balance were decreased
(Table 2).   Fibre-B raw and saute did not affect fecal Ca
excretion but Ca intake was decreased by the fibre. Therefore both the raw and saute carrot residue extracted by 85%
methanol significantly decreased Ca absorption, and also
decreased Ca balance. On the other hand, NDF raw and saute
did not affect absorption and balance of Ca. In the fibre-B
and NDF groups cooking did not influence absorption and
balance of Ca. The fibre-A group showed that both absorption and balance of Mg changed similarly to absorption
and balance of Ca, that is, fibre-A raw significantly
decreased both absorption and balance of Mg. But both
absorption and balance of Mg in fibre-B and NDF group
were mostly similar to the values of the control-2 group,
and were not affected by cooking.

In fibre-A it was clear that cooking affected Ca and
Mg availability, but fibre-B or NDF had no effect from
cooking on mineral availability. Fibre-A might contain
more of the other components except fibre than fibre-B,
since fibre-B was the residue extracted from fibre-A with
85% methanol. Therefore the other components might be
changed by cooking, and the change of other components
resulted in the cooking effect on Ca and Mg availability.
But further studies will be necessary to know these
results completely.

REFERENCES

1. J.Herranz, C.V. Valverde and E.R. Hidalgo, J. Food Sci. 1983,
    48, 274.
2. L.M. Brandt, M.A. Jeltema, M.E. Zabik and B.D.Jeltema,
    J.Food Sci., 1984, 49, 900.
3. A.A. McConnell, M.A. Eastwood and W.D. Michell, J. Sci. Food Agric.
    1974, 25, 1457.

EFFECTS OF CASEIN AND SOYBEAN ISOLATE ON THE BIOAVAILABILITY OF
MAGNESIUM. A BALANCE STUDY IN RATS

E.J. Brink, P.R. Dekker, E.C.H. van Beresteyn
Netherlands Institute for Dairy Research,
P.O. Box 20, 6710 BA Ede,
The Netherlands

1 INTRODUCTION

Little is known about the effects of nutritional factors on the
bioavailability of Mg. Some investigators (1,2) showed that casein
and soybean isolate did not have different effects on the
bioavailability of Mg. However, in these studies Mg-bioavailability
was evaluated only by the Mg-levels in plasma, femur and kidneys;
intestinal absorption, urinary excretion and retention were not
measured. Therefore, balance studies in rats were performed to
investigate the effects of casein versus soybean isolate on the
bioavailability of Mg.

2 METHODS

Forty-two male Wistar rats, six weeks old and with body weight
approximately 136 g were randomly divided into six equal groups.
For four weeks they were fed ad libitum semisynthetic diets
containing 20 % casein or 20 % soybean isolate and a low (200 ppm),
normal (400 ppm) and high (600 ppm) level of Mg. Animals were kept
individually in stainless steel metabolic cages under temperature and
light controlled conditions. Food consumption was recorded daily and
body weights were measured weekly. After two and four weeks of
feeding the diets, feces and urine were collected for four days. At
the end of the feeding period blood was drawn under slight ether
anaesthesia by orbita puncture. After liver perfusion the rats were
sacrificed. Femur, kidneys and liver were removed for analyses. Mg
was analysed by atomic absorption spectrophotometry in plasma
and urine, and in feces, femur, kidneys and liver after ashing. In
addition plasma alkaline phosphatase and urinary hydroxyproline
excretion were determined.
  Bioavailability of Mg was evaluated by comparing the intestinal
absorption, urinary excretion and Mg-content in femur and plasma.

Results were statistically treated by analysis of variance and differences between group means by Scheffé's test.

3 RESULTS

The experimental diets did not differ in the analysed content of minerals except for Mg (Table 1). Body weight gain, food consumption and food efficiency were not significantly different for rats fed the different experimental diets (Table 2). Table 3 shows that the minimum requirement of Mg in this study appeared to be approximately 200 ppm because at this dietary level of Mg urinary excretion was low (0.38 mg/d) and intestinal absorption (% intake) high.

Independently of the dietary Mg level intestinal absorption was significantly higher on the casein diets as compared to the soybean isolate diets. Differences were reflected in urinary Mg excretion and content of Mg in femur. Plasma Mg concentration was significantly higher on the casein diet only at the lowest level of Mg (200 ppm). Increasing the level of Mg in the diet resulted in an increase of absolute intestinal absorption, urinary excretion and Mg content of the femur and plasma, while intestinal absorption expressed as a percentage of intake decreased.

Urinary excretion increased and intestinal absorption (% intake) decreased with age. Plasma alkaline phosphatase was significantly higher on the casein diets, and was independent of the Mg level. Urinary hydroxyproline excretion was significantly higher on the casein diet as compared to the soybean isolate diet only at the lowest level of Mg (200 ppm). There was no effect of diet on the Mg content of kidneys or liver.

Table 1 Analysed mineral content of the experimental diets

	casein[1])			soybean isolate[1])		
	dietary Mg level (ppm)			dietary Mg level (ppm)		
	200	400[2])	600	200	400[2])	600
Mg (%)	0.025	0.043	0.075	0.022	0.044	0.065
Ca (%)	0.58	0.57	0.57	0.59	0.57	0.57
P (%)	0.31	0.31	0.31	0.32	0.31	0.31
Na (%)	0.22	0.22	0.22	0.27	0.26	0.26
K (%)	0.49	0.50	0.49	0.50	0.48	0.48
Zn (%)	0.012	0.012	0.012	0.012	0.012	0.013

[1]) protein 20 %, DL-methionine 0.3 %, dextrose 40 %, palm oil 15 %, wheat starch 15 %, cellulose 5 %, vitamins 1 %, minerals 3.5 %.
[2]) amount according to the AIN-76

Table 2 Body weight gain, food consumption and food efficiency (x ± SEM, n = 7)

	casein			soybean isolate		
	dietary Mg level (ppm)			dietary Mg level (ppm)		
	200	400	600	200	400	600
body weight gain (g/4 weeks)	158±6	148±6	149±6	154±6	148±6	145±4
food consumption (g/4 weeks)	546±11	524±17	508±13	499±13	501±5	509±9
food efficiency (g/g)	0.31±0.03	0.30±0.02	0.31±0.02	0.32±0.03	0.31±0.03	0.30±0.03

Table 3 Parameters of magnesium bioavailability (x ± SEM, n = 7)

	casein dietary Mg level(ppm)			soybean isolate dietary Mg level (ppm)			main effect[1]) protein	Mg level
	200	400	600	200	400	600	p	p
intestinal absorption[2])	3.25±0.08	5.15±0.14	8.06±0.27	2.36±0.08	4.57±0.16	6.45±0.26	<0.01	<0.01
intestinal absorption[3])	69.5±1.3	65.9±2.0	60.4±1.6	62.5±2.1	58.0±2.1	55.2±1.5	<0.01	<0.01
urinary excretion[2])	1.40±0.06	3.24±0.10	5.53±0.14	0.70±0.09	2.24±0.10	3.29±0.23	<0.01	<0.01
femur Mg content (mg/g ash)	6.93±0.14	7.37±0.08	7.64±0.08	6.22±0.14	7.16±0.12	7.57±0.12	<0.01	<0.01
plasma Mg (mg/d)	1.86±0.09	1.99±0.08	2.18±0.14	1.62±0.10	1.98±0.09	2.12±0.07	n.s.	<0.01

[1]) one way analysis of variance
[2]) values from week 4, mg/d
[3]) values from week 4, % intake

4 DISCUSSION

The most sensitive model to investigate the bioavailability of Mg is a model in which the Mg is given at a level near or below the minimum requirement. In this study the minimum requirement of Mg appeared to be 200 ppm. This is in agreement with other studies (2,3).

From our results it can be concluded that the bioavailability of Mg is increased on the casein diets as compared to the soybean isolate diets. In addition bone turnover appears to be higher on the casein diets as measured by plasma alkaline phosphatase and urinary hydroxyproline excretion. These results are in contrast with other studies in which the variables used to evaluate bioavailability of Mg were different from our study (1,2) or in which the diets contained excessive amounts of Mg (1).

It should be noted that soybean isolate contains a significant amount of phytate. Some reports have indicated that the amount of soybean protein in the diet will suppress the utilization of minerals and trace elements due to the presence of phytate (4,5).

Whether the effects of the protein source on the bioavailability of Mg, as measured in this experiment are due to phytate or to the protein itself remains to be studied.

REFERENCES

1. R.M. Forbes, K.E. Weingarter, H.M. Parker, R.R. Bell and J.W. Erdman, J. Nutr., 1979, 109, 1652.
2. G.S. Lo, F.H. Steinke and D.T. Hopkins, J. Nutr., 1980, 110, 829.
3. P.W.F. Fisher and A. Giroux, J. Nutr., 1987, 117, 2091.
4. B.L. O'Dell and A.R. de Boland, J. Agr. Food Chem., 1976, 24, 804.
5. J.G. Reinhold, Proc. 9th Int. Cong. Nutr. Mexico 1972, A. Chavez, H. Bourges and S. Basta (eds), Kargers, Basel, 1985, 115.

ASSESSING THE AVAILABILITY OF DIETARY PHOSPHORUS FOR
SHEEP.

N.F. Suttle, R.A. Dingwall and
C.S. Munro,
Department of Biochemistry,
Moredun Research Institute,
408 Gilmerton Road,
Edinburgh, EH17 7JH

1.   INTRODUCTION
     There is a dearth of information on the nutritive
value of organic and inorganic food sources of phosphorus
(P) which reflects the inappropriateness rather than
the scarcity of experimentation (1). The major determinants of the nutrient value of P sources for ruminants
are concentration and absorbability. Absorbabilities
have recently been reported for 12 different feeds
using laborious but sensitive radioisotope methods (2).
This paper reports the use of similar techniques to
evaluate two inorganic sources, rock phosphate (RP) and
'dicalcium phosphate' (DCP, $CaHPO_4$) and addressing and
value in vitro extraction for routine quality control.

2.   MATERIALS AND METHODS
     Seven adult ewes were given a pelleted, complete
diet low in P, 0.5g/kg DM, apart from the minerals
under test which added 3g P/kg DM. Each sheep was given
RP and DCP separately in sequences allocated at random.
The pelleted diet consisted of (g/kg: dried sugar beet
pulp, 536, oat husk, 185, starch, 93, molasses, 56, urea,
23, vegetable oil, 19, $NaHCO_3$, 14, Na_2SO_4, 28, with
added trace elements and vitamin A, D & E and a pellet-
ing agent ("Pristearine", 19). Sheep accustomed to
metabolism crates were offered 0.6kg (air dry) of each
feed/d for 7 days. 32P was then given by intravenous
injection, and stable and radioisotope balances
conducted by making total collections of urine and
faeces for a further 8-10d. Specific activity (SA) of
P in plasma was measured in deproteinised samples and
the endogenous contributions to faecal P calculated by

268

isotope dilution from the ratio of areas under the SA $\underline{v}$
time curves for faeces and plasma (2). In vitro availability was assessed by extraction in citric acid (3):
1g of RP or DCP, containing 120 and 189mg P 'respectively'
was extracted in 100ml 2% w/v citric acid for 2 to 48h
with occasional shaking. The RP had been fed in a coarse
form: dry sieving showed that only a small fraction
(0.026) passed a 100μm sieve and only 0.47 passed a 200μm
sieve. A milled sample was therefore prepared and
extracted. Five feeds (2) and two poultry wastes (4) for
which P absorption had been measured in vivo were
extracted without prior milling to see whether their
values could be assessed more simply.

RESULTS

The in vivo trial gave contradictory results. The
less absorbable source (RP) gave a significantly higher
positive balance in adult animals that should have been
in equilibrium (Table 1). There were significant differences in P metabolism, particularly in urinary P
excretion (p<0.01) between individual sheep. The in vitro
extraction indicated a lower availability for RP. DCP
dissolved quickly and totally in citric acid but only
0.17, 0.44 and 0.65 of the P in RP had been extracted
after 2, 24 and 48h, respectively. Milling RP increased
fractional extraction to 0.44, 0.65 and 0.73 after 2, 24
and 48h respectively. The comparison between in vitro
and in vivo methods for foods indicates poor agreement
(Table 2).

Table 1. Effect of P source on P metabolism in lambs (g/d)

P Source	Absorption	Excretion Faecal endogenous	Urinary	Retention
DCP	1.559	0.476	1.157	-0.076
RP	1.032	0.282	0.463	0.287
se	0.107	0.089	0.069	0.098

Table 2. Comparison of in vitro (A) and in vivo (B)
availability coefficients

	Broiler waste	Battery waste	Clover hay	Grass hay	Rapeseed meal	Soyabean meal	Rice bran
A	0.27	0.19	0.18	0.19	0.47	0.91	0.12
B	0.73	0.73	0.71	0.64	0.69	0.71	0.63

DISCUSSION

The *in vivo* coefficient for absorption from RP
(0.66) requires a correction. It is unlikely that absorbable P from RP is more efficiently used than that from
DCP; rather that some P from RP was retained in the
alimentary tract and not absorbed. Soil particles of
similar size and specific gravity to those of RP pass
very slowly through sheep (5). If only half of the 'retained' P, trapped in RP particles, was absorbed prior
to their passage from the animal, the absorption
coefficient would be reduced to 0.55: the corrected value
indicates that such materials should be given about 2/
3rds of the value of DCP. Variation in availability due
to particle size should be reduced by milling and citric
acid extraction could be used to routinely monitor the
quality of RP.

The *in vitro* method did not predict the *in vivo*
value of 'non-mineral' sources of P. While this is not
surprising for foodstuffs which are extensively degraded
in the rumen, it is noteworthy for the poultry wastes
which would contain mostly inorganic P. The *in vivo* data
support the use of absorption coefficients for assessing
the nutrient value of P sources for ruminants provided
that the design of the experiment minimises individual
animal bias. The high absorption of P from DCP indicates
that assessments of the feed were not greatly complicated
by the animal adapting to a plentiful supply by
absorbing P inefficiently.

REFERENCES

1. Suttle, N.F. (1986) Proc. XIIIth Int. Cong. Nutr,
Brighton U.K. p 232-237.

2. Field, A.C., Woolliams, J.A., Dingwall, R.A. and
Munro, C.S. (1984). J. agric. Sci. Camb. 103, 283-291.

3. Guegen, L. (1970) Bull. Soc. Scient. Hyg. Alim.
Assoc. fr Tech. Alim Anum. Zoot. 58, 115.

4. Field, A.C., Munro, C.S. and Suttle, N.F. (1977) J.
agric. Sci. Camb. 89, 599-604.

5. Brebner, J.(1986)PhD. Thesis.   Imperial College,
London.

We acknowledge the support of Dalgety Agriculture Ltd.

FACTORS INFLUENCING THE BIOAVAILABILITY OF PHYTATE PHOSPHORUS TO CHICKENS

Hardy M. Edwards, Jr., Pierre Palo,
Somchit Sooncharernying and Michael A. Elliott

Department of Poultry Science
University of Georgia
Athens, Georgia 30602 USA

1 INTRODUCTION

Reviews[1,2] of the utilization of phytate phosphorus by poultry have emphasized the effects of calcium, vitamin D_3 and phytase content of the diet on phytate utilization. Studies from this laboratory[3] showed that Single Comb White Leghorn chickens retained a much higher amount of the phytate phosphorus from the feed than broiler chickens. Further studies[4] quantified the effects of both dietary calcium and phosphorus on the retention of phytate phosphorus when the diets were primarily composed of corn and soybean meal. Additional observations have been made on the effects of age of bird, sex, period of life cycle and a synthetic zeolite on phytate phosphorus retention by chickens fed corn-soybean meal diets.

2 MATERIALS AND METHODS

Experiment 1 was conducted with broiler chickens 8-9 weeks of age and the retentions were from total balance studies. Experiment 2 was conducted with laying Single Comb White Leghorn hens and the retentions were obtained by Cr_2O_3 balances. Experiment 3 was conducted with broiler chickens at 1, 2 and 3 weeks of age, the retentions were obtained by Cr_2O_3 balances. All studies were conducted with corn-soybean meal diets. The phytate phosphorus in feed and feces were determined by the method of Common.[5]

3   RESULTS AND DISCUSSION

The results of experiment 1 indicate that male broilers retain significantly more phytate phosphorus than females at either high or low dietary calcium levels (Table 1).

The high calcium content of the diet of laying hens, Experiment 2, caused increased retention of phytate phosphorus early in the egg laying cycle, but retention of phytate phosphorus was apparent in hens fed the high or low calcium diets by 187 to 211 days of age (Table 2).

The broiler chickens in Experiment 3 at 1, 2 and 3 weeks of age retained 35%, 47% and 59%, respectively, of the phytate phosphorus in the diet.

These studies clearly show that age and sex as well as calcium and phosphorus content of the diet have a significant effect on the amounts of phytate phosphorus that chickens utilize from a corn-soybean meal type diet.

Table 1. Effect of sex and calcium on phytate phosphorus retention.

Dietary Ca	Sex	Phytate phosphorus retention
%		%
.32	M	62.0
1.01	M	38.7
.32	F	36.3
1.01	F	18.1
ANOV Ca		<.001
Sex		<.001

Table 2. Effect of dietary calcium and age of laying hen on retention of phytate phosphorus.

Age of hen Days	Phytate phosphorus retention	
	1.8% Ca diet	2.8% Calcium diet
	%	%
151	19.7c,x	54.4a,y
162	35.0a,x	46.0b,x
163	37.7a,x	57.5a,y
164	32.8ab,x	44.9b,x
187	36.5a,x	14.9c,y
211	26.1bc,x	11.5c,x

Values a,b,c in the vertical row or x,y in the horizontal row having the same superscript are not significantly different (P<.05).

REFERENCES

1. T.S. Nelson, *Poul. Sci.*, 1967, 46, 862.
2. S.H. Hayes, et al., *J. Anim. Sci.*, 1979, 49, 992.
3. H.M. Edwards and J.R. Veltmann, *J. Nutr.*, 1983, 113, 1568.
4. H.M. Edwards, *Poul. Sci.*, 1983, 62, 77.
5. R.H. Common, *Analyst*, 1940, 65, 79.

DIFFERENT BIOAVAILABILITY OF PHOSPHORUS AS THE BASIS FOR A CONTROLLED PHOSPHORUS INTAKE

C. Strobel and R. Kluthe

Section of Nutritional Medicine and Dietetics
Medical University Hospital
Freiburg im Breisgau, FRG

1. INTRODUCTION

The common daily phosphorus(P)-intake in the FRG and in many other western countries is about 1600 mg/day. This is nearly twice the recommended dietary allowance of 800 mg P/day[1,2]. Some authors[3,4] assume this difference between real and recommended P-intake has adverse effects on bone metabolism. The high P-intake, together with the usual low Ca-intake, may lead to secondary hyperparathyroidism and - in the long run - to osteodystrophy.

For patients with renal insufficiency there is no doubt about the hazard of a high P-intake. According to Crooks and Coburn[5] the P-supply for these patients should be below 800-900 mg/day. Since P is a constituent of all cells and therefore present in all natural food, partly in considerable amounts, it is difficult to compose a P-restricted diet. There are a few data in the literature[6,7] indicating different bioavailability of P from different foodstuffs. The question is whether this could be used for a critical examination of the P-intake of healthy persons as well as for a rational diet in renal insufficiency. To evaluate the bioavailability of P from foodstuffs and from diets we performed two balance studies with healthy volunteers.

2. BALANCE STUDY I

Experimental Design

In the first balance study 10 healthy volunteers (8 ♀, 2 ♂) 20 to 28 years old participated. During the 24 days of the experiment they received a basal diet containing 98 ± 9 kJ,

0.9 ± 0.1 g protein, 15 ± 1 mg P and 7 ± 3 mg Ca per kg
body weight and day. To this basal diet different supplements constant in energy and Ca (49 ± 5 kJ and 14 ± 1 mg Ca
per kg body weight and day) were added according to the
following scheme:

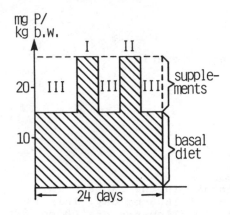

period I/II: one of the following foodstuffs as P-source
equivalent to 11 ± 1 mg P/kg
b.w./day:
- whole rye bread
- cow's milk, 3.5 % fat
  i.d.m.
- bread, wheat+rye, low extraction flour
- cheese, gouda, 40 % fat
  i.d.m.
- meat, pork

period III:
P-free oligosaccharides

To achieve a constant energy supply oligosaccharides were
added to the milk- and cheese-supplements. For a constant
Ca-supply Ca-citrate was added to each period III, to the
whole rye bread- and to the wheat+rye bread-supplements.
The protein intake varied with the supplements. The first
period III lasted 8 days, all other periods 4 days. From
the 5th day on the volunteers collected 24 h-urine and
complete faeces.

Results

The "apparent absorption" of P (= (intake - faecal output)
: intake x 100) from each supplemented foodstuff was calculated via the faecal excretion of the supplemented P:
- whole rye bread (n = 8)   29 ± 22 %
- cow's milk, 3.5 % fat i.d.m. (n = 7)   64 ± 19 %
- bread, wheat+rye, low extraction (n = 2)   72 ± 6 %
- cheese, gouda, 40 % fat i.d.m. (n = 2)   62 ± 20 %
- meat, pork (n = 1)   69 %

3. BALANCE STUDY II

Experimental Design

In the second balance study we transformed the results of
balance study I into acceptable diets. 6 healthy volunteers
(5 ♀, 1 ♂) 24 to 37 years old participated. The experiment

consisted of 3 consecutive periods 10 days each with a constant supply of energy, P and Ca (139 ± 22 kJ, 20 ± 3 mg P and 28 ± 4 mg Ca per kg body weight and day). The 3 periods differed as follows:
- "normal" diet,
- "milk-cheese diet": 2/3 of the P was supplied by milk and milk products ,
- "cereal diet": 2/3 of the P was supplied by cereals and cereal products (whole grain).

The protein intake varied with the 3 diets (1.1 ± 0.2 g, 1.0 ± 0.2 g, and 0.7 ± 0.1 g respectively). A constant Ca-supply was achieved by the supplementation of the "normal" diet and the "cereal diet" with Ca-citrate. Throughout the study the volunteers collected 24 h-urine and complete faeces.

Results

The "apparent P-absorption" (n = 6) during the three periods was:

-	"normal" diet	52 ± 9 %
-	"milk-cheese diet"	52 ± 6 %
-	"cereal diet"	36 ± 4 %

4. CONCLUSIONS

There are distinct differences in the "apparent absorption" of P from different foodstuffs and consequently from different diets. This is in our opinion a considerable aspect for
1. the evaluation of the P-intake of healthy persons and
2. the composition of a P-defined diet for patients with renal insufficiency.

REFERENCES
1. DGE, `Empfehlungen für die Nährstoffzufuhr`, Umschau-Verlag, Frankfurt am Main, 4. Auflage, 1985, pp. 31.
2. National Research Council, `Recommended Dietary Allowances`, National Academy of Sciences, Washington, D.C., 9th edition, 1980, pp. 133.
3. R.R. Bell, H.H. Draper, D.Y.M. Tzeng, H.K. Shin and G.R. Schmidt, J. Nutr., 1977, 107, 42.
4. D.E. Yuen and H.H. Draper, J. Nutr., 1983, 113, 1374.
5. P.W. Crooks and J.W. Coburn, Blood Purification, 1985, 3, 27.
6. J.E. Tewell, H.E. Clark and J.M. Howe, J. Am. diet. Ass., 1973, 63, 530.
7. W.-H. Moon, J.L. Malzer and H.E. Clark, J. Am. diet. Ass., 1974, 64, 386.

TISSUE MINERAL UPTAKE AS A MEASURE OF SUPPLEMENTAL INORGANIC TRACE MINERAL BIOAVAILABILITY IN LIVESTOCK AND POULTRY

C. B. Ammerman, P. R. Henry and R. D. Miles

Departments of Animal Science and Poultry Science
University of Florida
Gainesville, FL 32611 USA

1 INTRODUCTION

The study of mineral bioavailability has been hindered through the years due to the lack of agreement concerning the definition of bioavailability and a suitable method of determination. Generally, bioavailability implies that portion of a dietary element which is absorbed and supports some physiological process. While it may be practical to measure a physiological process such as glutathione peroxidase activity to assay for Se bioavailability, the task would be very complex for elements such as Mn or Zn which are known to be involved in numerous enzyme systems. It is recognized generally that absorption of an element is maximized when that element is deficient in the animal's diet. However, for many elements the use of purified diets is necessary to create diets which are deficient. These diets are expensive, often unpalatable, especially for ruminants, and their use often alters normal absorption and metabolism of the element in question as well as other dietary nutrients. In some parts of the world it is simply impossible to obtain test diets which are deficient.

The response of tissue mineral concentration to dietary supplementation of the same element is illustrated in Figure 1.[2] If the responses to an unknown source and a soluble test source are linear, comparisons may be made by slope ratio techniques. In the assay method proposed, graded levels of the element of interest are added to natural, commercial-type diets and fed for a short period of time. The greatest level fed is that which is just below the level at which feed

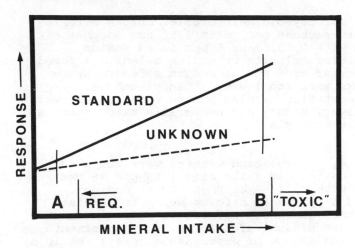

Figure 1. Predicted tissue mineral
response to dietary addition of a
mineral

refusal would be expected to occur and is indicated by
the letter "B" in Figure 1. True differences would be
easier to detect with fewer animals at this point
compared with point "A", which is below the animal's
requirement for the element. The following experiments
were conducted to estimate the bioavailability of
inorganic Mn and Se sources for sheep and chicks.

2 EXPERIMENTAL PROCEDURE

In Exp. 1, 0, 1000, 2000 and 4000 ppm Mn as
reagent grade Mn sulfate, monoxide or carbonate were
supplemented to a corn-soybean meal diet (116 ppm Mn
DMB) and fed to 120 male broiler chicks for 22 d. Bone
and liver were analyzed for Mn. In Exp. 2, 105 day-old
male broiler chicks were fed a corn-soybean meal diet
(35 ppm Mn DMB) supplemented with 0, 40, 80 or 120 ppm
Mn as reagent grade Mn sulfate or monoxide for 21 d.
Bone, liver and kidney were analyzed for Mn.

In Exp. 3, 192 day-old male broiler chicks were fed the basal corn-soybean meal diet (.18 ppm Se DMB) supplemented with 0, 3, 6 or 9 ppm Se as sodium selenite, calcium selenite or sodium selenite + fumed amorphous carrier or 6 ppm as sodium selenate or Se metal. Chicks were fed 1 week, then plasma was collected by anterior cardiac puncture and chicks were killed and liver, kidney and pectoralis major muscles removed for Se analysis.

In Exp. 4, 28 crossbred wethers were fed a corn-soybean meal-cottonseed hulls diet (.18 ppm Se DMB) supplemented with 0, 3, 6 or 9 ppm Se as sodium selenite, and 6 ppm Se as calcium selenite, sodium selenite + fumed amorphous carrier or sodium selenate. Sheep were fed the basal diet for a 10-d adjustment period, then fed 1200 g of experimental diets for 10 d. Liver, kidney and serum were analyzed for Se.

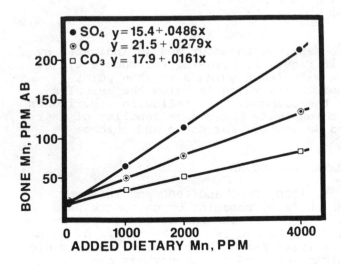

Figure 2.   Effect of source and level of dietary Mn on bone Mn concentration of chicks - Exp. 1[3].

3 RESULTS

As illustrated in Figure 2, bone Mn concentration in
Exp. 1 increased linearly as dietary Mn from all
sources increased; however, birds fed Mn sulfate had
greater ($P < .05$) bone Mn concentrations than those fed
Mn oxide or carbonate. Liver Mn concentrations were
also lower ($P < .01$) in birds fed carbonate compared
with the other Mn sources. Based on linear and multiple
linear regression and the average increase in bone and
liver Mn concentration, Mn oxide and carbonate had
relative values of 70 and 39 compared with 100 for
Mn sulfate.

In Exp. 2, bone, kidney and liver Mn
concentrations increased linearly ($P < .001$) as dietary
Mn increased; however, kidney was found to be more
sensitive to dietary Mn than was liver. Based on
linear and multiple linear regression and average
increase in bone, liver and kidney Mn concentration,
oxide has a relative availability of 67% to that of
sulfate. Thus, availability of oxide compared with
sulfate was similar when calculated from experiments
when low (40-120 ppm) or high (1000-4000 ppm) dietary
concentrations of Mn were fed.

In Exp. 3, Se concentrations in all tissues
increased linearly ($P < .01$) as dietary concentrations
increased. Based on linear and multiple linear
regression and average increase in plasma, muscle,
liver and kidney Se concentrations, relative
availability estimates were 100, 89, 86, 101 and 75 for
sodium selenite, calcium selenite, sodium selenite +
carrier, sodium selenate and Se metal. Availability of
Se in Se metal was lower ($P < .05$) than that from other
sources.

Liver Se concentrations in sheep fed 0, 3, 6 or 9
ppm Se as sodium selenite were 1.3, 4.2, 7.0 and 10.5
ppm (dry basis) and kidney Se concentrations were 3.0,
4.9, 6.0 and 12.3 ppm (dry basis), respectively (Exp.
4). Serum Se concentration increased from .09 μg/ml in
sheep fed the basal diet to .16, .22 and .35 ppm as
dietary Se increased. Based on linear and multiple
linear regression and average increase in liver, kidney
and serum Se concentration, calcium selenite, sodium
selenite + carrier and sodium selenate had estimated
availabilities of 101, 90 and 133% that of sodium
selenite. Due to variability these values were not
different ($P > .10$).

Short term, high level supplementation of Mn and
Se resulted in tissue mineral deposition of the
elements which was useful for estimation of
bioavailability of inorganic sources.

REFERENCES

1.   H.T. Peeler, J. Anim. Sci., 1972, 35, 695.
2.   P.R. Henry, C.B. Ammerman and R.D. Miles, Poul.
     Sci., 1986, 65, 983.
3.   J.R. Black, C.B. Ammerman, P.R. Henry and R.D.
     Miles, Poul. Sci., 1984, 63, 1999.

SELENIUM IN THE DIET OF CHILDREN WITH PHENYLKETONURIA

J. Barrett, C. Patterson, C. Reilly, U. Tinggi

Department of Public Health and Nutrition
Queensland Institute of Technology
and
S. Latham and A. Marrinan

Royal Children's Hospital
Brisbane, Australia

1 INTRODUCTION

There have been several reports that children with
phenylketonuria (PKU) who are maintained on a low
phenylalanine diet may be at risk of inadequate intake
of essential trace elements[1]. This deficiency is due
to a limited intake of whole protein foods, the main
source of trace elements in normal diets. Supplements
containing Fe, Zn, Cu and Mn have been used to increase
intake but deficiencies of Se continue to be reported
in PKU children[2]. While some investigators advocate
the use of an Se supplement, others have urged caution
because of the potential toxicity of the element[3].

The study reported here was designed to
investigate the Se status of children attending the PKU
Clinic at the Royal Children's Hospital, and to look at
total intake as well as the distribution of the element
between components of the diet, with a view to
increasing availability and intake of the element.

2 METHODS

A three day weighed food intake record was kept for 20
PKU children and 20 of their siblings. Samples of food
consumed were collected for laboratory analysis.

Blood samples of patients and siblings were
analysed for Fe, Zn, Cu, Mn by atomic absorption
spectrophotometry, Cr by Zeeman polarised AAS and Se
both by vapor generation AA and spectrofluorimetric
technique.

Gluthathione peroxidase was determined in whole blood by a spectrophotometric precedure.

Food samples were acid digested in preparation for trace element determination by the above instrumental methods.

3   RESULTS AND DISCUSSION

No significant differences were found for Fe, Zn, Cu, Mn or Cr levels in plasma of PKU children and their siblings, but were for Se and gluthathione peroxidase, as is shown in Table 1.

Dietary intake of Se (Table 2) was significantly lower in PKU children compared to siblings and failed to meet the proposed (Australian) RDI of 25-85 µg. Though no overt clinical symptoms of Se deficiency were noted, the possibility of long term effects cannot be ruled out and ways of increasing intake of Se by the PKU children are being considered. While Lipson[4] and others have used Se supplements to do this, the potential toxicity of the element must be recognised and the possibility of improving intake by dietary means investigated.

Table 2 shows that while normal children receive the bulk of their Se in cereals, meat, fish and dairy products, the only foods reasonably rich in Se available to PKU children are certain cereals which are low in protein. Usually these also have low levels of trace elements,including Se. However, the Se content of foods reflects levels of the mineral in soil on which they are produced. Wheat from high Se areas has been used to increase dietary Se intakes in Finland[5] and New Zealand[6]. While Se-rich wheat would be unsuitable for use in the PKU diet because of its protein content, theoretically maize or other cereals, as well as vegetables low in phenylalanine, which were grown on high Se soils, could be used to increase dietary intake of Se. Certain regions of East and South Australia have elevated soil Se where herbage and cereals have relatively high Se contents. It is proposed that appropriate foodstuffs from these regions be used to provide a PKU diet in which availability, including total content of Se, will be increased to meet the nutritional needs of the children without having to use Se supplements. The possibility of using hydroponically-grown crops in which an Se-rich culture medium has been used, is also being considered.

Table 1 Plasma Selenium and Red Cell Gluthathione Peroxidase
(mean SD)

Subjects	Plasma Se	Red Cell GSHpx
(N)	μmol 1^{-1}	IU/gHb
PKU:		
mean ± SD	0.41 ± 0.19 (16)	14.24 ± 5.54 (19)
range	0.14 - 0.77	7.9 - 27.8
Siblings:		
mean ± SD	0.98 ± 0.15 (12)	22.65 ± 5.22 (16)
range	0.83 - 1.29	14.3 - 32.0

Table 2 Selenium Content and Estimated Daily Intake

Food	Se Content	PKU (n=10)		Siblings (n=10)	
		Amount	Se Intake	Amount	Se
	μg g^{-1} (range)	g/day	μg/day	g/day	μg/day
Cereals	0.09(0.06-0.12)	71	6.4	174	15.7
PKU Bread	0.006	66	0.40	-	-
Meat,Fish	0.21(0.14-0.26)	-	-	74	15.5
Milk,Cheese	0.06(0.05-0.12)	16	1.0	255	15.3
Fruit	0.003 (0.002-0.003)	146	0.44	94	0.28
Vegetables	0.005 (0.001-0.002)	117	0.59	108	0.54
	Total Se Intake (Approx.):		8.83		47.3

REFERENCES

1.   F.W. Alexander, B.E. Clayton and H.T. Delves,
      Quart. J. Med., 1974, 43, 89.
2.   P.J. Aggett and N.T. Davies, J. Inher. Metab. Dis., 1983, 6,
      (Suppl. 1) 22.
3.   C.F. Thomson, C.E. Burton and M.F. Robinson, Br. J. Nutr.,
      1978, 39, 579.
4.   A. Lipson et. al., Aust. Paediatr. J., 1988, 24, 128.
5.   O.A. Levander et. al., Am. J. Clin. Nutr., 1983, 37, 887.
6.   J.H. Watkinson, Am. J. Clin, Nutr., 1981, 34, 936.

INTERACTION OF HEAVY METALS ON THE AVAILABILITY OF
SELENIUM COMPOUNDS TO ARTEMIA SALINA

H. Deelstra, P. Van Dael, R. Van Cauwenbergh and
H. Robberecht

Department of Pharmaceutical Sciences
University of Antwerp
B-2610 Wilrijk, Belgium

1 INTRODUCTION

The uptake of selenium from food largely depends upon its
chemical form. The influence of organic and inorganic
mercury and cadmium upon selenite and selenomethionine
absorption has been studied using Artemia salina as a
model. Dry cysts of Artemia salina can be cultivated and
hatched to adult shrimps quite easily and very quickly[1].

2 MATERIALS AND METHODS

Chemicals

    Sodium selenite and selenomethionine were purchased
from Sigma Chemical Co. St.Louis (USA) and made up to
stock solutions of 1000 ppm.
Cadmium nitrate, cadmium acetate, mercury (II) chloride,
and nitric acid were purchased from Merck, Darmstadt (FRG).
Mercury (II) acetate was obtained by Riedel-De Haen A.G.,
Hanover, (FRG). All heavy metals were made up in stock
solutions of 1000 ppm.

Artemia Salina

    Artemia cysts (Sanders Brine Shrimp Co., Ogden, USA)
were provided by the Artemia Reference Center at the
State University of Ghent (Belgium). The nauplii were
hatched after aerating the cysts for 24 h at 30°C, and
transferred into conical tubes containing specific
concentrations of selenium and heavy metals. After 20 h
of aeration they were hatched, filtered, washed with
deionised water and dried at 60°C.

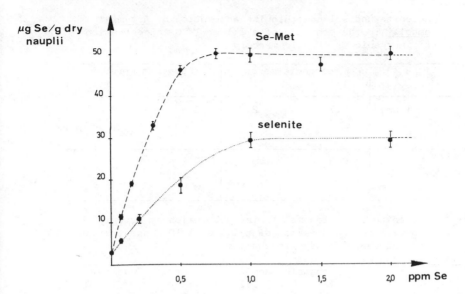

<u>**Figure 1**</u>   Absorption of selenomethionine and selenite
          by <u>Artemia nauplii</u>

<u>Selenium analysis</u>

The dried <u>Artemia nauplii</u> were digested with nitric
acid and the selenium content measured with a flameless
atomic absorption spectrometer (Perkin Elmer 4000 and
HGA 500) as described elsewhere [2].

3 RESULTS AND DISCUSSION

The absorption of selenite respectively selenomethionine
by Artemia is represented in Figure 1.   It is clear that
the <u>Artemia salina</u> has a higher selenium tissue level
after supplementation with selenomethionine rather than
selenite.   This observation is confirmed by numerous
experiments in the literature [3].

The results for selenium absorption in the presence
of different mercury or cadmium compounds are shown in
Tables 1 and 2.   Thus mercury added as chloride shows
a doubling of the Se-tissue levels in the presence of
selenite 1:10 ratio, while in presence of selenomethionine
the level is reduced to more than a half.   When cadmium
is added as nitrate, the Se-tissue level is higher in
presence of the seleno-amino acid compared to selenite.

Table 1   Selenite and selenomethionine absorption by <u>Artemia</u>
           <u>nauplii</u> in the presence of a 1:1 or 1:10 concentration
           of inorganic or organic mercury

| | | Inorganic mercury | | Organic mercury | |
		1:1	1:10	1:1	1:10
selenite	1 ppm	0.7*	2.7	0.3	–
	1.5 ppm	1.0	2.2	0.4	0.4
Se-Met	1 ppm	0.5	0.6	0.5	–
	1.5 ppm	0.4	0.6	0.5	0.8

Table 2   Selenite and selenomethionine absorption by <u>Artemia</u>
           <u>nauplii</u> in the presence of a 1:1 or 1:10 concentration
           of inorganic or organic cadmium

| | | Inorganic cadmium | | Organic cadmium | |
		1:1	1:10	1:1	1:10
selenite	1 ppm	0.5*	1.1	1.0	0.9
	1.5 ppm	–	–	1.2	0.6
Se-Met	1 ppm	0.8	2.3	0.3	0.3
	1.5 ppm	–	–	0.4	0.1

*expressed as ratio of selenium-absorption in the presence of
mercury (or cadmium)/selenium absorption in the absence of the
same metal.

Addition of mercury acetate reduces the tissue selenium
levels in the presence of selenite and selenomethionine.
The same trend is observed for cadmium acetate only in
the case of the seleno-amino acid and tissue selenium
values are not very pronounced.   The interactions of
selenium compounds with mercury and cadmium compounds
appear   complicated;   although various mechanisms have
been proposed these still require confirmation[4].

        4   REFERENCES

1. P. Sorgeloos, 'The brine shrimp Artemia', Vol.3, Universa Press,
    Wetteren, Belgium, 1980.
2. M.A. Deschuytere, Ph.D. Thesis, University of Antwerp, 1987.
3. G.F.Combs & S.B.Combs, 'The role of selenium in nutrition',
    Academic, New York, 1986, p. 187.
4. G.F.Combs & S.B.Combs, 'The role of selenium in nutrition',
    Academic, New York, 1986, p.242.

THE INFLUENCE OF A ZINC- CALCIUM- OR IRON- DEFICIENT DIET ON THE RESORPTION AND KINETICS OF CADMIUM IN THE RAT.

Kollmer, W.E. and Berg, D.

Institut für Strahlenbiologie
Gesellschaft für Strahlen- und Umweltforschung Neuherberg

INTRODUCTION

Metabolic interactions between cadmium and several of essential elements have been described [1]. Its ultimate level in the organs at risk is subject to a number of influences, the resorption in the intestine being only one of them. A dietary deficiency of Ca or Fe leads to an increased accumulation of Cd especially in the kidneys [1]. This is at least partially due to an increased resorption. Zinc deficiency also produces elevated levels of Cd in the kidneys and liver [1], but its specific influence on Cd resorption is less well documented [1]. This experiment compares the influence of Zn-, Ca- and Fe-deficiency on Cd resorption and on the levels in different organs and demonstrates that the determination of "bioavailability" at different sites of the body may yield different results.

MATERIAL AND METHODS

Experimental animals were 32 adult male rats of 169 ± 3g body weight at the beginning of the experiment. The animals were fed a pelleted semipurified diet containing 30 µg Zn, 9500 µg Ca, and 180 µg Fe per g in the controls. In the dietary deficient groups it contained only <2µg Zn, or 799 µg Ca or 6 µg Fe per g respectively. Three weeks afterward 3 mg Cd per litre drinking water was supplied to all animals up to the end of the experiment. After 12 days of Cd supply all animals were transferred to single cages with a wire grid bottom and 4 in each group received 3,7 MBq radioactive Cd 109 in 2 ml of the drinking solution by way of a stomach tube. The administered radioactivity was determined by whole body measurement immediately after the intubation. A follow up of the whole body retention was made by repeated measurements. From these the intestinal resorption

Table 1 Resorption and ^{109}Cd in tissues relative to the
        dose 31d after the administration of the tracer

	% of dose RESORBED	% of the dose x 10^{-3} per g freshw. LIVER	KIDNEY	TIBIA	ERYTHROC.
Controls. (N=3)	0.5±0.1	7.1± 0.2	26± 8	0.3±0.1	0.06±0.02
Zn def. (N=4)	*1.2±0.2	*17.4± 3.1	*69±12	*1.2±0.3	*0.24±0.04
Ca def. (N=4)	*1.2±0.1	*18.8± 3.1	*154±23	*1.8±0.3	*0.18±0.06
Fe def. (N=4)	*4.7±0.6	*152.0±20.0	*194±20	*6.6±0.9	*1.80±0.60

*) statistically significant 2p<0.05 relative to controls

Table 2 Levels of stable Cd in liver and kidney after 43 d
        of exposure to 3 µg Cd/ml in the drinking water

	µg Cd/g freshweight LIVER	KIDNEY	% of the controls LIVER	KIDNEY
Controls. (N=8)	0.15±0.03	0.60± 0.07	100	100
Zn def. (N=8)	0.13±0.02	0.51± 0.07	86	85
Ca def. (N=8)	*0.57±0.05	*5.84± 0.59	380	973
Fe def. (N=8)	*1.79±0.16	*4.37± 0.32	1193	728

*) statistically significant 2p<0.05 relative to controls

Table 3 ^{109}Cd in tissues relative to the resorbed amount
        31d after the administration of the tracer

	% of the resorbed amount per g freshweight LIVER	KIDNEY	TIBIA	ERYTHROC.
Controls. (N=3)	1.4±0.1	5.3± 0.3	0.053±0.011	0.012±0.002
Zn def. (N=4)	1.5±0.1	6.0±0.4	*0.101±0.006	*0.020±0.002
Ca def. (N=4)	1.5±0.2	*12.7±1.2	*0.152±0.013	0.013±0.005
Fe def. (N=4)	*3.2±0.3	*4.2±0.5	*0.140±0.017	*0.040±0.017

*) statistically significant 2p<0.05 relative to controls

was calculated. All animals were killed by bleeding under CO_2 anaesthesia 31 days after the radioactive dose i.e. after 43d supplying stable Cd in the drinking water. The liver, the right kidney and the tibia were recovered and their Cd 109 content measured by γ-spectrometry. Erythrocytes were obtained by centrifuging heparinized blood.The radioactive measurements were corrected for background and decay and the results recorded on a per gram basis of the fresh weights. In the liver and kidney samples Cd was analysed by flameless AAS. The statistical significance was examined by Students t-test after the F-test.

RESULTS AND CONCLUSIONS

At the end of the experiment the body weights of the controls and the Fe-deficient animals were 353 ± 5 and 362 ± 12 g, while those of the Zn- and the Ca-deficient ones were only 313 ± 5 and 307 ± 11 g. Liver and kidney weights were not influenced.The intestinal resorption of Cd was increased under the influence of Zn-, Ca- and Fe-deficiency (Tab.1). The influence of Fe-deficiency on resorption was more efficient than those of Zn and Ca. The retention of tracer in liver, kidney, tibia and erythrocytes as well as the level of stable Cd in liver and kidney was not always proportional to the fractional resorption. This must be attributed to a specific influence of each of the deficiencies on the distribution of Cd within the body. Due to the lower body weights in the Zn- and Ca- deficient groups at the end of the experiment it may be assumed that their water and feed consumption and consequently their Cd intake and levels in the organs might have been decreased. Nevertheless stable Cd in liver and kidneys was higher in the Ca deficient group than in the controls. In the Zn deficient one this was not the case (Tab.2). Thus the assumed lower intake of Cd may have been compensated (Zn def. group) or even overcompensated (Ca def. group) by the increased resorption. From comparing stable (Tab. 2) and tracer (Tab. 3) Cd data it may be concluded that in Ca deficiency Cd is specifically enhanced in the kidney while in Fe deficiency this is the case in the liver. The higher level of the tracer in the tibia of all the dietary deficient groups may be due to a higher uptake or a slower turnover of Cd in bone relative to the controls. In the Zn deficient rats Cd 109 was also high in the erythrocytes.

REFERENCES

1. G.F. Nordberg, T. Kjellström, M. Nordberg, 'Cadmium and Health' L. Friberg, C.G. Elinder, T. Kjellström, G.F Nordberg, CRC Press, Boca Raton, 1985, Vol 1, 103.

TOXICOKINETIC STUDIES OF FLUORIDE IN RABBITS

M. Nedeljković, V. Matović and M. Maksimović

Department of Toxicological Chemistry, School of
Pharmacy, University of Belgrade and Military
Technical Institute - Belgrade Yugoslavia

1 INTRODUCTION

Fluoride is widely distributed in nature. The beneficial
effects of fluoride ion, especially in reducing dental
caries, are well known. However, excessive fluoride
intake can cause adverse or toxic effects. Fluoride may
gain access to the body from the ingestion of water and
food containing increased levels of this ion, originated
from the regions naturally rich in fluorides or contaminated as a result of the manufacturing of superphosphate,
aluminum, steel, etc. A very important route of absorption
is also via the lungs. Incidental sources include ingestion of food contaminated with fluorides used as insecti-
cides and rodenticides.

The aim of this experiment was to define absorption,
distribution and elimination of orally administered sodium
fluoride in rabbits using a suitable pharmacokinetic
model.

2 MATERIALS AND METHODS

Fluoride kinetics were investigated in eight rabbits
Oryctolagus cuniculus-Belgian hare, weighing 2.2-2.7 kg.
Aqueous solution of sodium fluoride was administered by
a ball-tipped animal feeding needle to give single
fluoride dose level of 2.105 mmol F^-/kg (40 mg F^-/kg)
body weight. Blood samples were taken from the ear
arteries 0.15, 0.25, 0.5, 1, 2, 3, 5, 8, 12, 24, 30 and
48 hours after fluoride administration.

The fluoride analyses in blood were carried out
with ion-selective electrode [1], and for preparation of

biological material, a modified procedure without mineralization, was applied.

Blood samples (5 ml) were dried at $55^{\circ}C$ in diffusion cells and treated with 1.5 ml 40% $AgClO_4$ and 1.5 ml 70% $HClO_4$. After microdiffusion, released fluorides were determined in TISAB buffer.

Blood fluoride concentrations <u>versus</u> time curve were analysed using a two-compartment model. All pharmacokinetic data were calculated according to Ritschel[3].

3 RESULTS AND DISCUSSION

The plot of log fluoride blood concentrations <u>versus</u> time following 2.105 mmol F⁻/kg (40 mg F⁻/kg) p.o. in 8 rabbits is shown in Fig.1.

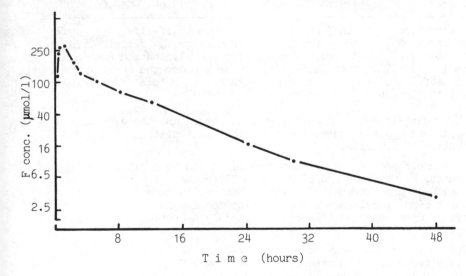

Figure 1 Log blood fluoride concentrations <u>versus</u> time following
an p.o. dose of 2.105 mmol F⁻/kg

The curve was bioexponential so that the two-compartment model was used for data analysis. The various pharmacokinetic parameters were calculated and are presented in Table 1.

The obtained results concerning absorption phase indicate that orally administered sodium fluoride to rabbits is absorbed rapidly. Peak blood levels were reached within less than one hour.

Table 1   Pharmacokinetic parameters of orally administered
          fluoride in rabbits

Pharmacokinetic parameters[a]	Mean ± SD	min - max
K_a, h^{-1}	4.3984 ± 2.4712	2.4148 - 8.8773
$t_{1/2a}$, h	0.20 ± 0.08	0.08 - 0.29
C_{max}, $\mu mol/l$	297.0 ± 47.2	244.0 - 382.4
t_{max}, h	0.88 ± 0.23	0.5 - 1.0
α, h^{-1}	0.3914 ± 0.152	0.2404 - 0.6295
$t_{1/2\alpha}$, h	2.0 ± 0.69	1.10 - 2.88
β, h^{-1}	0.0912 ± 0.0353	0.057 - 0.1663
$t_{1/2\beta}$, h	8.44 ± 2.62	4.17 - 12.15
AUC, $\mu mol/l/h$	2891.4 ± 643.1	2076.0 - 3947.8
Cl_{tot}/F, l/h/kg	1.38 ± 0.31	0.99 - 1.88
Vd/F, l/kg	15.85 ± 2.62	10.04 - 17.66

[a] K_a absorption rate constant, $t_{1/2a}$ absorption half-life, C_{max} peak plasma level, t_{max} time to reach peak plasma level, α distribution rateconstant, $t_{1/2\alpha}$ distribution half-life, β elimination rate constant, $t_{1/2\beta}$ elimination half-life, AUC area under the curve from zero to infinite, Cl_{tot} total body clearance, V_d volume of distribution, F absolute bioavailability.

The mean distribution half-life was 2 hours and the elimination half-life was ca 8.5 hours, showing rather fast distribution and elimination of fluoride.

The rapid decrease of fluoride in blood can be explained by its incorporation into bone and distribution throughout the body, in both intracellular and extracellular water. Sodium fluoride is a soluble salt that readily releases its toxic fluoride ion in the gastrointestinal tract. Once absorbed, fluoride is rapidly excreted through the kidney.

The obtained pharmacokinetic parameters of sodium fluoride in rabbits after oral administration of 2.105 mmol F^-/kg (40 mg F^-/kg body weight) agree with the investigations carried out in humans[4].

REFERENCES

1. J. Tušl, Clin.Chim.Acta, 1970, 27, 216.
2. D. Soldatović and M. Nedeljković, Food and Nutrition, 1969,
    X, 8, 448.
3. W.A. Ritschel, 'Graphic Approach to Clinical Pharmacokinetics',
    J.R. Prous Publishers, Barcelona, 1984, p.78.
4. J. Ekstrand, 'Studies on the Pharmacokinetics of Fluoride in
    Man', Stockholm Karolinska Institutet and Karolinski Hospital, 1977.

INFLUENCE OF PECTIN ON THE AVAILABILITY OF TOXIC AND ESSENTIAL MINERALS IN LEAD EXPOSED PERSONS

R. Macholz, E. Walzel and M. Kujawa

Central institute of Nutrition,
Academy of Sciences of the GDR,
Potsdam-Rehbruecke,
German Democratic Republic

1 INTRODUCTION

Host variables, dietary variables and metabolic variables affect the bioavailability of trace elements. Interaction of the trace elements with complexing agents are most important. Trace elements from plant material exhibit a lower bioavailability in most cases than from animal sources. Polysaccharides like pectin bind minerals in physiological and toxic doses. Trace element ingestion and/or elimination can be enhanced by pectin of different degrees of esterification. The effect of a pectin containing diet on Cd and Pb elimination in exposed workers was investigated.

2 MATERIAL AND METHODS

Volunteers: 10 male workers, (No. 1 - 10) average age 30 years, (25 - 40 y), and average exposure duration 8 years (4 - 15 y) were without drug influences and free from metabolic diseases during the test period.

Test periods: 12 weeks (3 sections)
1 - 3 week (VaA) control (food intake normal)
4 - 9 week (VaB) daily intake of about 8 g pectin as bar
10-12 week (VaC) control
In each case ⅓ of the bar was ingested before the meal.

Composition of the pectin bar:
24% pectin (degree of esterification 39.6%) with 16.5% pectin (degree of esterification 62.5%) and 7.5% Mg/K-polygalacturonate (4.3% Mg/2.3% K)

```
Examinations:  urine (in the morning) 2 times/week
               faeces                  1 times/week
               blood                   1 times/week
```

Determinations: after wet or dry digestion by AAS,
Perkin Elmer model 2380, delta-ALA in urine, reaction
with acetylacetone, p-dimethylaminobenzaldehyde, at 555nm.

3 RESULTS

1. The blood lead level was reduced for ca.30% at
    9 persons (Fig. 1).
    A similar course of the renal excretion of delta-ALA
    was only detectable at 3 volunteers (Fig. 2).

2. The renal Pb-excretion increased up to 130%
    (from 55 to 127 ng Pb/ml urine) (Fig. 3).

3. No significant alteration of the blood Cd-content
    observed, but the renal Cd-excretion was reduced.

4. Negligible losses of essential trace elements were
    found.

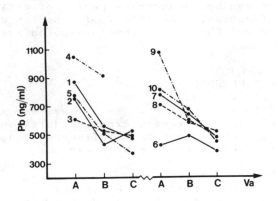

Figure 1:   Lead Concentration in Blood

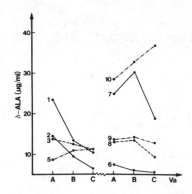

Figure 2:   δ-ALA Content

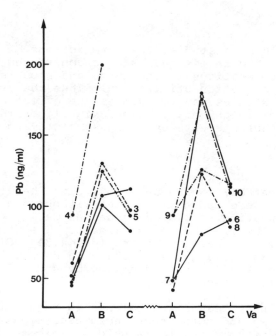

Figure 3:   Pb-excretion <u>via</u> Urine

4 CONCLUSIONS

As a result of our investigations we recommend pectin,
especially highly esterified pectins from vegetables,
with normal food intake, for people exposed to lead.

EFFECT OF DIETARY ANIONS ON MINERAL BIOAVAILABILITY

J.L. Greger, N.M. Lewis, M.S.K. Marcus, A.R. Behling and
S.M. Kaup

Department of Nutritional Sciences
University of Wisconsin
Madison, Wisconsin 53706

1. INTRODUCTION

Many investigators have studied the interactions of
dietary cations. Few investigators have considered the
significance of alterations in the types and amounts of
inorganic anions on cation utilization. Thus the overall
purpose of these studies was to examine the effect of
dietary variations in anions, particularly Cl, on the
utilization of other elements by human subjects and rats.

2. METHODS

During a 56-day metabolic balance study, eight healthy
men (23-30 years) were fed a mixed diet without and with
calcium supplementation ($\approx$ 870 mg Ca/day as $CaCl_2$,
$CaCO_3$ or milk). The diets were isocaloric. The
nutritionally balanced basal diet provided 4.31 g Cl,
3.49 g K, 3.01 g Na, 1.26 g P and 0.70 g Ca daily. The
diets supplemented with $CaCl_2$ and milk provided 5.79
and 5.14 g Cl daily, respectively.

Fecal and urinary losses and balance in regard to Cl,
Na, K, P, Ca and Mg and total renal acid excretion (the
sum of excretion of ammonia, titratable organic acids and
acid buffered by phosphate) were monitored throughout the
study (1).

The effects of variations in level and type of
chloride salts fed were examined in a 58-day study with
male, weanling Sprague-Dawley rats. Thirty rats were fed
one of five diets: a semi-purified basal diet similar to
AIN 76 formulation containing 2.0 mg Cl/g diet or that

diet supplemented with 0.4 mEq Cl/g diet as NaCl, KCl, a combination of lysine-Cl and $CaCO_3$, and $MgCl_2$. The Cl-supplemented diets provided 15.7 mg Cl/g diet.

Growth and water intake of rats were monitored throughout the study. Urinary excretion and tissue levels of Cl, Na, P, Ca and Mg were determined (2).

3. RESULTS

Human Study

Urinary excretion of Cl paralleled Cl intake by human subjects (Table 1). The ingestion of supplemental Ca as $CaCl_2$ rather than as $CaCO_3$ or milk significantly increased renal excretion of ammonia, titratable organic acid, total acid and Ca. Urinary excretion of Mg was greater when $CaCl_2$ rather than $CaCO_3$ was fed. Urinary excretion of Na and K paralleled intake of these elements. Alterations in the anions fed with Ca did not affect plasma levels or balance in regard to the elements studied during the 14-day balance periods.

Rat Study

Rats fed excess Cl excreted 5 to 15-fold more Ca in urine than those animals fed moderate amounts of Cl (Table 2). However, only the animals fed $MgCl_2$ had significantly depressed concentrations of Ca in bone. Urinary excretion of Mg, Na and K was not significantly affected by the level of chloride consumed. Rats fed NaCl and KCl excreted more P in urine than rats fed $MgCl_2$ or Ca with Cl.

The mechanisms by which chloride affected urinary calcium excretion are not known. Endogenous creatinine clearance was not affected by chloride intake but kidneys

Table 1. Urinary excretion of Cl, acid, and Ca by humans

Dietary Treatments	Urine Cl (g/d)	Urine Cl (% intake)	Urine total acid mEq/d	Urine Ca (mg/d)	Urine Ca (% intake)
Basal	4.26 ± 0.14^c*	96	45.0 ± 2.1^c	181 ± 28^d	26
$CaCl_2$	5.80 ± 0.14^a	95	60.0 ± 2.2^a	275 ± 31^a	17
$CaCO_3$	4.39 ± 0.11^c	98	32.0 ± 1.4^d	251 ± 29^b	16
Milk	5.16 ± 0.12^b	99	53.3 ± 2.3^b	228 ± 28^c	15

* Mean ± SEM (n=8) Means in [a] column that do not share a common superscript letter are significantly (p<0.05) different.

Table 2. Urinary excretion of Ca, Cl, and solids and bone Ca concen-
          trations of rats fed various levels and types of Cl salts

Dietary Treatments	Urine Ca (mg/d)	Bone Ca (mg/g)	Urine Cl (mg/d)	Urine Solids (g/d)
Basal	0.3 ± 0.1^{c}*	155 ± 2^{a}	13 ± 1^{c}	0.74 ± 0.04^{c}
NaCl	2.8 ± 0.7^{ab}	151 ± 3^{a}	241 ± 13^{a}	1.22 ± 0.08^{a}
KCl	1.7 ± 0.6^{bc}	$151\pm a^{a}$	208 ± 11^{b}	1.23 ± 0.06^{b}
Ca & Cl	1.8 ± 0.2^{bc}	150 ± 2^{a}	204 ± 7^{b}	1.22 ± 0.04^{a}
$MgCl_2$	4.4 ± 0.1^{a}	135 ± 3^{b}	193 ± 10^{b}	1.01 ± 0.05^{b}

*Mean ± SEM (n=8) Means in a column that do not share a common
superscript letter are significantly ($p<0.05$) different.

(g/100 g body weight) of rats fed excess Cl tended to be
enlarged. The increased excretion of Cl in urine by rats
fed excess Cl was accompanied by increased excretion of
total urine volume and urine solids. Urinary Cl accounted
for only 40-67% of the increase in urine solids when
supplemental Cl was fed.

    Although all rats fed excess Cl excreted more urine,
only rats fed NaCl consumed significantly more water.
Moreover, ingestion of excess Cl did not affect Cl levels
in plasma, liver, kidney or bone.

    4. DISCUSSION

Little is known about the typical Cl content of Western
diets. Thus the significance of interactions between Cl
and Ca in humans has not been adequately assessed.
Alterations in Cl intake are apt to alter acid-base balance
and could ultimately affect bone metabolism.

REFERENCES

1. N.M. Lewis, M.S.K. Marcus, A.R. Behling and J.L.
    Greger, Am. J. Clin. Nutr., 1988, 48 (In Press).

2. M.S. Marcus, S.K. Kaup, N.M. Lewis and J.L. Greger,
    FASEB J., 1988, 2, 746 (abstract).

The Bioavailability of Organic Nutrients and Energy

BIOAVAILABILITY OF FOOD CARBOHYDRATES AS RELATED TO ANALYTICAL METHODS

N.-G. Asp

Chemical Centre, Department of Applied Nutrition
Lund University, Box 124, S-221 00 Lund, Sweden

1 INTRODUCTION

With the exception of some rare sugars, e.g. xylose, food carbohydrates that are absorbed in the intestinal tract are further utilized in the metabolism. Therefore, their bio-availability will be discussed in terms of availability for intestinal absorption.

There are three different and nutritionally important aspects of bioavailability of food carbohydrates: a) rate of small-intestinal absorption, b) extent of small-intestinal absorption, i.e. digestibility, and c) extent (and rate) of colonic fermentation of unabsorbed carbohydrates. Furthermore, the availability for fermentation by dental plaque bacteria is of importance for their cariogenic properties.

Progress in this field during the last few years has lead to a profound revision of concepts regarding the nutritional importance of various food carbohydrates. It has also created a need of analytical methods for a nutritionally relevant classification. This paper reviews mainly the first two aspects of carbohydrate bioavailability.

Quantitatively important food carbohydrates

The principal digestible dietary carbohydrates are the polysaccharide starch from cereals and tubers ; the disaccharides sucrose from added refined sugar, as well as fruits, berries and vegetables, and lactose from milk products ; the monosaccharides glucose and fructose from fruits, berries and vegetables (1). The undigestible poly-saccharides are included in the dietary fibre concept, the

main. components being cellulose, hemicelluloses, pectins
and hydrocolloids (2). The raffinose family of α-galactosides in leguminous seeds, and fructans in cereals and some
vegetables are examples of undigestible oligosaccharides.
The carbohydrate content in various types of diets has been
investigated using the duplicate portion technique (3).

      2 RATE OF ABSORPTION   -   GLYCEMIC RESPONSE

Current dietary guidelines in Western countries include a
recommendation to increase the intake of starchy foods at
the expense of fat and low molecular weight refined carbohydrates (4). A rationale for this is the assumption that
the polymeric starch is more slowly digested and absorbed
than low molecular weight carbohydrates. However, although
frequently cited in textbooks of nutrition, this view has
no experimental support, and it is remarkable that it was
not disproved experimentally until about 10 years ago (5).
It was also shown that the glycemic response to low molecular weight carbohydrates in foods was variable and dependent on such factors as dietary fibre content and structural
integrity of the foods (6).

Physiological importance of the glycemic response

     A prime therapeutic goal in the treatment of diabetes
is to normalize blood glucose levels and glucose metabolism. It is, therefore, natural that the classification of
carbohydrates into "slow" and "rapid" ones regarding the
glycemic response has been discussed mainly when defining
an optimal diabetic diet. Slow carbohydrates would be important for avoiding blood glucose fluctuations and for
diminishing the insulin requirement.

     However, slow carbohydrates would be advantageous also
in the prevention and treatment of other nutritionally
related disorders - including obesity, hyperlipidemia and
hypertension - with concommittant high risk especially for
cardiovascular complications. There is increasing evidence
for a central role of hyperinsulinemia in these disorders
(7). Choice of "lente" foods (8) would be an important
feature of a nutritious diet also in the future, but the
basis for such a classification has changed dramatically.

Overview of digestion and absorption of carbohydrates

     The digestion of dietary starch begins during chewing,
when the salivary amylase is mixed into the food. This is
an α-amylase, cleaving the α-1,4 linkages of amylose and

amylopectin randomly.

The pancreatic α-amylase completes the luminal starch digestion, leaving a mixture of oligosaccharides - maltose, maltotriose, and dextrins including the α-1,6 linkages of the branching points of amylopectin. These hydrolysis products, as well as the dietary disaccharides, are then hydrolysed to monosaccharides by the disaccharidases, attached by an anchor protein to the brush border membrane of the small-intestinal enterocytes (9). Before reaching these enzymes, the oligosaccharides have to diffuse through an unstirred water layer covering the mucosal epithelial cell surface. The mucins secreted by goblet cells are an important component of this surface layer, as well as the glycoproteins linked to the brush border membrane and referred to as the glycocalyx.

The monosaccharides are transported through the brush border membrane by carrier mechanisms spatially closely related to the disaccharidases. There are probably two different carriers for glucose and galactose, that are sodium dependent, i.e. transport against a concentration gradient is driven by co-transport of sodium ions. Fructose is transported by a separate, sodium independent pathway (10).

The monosaccharide absorption seems to be the rate limiting step in the digestion/absorption of carbohydrates in solution. This has been demonstrated by measuring disappearance rates of various carbohydrates in intestinal perfusion experiments, both in experimental animals and in man, and by showing similar glycemic responses by feeding solutions of starch, starch hydrolysates and glucose (5). Only when the lactase activity approaches levels character-istic of primary low lactase activity, it becomes rate limiting for lactose absorption (11).

When carbohydrates occur naturally in foods, the situation is more complex. Steps during which the rate of digestion and/or absorption may be influenced by food constituents or structural properties of the food include chewing, gastric emptying, small-intestinal mixing and transport, effects on the unstirred water layer thickness, inhibition of amylase, inhibition of disaccharidases, inhibition of monosaccharide transport, effects on mucosal morphology, and gastro-intestinal hormone release.

Measurement of the glycemic response - the glycemic index

The glycemic response after a carbohydrate containing

test meal is usually measured by capillary or venous blood
sampling every 10-15 min during the first hour and with
longer intervals during the following hours (12). Continuous venous blood glucose monitoring has been used in some
studies, including those from our group (13). It allows a
more detailed study of various phases of the blood glucose
curve, but is not necessary for the classification of foods
regarding their glycemic response.

The blood glucose level is the result of a dynamic
equilibrium between intestinal carbohydrate absorption,
liver glycogen formation/breakdown, gluconeogenesis, and
peripheral glucose uptake. This, in turn, is determined by
the insulin response and the peripheral insulin sensitivity
and by a number of other hormones. Thus, the glycemic
response is influenced by many factors in addition to the
rate of intestinal carbohydrate absorption. It cannot
therefore be used as an absolute measure.

To overcome some of these difficulties, Jenkins' group
introduced the glycemic index (GI), defined as the incre-
mental area under the glucose curve during 2 hours after a
test meal, divided by the area after a control meal in the
same individual (12). A large number of foods have now
been classified according to their GI (14). The GI obtained by testing healthy volunteers is correlated with that
obtained in diabetics, although with a different amplitude
of response. The GI obtained with single food items seems
to predict GI of mixed meals (14).

In non-diabetic subjects, measurement of the insulin
response may be more sensitive in differentiating foods.
Thus, incorporation of sugar beet fibre into a breakfast
meal diminished the glycemic response in type II diabetics
(13), but not in healthy volunteers, who showed instead a
diminished insulin response (15).

In vitro techniques for predicting glycemic response

The rate of starch degradation with α-amylase *in vitro*
correlates with the glycemic response of variously processed cereals, especially when preceded by a pepsin step (16).
A technique measuring the liberation of oligosaccharides
from a dialysis bag containing a food sample and human
digestive juices has shown a correlation with the glycemic
index (17). Such techniques are especially useful when comparing, for instance, variously processed, but otherwise
similar foods.

Dental plaque fermentation

Acid production through fermentation of carbohydrates in dental plaque is important in the pathogenesis of caries. Low molecular weight sugars - especially monosaccharides and sucrose - are readily available. However, there has been an increased interest in starch as a potentially cariogenic carbohydrate. We found a good correlation between in vitro susceptibility to α-amylase of the starch in variously processed cereals, and drop in dental plaque pH after rinsing the mouth with suspensions of the samples (18).

3 DIGESTIBILITY - DIETARY FIBRE

Carbohydrate digestibility is the basis of the dietary fibre concept, and the definition as polysaccharides and lignin that are not digested by indigenous enzymes of the human gastro-intestinal tract (19) has been widely accepted. This definition is the basis for a nutritionally relevant initial classification of carbohydrates. Although not a carbohydrate, there are reasons to include lignin in the dietary fibre concept : it is undigestible and it has a close structural and functional relationship to the main dietary fibre polysaccharides.

Starch has generally been regarded as completely digested in the small intestine, at least when fully gelatinized. It is now well documented that certain starch fractions are undigestible in the small intestine, but fermented in the large bowel, similarly to non-starch polysaccharides (20). This complicates the definition and analysis of dietary fibre (see below).

Some oligosaccharides, such as the raffinose family of α-galactosides, are undigestible due to the absence of α-galactosidase activity in the small intestine. Cereal fructans, that have recently been characterized, show a similar behaviour (21).

Due to the widespread occurrence of primary low lactase activity, it can be argued whether lactose should be regarded as a digestible carbohydrate. There is generally a residual lactase activity capable of hydrolysing small or moderate amounts of lactose (22). Furthermore, a high milk consumption is uncommon in populations with low lactase activity. In practice, therefore, lactose can generally be regarded as a digestible carbohydrate.

Measurement of digestibility

　　Balance studies in man or experimental animals have
the disadvantage of not being able to distinguish between
small-intestinal absorption and fermentation. Therefore,
the following four techniques have been used recently to
study digestibility in vivo:
　　The ileostomy model. Studies on subjects operated
on with an ileostomy allows direct measurement of carbohydrates and other nutrients leaving the small intestine.
Short balance periods (1-2 days) can be used. With this
technique, the main non-starch polysaccharides have been
demonstrated to be practically undigestible in man (23,24).
　　Antibiotic suppression of the intestinal flora.
Balance experiments with rats receiving broad spectrum
antibiotics to suppress the instestinal flora offer a useful alternative to germfree rats. Easily fermented non-
starch polysaccharides, as well as "resistant starch" have
been recovered quantitatively in faeces in such experiments
(25,26).
　　Breath hydrogen excretion. Hydrogen is formed during
fermentation of carbohydrates in the large intestine.
This is the basis for breath hydrogen determination to
measure carbohydrate malabsorption as well as small-
intestinal transit (27).
　　In vitro techniques. Measurement of carbohydrates
that resist digestive enzymes is the basis for analysis
methods for dietary fibre and will be dealt with below.

　　　4 FOOD PROPERTIES INFLUENCING THE RATE AND EXTENT
　　　　OF CARBOHYDRATE DIGESTION AND ABSORPTION

Although much research is still needed to describe in
detail the factors influencing the glycemic response and
digestibility of food carbohydrates, some features can be
distinguished as important.

Determinants of carbohydrate digestion and absorption
　　Gross and cellular structure. The low GI of rice is
related to its particle size. Milling to flour increases
the GI considerably, approaching the level of potatoes
(28). Similarly, pumpernickel type bread and bulgur show a
lower GI than bread baked with flour (29). Mashing apples
to puré increases the GI (6). An intact cellular structure
in leguminous seeds also after boiling seems to be an important factor explaining the very low glycemic response to
these foods (30).
　　Dietary fibre. It is well documented that soluble,
viscous types of dietary fibre, such as guar gum and pec-

tin, reduce the glycemic response when incorporated into a meal. Mechanisms that have been demonstrated include delay of gastric emptying and inhibition of mixing and transport of the small-intestinal content, as well as diffusion over the intestinal mucosal cell surface (5, 31). The soluble viscous rye pentosans and ß-glucans are probably important for the lower glycemic response to rye bread than to wheat bread (32).

Starch gelatinization. Native starch granules are hydrolysed very slowly by amylases, and produce a very low glycemic response. Gelatinization during heating increases the susceptibility of starch to amylases. There is a close correlation between degree of starch gelatinization and glycemic response in vivo (33), and much of the difference in glycemic response between variously processed cereal foods can be explained in terms of differences in degree of gelatinization. However, even fully gelatinized products may differ when processed by different methods (16).

Amylose/amylopectin ratio. The glycemic response to various types of rice has been negatively correlated with the amylose/amylopectin ratio (34), which is possibly related to amylose-lipid complexes.

Starch/lipid complexes. The inclusion complexes of amylose and polar lipids display a low susceptibility to amylases in vitro and give a lower glycemic response than free amylose in vivo (35).

Starch/protein interactions. The presence of protein structures encapsulating starch has been reported to limit the rate of enzymic starch degradation (36). Addition of a protease step in an in vitro assay of the rate of enzymic starch degradation improved the correlation with the glycemic response in vivo (16). Starch/protein interactions have been suggested to influence both starch digestibility and glycemic index of bread (37), but further studies are needed to substantiate the presence of such interactions.

Retrogradation. The recrystallization of starch molecules during cooling and storage is referred to as retrogradation. We found no effect of amylopectin retrogradation on the susceptibility of starch in whole grain wheat bread to amylase (38). On the other hand, retrogradation of amylose seems to be the main mechanism behind "resistant starch" formation (39).

Enzyme inhibitors. Various antinutrients such as polyphenols, phytic acid and lectins, which are present mainly in leguminous seeds, have been reported to inhibit in vitro starch hydrolysis and to lower the glycemic index (40). Tannic acid significantly inhibits both amylases and intestinal maltase activity (41).

5 DIETARY FIBRE ANALYSIS

There are two basically different ways of measuring dietary
fibre: 1) The gravimetric methods, in which an undigestible
residue is measured and corrected for non-fibre material,
and 2) the component analysis methods, in which dietary
fibre constituents are measured more or less specifically
and summed up to a total fibre value. Modern methods have
been reviewed elsewhere (2,42).

   In the present controversy whether to use a gravimetric method or a component analysis method for the
purpose of measuring total dietary fibre (43,44), it is
often overlooked that these approaches are quite different
regarding wealth of details and need of analytical equipment and skill. Because we usually do not add individual
amino-acids to obtain total protein, or individual fatty
acid to obtain total fat, there is no need for determining
individual dietary fibre monomers to obtain total fibre.
The enzymic gravimetric method of the AOAC (45) has proved
useful for the proximate analysis of foods. This and similar methods (46) can be used also for the separate assay
of soluble and insoluble fibre, and show good agreement
with component analysis methods measuring resistant starch
and lignin as dietary fibre (47). The exclusion of these
components from the dietary fibre concept, as advocated by
Englyst et al. (43), would be a step backwards to a more
limited and nutritionally less meaningful concept and
measurement of dietary fibre.

6 PROXIMATE ANALYSIS AND LABELLING OF CARBOHYDRATES

Determination of dietary fibre with an enzymic, gravimetric
method (45,46) provides a possibility to make a primary
classification into digestible (available) and undigestible
carbohydrates. For most foods, this gives nutritionally
relevant information.

REFERENCES

1. D.A.T. Southgate, 'Determination of Food Carbohydrates'
    Applied Science Publishers Ltd, London, 1976.
2. N.-G. Asp, Molec. Aspects Med., 1987, 9, 17.
3. M. Abdulla et al., Am. J. Clin. Nutr., 1983, 40, 325.
4. A.S. Truswell, Am. J. Clin. Nutr., 1987, 45, 1060.
5. M.L. Wahlqvist, Am. J. Clin. Nutr., 1987, 45, 1232.
6. G.B. Haber et al., Lancet, 1977, ii, 679.
7. R.W. Stout, Lancet, 1987, i, 1077.

8. D.J.A. Jenkins, Diabetes Care, 1982, 5, 634.
9. A. Dahlqvist and G. Semenza, J. Pediatr. Gastroenterol. Nutr., 1985, 4, 857.
10. U. Hopfer, 'Physiology of the Gastrointestinal Tract', Ed. L. R. Johnson, Raven Press, New York, 1987, p.1499.
11. E. Gudmand-Höyer and S. Jarnum, Scand. J. Gastroent., 1968, 3, 129.
12. D.J.A. Jenkins et al., Am. J. Clin Nutr., 1981,34, 362.
13. B. Hagander et al., Diabetes Research, 1986, 3, 91.
14. D.J.A. Jenkins et al., 'Dietary Fiber. Basic and Clinical Aspects', Ed. G.V. Vahouny, D. Kritchevsky, Plenum Press, New York and London, 1986, p. 167.
15. B. Hagander, Human Nutr./Applied Nutr.,1988, in press.
16. J. Holm et al., J. Cereal Sci., 1985, 3, 207.
17. D.J.A. Jenkins, Diabetologia, 1982, 22, 450.
18. J. Holm, Thesis, Univ. of Lund, Chemical Centre, 1988.
19. H.G. Trowell et al., Lancet, 1976, i, 967.
20. J.H. Cummings and H.N. Englyst, Am. J. Clin. Nutr., 1987, 45, 1243.
21. U. Nilsson and I. Björck, J. Nutrition, 1988, in press.
22. N.-G. Asp and A. Dahlqvist, Enzyme, 1974, 18, 84.
23. A.-S. Sandberg et al., Br. J. Nutr., 1981, 45, 283.
24. A.-S. Sandberg, Näringsforskning, 1983, 27, 37.
25. I. Björck et al., J. Cereal Sci., 1986, 4, 1.
26. I. Björck et al., J. Cereal Sci., 1987, 6, 159.
27. F. R. Steggerda, Ann. N. Y. Acad. Sci., 1968, 150, 57.
28. K. O'Dea et al., Am. J. Clin. Nutr., 1980, 33, 760.
29. D.J.A. Jenkins et al., Am. J. Clin. Nutr., 1986,43,516.
30. P. Würsch et al., Am. J. Clin. Nutr., 1986, 43, 25.
31. B. Elsenhans et al., Clin. Sci., 1980, 59, 373.
32. B. Hagander et al., Diab. Research Clin. Practice, 1987, 3, 85.
33. J. Holm et al., Am. J. Clin. Nutr., 1988, 48, in press.
34. M.S. Goddard et al., Am. J. Clin. Nutr., 1984, 39, 388.
35. J. Holm et al., Stärke/Starch, 1983, 35, 294.
36. P. T. Slack et al., J. Inst. Brew., 1979, 85, 112.
37. D.J.A. Jenkins et al., Am. J. Clin. Nutr., 1987,45,946.
38. M. Siljeström et al., Cereal Chem., 1988, 65, 1.
39. C. Berry, J. Cereal Sci., 1986, 4, 301.
40. L.U. Thomson and J.H. Yoon, J. Food Sci., 1984,49,1228.
41. I.M. Björck and M.E. Nyman, J. Food Sci., 1987,52,1588.
42. N.-G. Asp and C.-G. Johansson, Nutr. Abstracts and Reviews. Reviews in Clin. Nutr., 1984, 54, 735.
43. H.N. Englyst et al., Am. J. Clin. Nutr., 1987, 46, 873.
44. N.-G. Asp, Am. J. Clin. Nutr., 1988, 48, 688.
45. L. Prosky et al., J.Assoc.Off.Anal.Chem., 1985, 68,677.
46. N.-G. Asp et al. J. Agric. Food Chem., 1983, 31, 476.
47. O. Theander and E. Westerlund, J. Agric. Food Chem., 1986, 34, 330.

PREDICTION OF ENERGY AVAILABILITY FROM THE COMPOSITION OF HUMAN DIETS CONTAINING VARIOUS QUANTITIES AND SOURCES OF UNAVAILABLE CARBOHYDRATES.

G. Livesey

AFRC Institute of Food Research
Colney Lane, Norwich, NR4 7UA

The extent to which dietary fibre and resistant starch
contribute to the availability of energy from human diets
is assuming great importance. Regulatory bodies need to
know the energy values of fibre and starches to enable
judgement on the accuracy of low-energy claims for
high-fibre and related products. This extends also to
low-calorie bulking agents. However, even for fibre in
diets of whole foods, (let alone fibre isolates provided
as supplements or low-calorie bulking agents) there is
uncertainty about energy value. Various studies attribute
different values. Partly this arises because of a lack of
distinction between apparent energy value which gives that
energy contributed to the energy value of the whole diet
from the fibre per se and which is derived from a nutrient
balance study with a single diet, and partial energy value
which combines in a single value the energy made available
from the fibre per se with the effects of the fibre on the
apparent availability of energy from other components of
the diet and which is derived from an energy balance study
with two diets differing in the quantity of fibre.
Different suggested energy values can also arise through
the use of different calculation procedures for analysing
raw energy balance data, with some procedures, although
correct in principle, being subject to large errors due to
magnification of measurement errors. Since apparent and
partial digestible energy values may differ for
unavailable carbohydrate (UC, a term used subsequently in
preference to dietary fibre because of the possibility of
some fibre analytical values including resistant starch),
the question of which, partial or apparent, value should
be used for the calculation of the energy value of foods.

An analysis of data taken or calculated from

published work shows that all plots of the digestibility
of dietary gross energy against the proportion of gross
energy intake due to UC, extrapolate back to 0.978 (sd
0.007, n=13 diet pairs) for the digestibility of energy
for a diet free of UC. The slopes of such plots are
always negative because the partial digestibility of
energy for UC is always less than that for other dietary
components. However, the slopes differ significantly
between studies (diets) and this cannot be attributed to
the use of different analytical methods for UC. The
different slopes could indicate the UC in each study
differed with different partial energy values. The slopes
(S) of these plots relate to the apparent digestibility of
UC (α) such that $S = (1.77-4.46\alpha)^{-1}$. An equation
predicting the digestible energy value of the whole diet
[DE (kJ)=0.978 gross energy (kJ)-17.2xSxUC (g) with S
predicted from α] performed better than previously
suggested equations (Atwater, British, Levy et al,
Southgate and Miller and Judd) on 17 diets with between 8
and 93g UC per day. This indicates that the energy value
of the whole diet is closely associated with or directly
influenced by the occurrence, utilization and effects (on
protein and fat utilization) of UC. That is, UC appears
to be the major determinant of the digestibility of energy
for whole diets and this justifies the use of partial
rather than apparent energy values for UC when calculating
whole dietary energy values.

It should be remembered that energy values for
different components of the diet are used in combination
with an aim to calculate the energy value of the whole
diet. Components, like UC which have effects on the
apparent digestibility of other dietary components would
require two energy factors if apparent digestible energy
values have to be applied; one to account for energy
available from the UC per se and another to account for
effects on the utilization of other dietary components.
Hence, it is appropriate to combine these into a single
factor, called the partial digestible energy value. An
alternative would be to apply the apparent digestible
energy values for UC and have values for fat and protein
continually adjusted in accordance both with the
quantities of UC ingested and with its effects on the
apparent digestibility of proteins and fat. This seems
too cumbersome to contemplate further.

Presently, in Britain and increasingly in other parts
of the world (e.g. USA, West Germany) the energy value for
UC is considered to be zero. This arises from the work of
Southgate and Durnin and is a partial energy value. There

is a small point of principle to be made. It is that partial digestible energy values for UC are not strictly compatible with the energy conversion factors for fat and protein, as used in the Atwater and British general systems of food energy assessment. This is because in principle, they should be used with apparent energy values for protein and fat appropriate for diets of zero intake of UC. Such data obtained by extrapolation from plots of apparent digestibility for fat or protein against UC intake give^2 values of 0.963 (se 0.05) and 0.931 (se 0.004) for fat and protein respectively. These compare with 0.95 and 0.95 for fat in the reports of Merril and Watt and Southgate and Durnin respectively and 0.92 and 0.90 for protein in these reports respectively. For fat this new apparent digestibility corresponds to a caloric conversion factor of 9.05 rather than Atwater's 8.93 (kcal/g) (both round to 9) but for protein a value of 4.1 rather than 4.0 kcal/g would seem more appropriate. The question now is what really is the partial digestible energy value for UC?

The partial digestible energy value for UC in diets (calculable as 17.2(1-absolute value of S) kJ/g) is not found to be constant at 0kJ/g a value implied in the British system of food energy assessment but ranges between -20 and +10 kJ/g. While this range can be attributed to differences in apparent digestibility of UC ranging between 0.5 and 0.8, (corresponding to apparent digestible energy values between 8.6 and 14 kJ/g), the cause of the differences in digestibility of UC between diets for groups of subjects (n>5) needs clarification. A partial explanation could be the different proportions of resistant starch in the analytic value for UC as well as the different non-starch polysaccharides some of which will be soluble and highly digestible and others which will be insoluble and have low digestibilities. It must be noted also that supplements or isolates of UC appear not to behave like UC in whole diets (due to food matrix effects?) and tend to have more similar but not identical partial and apparent energy values because of small effects on losses of protein and fat to faeces.

1.   Livesey, G. (1988). Food energy values - old values and new perspectives. British Nutrition Foundation Bulletin 13, 9-28.
2.   Livesey, G. and Davies, I.R. (1987). Caloric value of fibre and guar gum. In: Low-calorie products (G. Birch and M. Lindley eds.) Applied Science Publishers: London.

USE OF BREATH HYDROGEN ANALYSIS IN THE STUDY OF STARCH ABSORPTION IN MAN

I.T. Johnson, E. Lund and J.M. Gee

Department of Nutrition and Food Quality
AFRC Institute of Food Research - Norwich Laboratory
Colney Lane, Norwich NR4 7UA

1 INTRODUCTION

Recent studies suggest that a significant proportion
of dietary starch escapes digestion in the human small
intestine and undergoes fermentation in the colon [1].
Some of this material is chemically resistant to
pancreatic enzymes because of the retrogradation of
amylose after gelatinisation [2]. Another fraction
appears to be starch which is physically protected
from hydrolysis by the food matrix. In this study the
quantity of starch reaching the colon after raw or
cooked test meals of oats was assessed by monitoring
breath hydrogen production in volunteers. The rate
and extent of starch hydrolysis in raw and cooked
rolled oats was also measured using a simulated
digestion technique in vitro.

2 METHOD

Breath Hydrogen Study

Eight healthy volunteers collected 25ml samples
of expired alveolar air in disposable syringes, at 30
min intervals, for approximately 10 h after waking.
On a single occasion each subject fasted until
lunchtime and then ate a self-selected snack meal.
The results of this run were used to define a baseline, which was subtracted from all experimental runs.
On 6 subsequent occasions each subject consumed 50g of
rolled oats, with 100ml skimmed milk and sucrose to
taste, either raw, or after boiling for 1 minute in
300ml of water. No other food besides the same self-
selected lunch was consumed during the collection
periods.

Breath-samples were analysed using a clinical breath-
hydrogen monitor and hydrogen concentration was
plotted against sampling time. Areas under the curves
were calculated, and each subject's breath hydrogen
production (ppm.h), for the 9 h following the test
breakfast, was estimated from the mean of the
triplicate runs. The significance of differences
between meals was assessed using a t-test for paired
observations.

Simulated Digestion Study

Samples of raw rolled oats (10g) were added to 100ml
of Krebs bicarbonate buffer, and either soaked at room
temperature or boiled for 5 min. Both samples were
then acidified (pH 2) with concentrated HCl, stirred
for 1 h at 37 , and homogenised. The samples were
then neutralised (pH 7.2) with NaOH. Porcine α-
amylase (ca, 65 units/ml) and pronase (ca, 5 units/ml)
were then added, and the solution was stirred
continuously for 180 min at 37 . A single sub-sample
for dry weight determination (oven dried; 85° o/n) and
duplicate samples for ethanol extraction (1.5ml. added
to 20ml 90% w/v ethanol), were removed at the time
intervals shown in Fig 1. The free sugar content of
each sample was determined using the anthrone method.

    3 RESULTS

The production of breath hydrogen by individual
subjects is compared in Fig. 1. There was a striking
variation in hydrogen output between individuals
consuming the same quantity of oats but seven of the
subjects produced less hydrogen in response to the
cooked test-meal. The mean difference, of
approximately 30%, was statistically significant (p
<0.02).

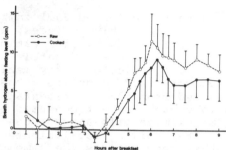

Figure 1. Breath hydrogen production

The time course for the enzymic degradation of cooked and raw rolled oats is shown in Fig. 2. The initial rate of starch hydrolysis in cooked oats was over twice that of raw oats, and the final extent of starch hydrolysis after 180 min (<u>ca</u>, 90%) was also approximately 2 fold higher.

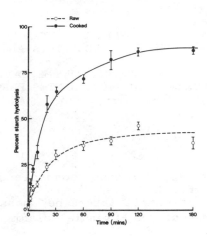

<u>Figure 2.</u> Simulated digestion of oat starch

4 CONCLUSION

The breath hydrogen technique provides an indirect measurement of carbohydrate fermentation, which is complicated by the contribution from non-starch polysaccharides and is evidently subject to wide individual variations. Nevertheless the results of the human trial were consistent with the evidence obtained <u>in vitro</u>. The starch component of rolled oats becomes more susceptible to amylolysis after gelatinisation, even under the relatively mild conditions used to prepare porridge. The quantity of carbohydrate reaching the colon after a meal of oats therefore depends partly upon the methods used to prepare it for consumption.

REFERENCES

1. A.M. Stephen, A.C. Haddad and S.F. Phillips, <u>Gastroenterol.</u>, 1983 <u>85</u>, 589.
2. S.G. Ring, J.M. Gee, M. Whittam, P. Orford and I.T. Johnson, <u>Food Chem.</u>, 1988, <u>28</u>, 97.

INFLUENCE OF COOKING TIME
ON PASTA STARCH CHARACTERISTICS AND NUTRITIONAL FEATURE

BARRY J.L., CLOAREC D., BORNET F., COLONNA P.,
GOUILLOU S., GALMICHE J.P., DELORT-LAVAL J.

GIS NUTRITION GLUCIDIQUE DE L'HOMME SAIN
1, Place Alexis Ricordeau 44000 NANTES FRANCE

INTRODUCTION

When cooked in standardized conditions, pasta starch is digested as follows:
- slowly digested in the small intestine, pasta starch leads to a low increase of post-prandial plasma glucose[1] and insulin responses
- as most of starchy foods, some starch reaches the end of the ileum and is then fermented in the colon[2].

The aim of this study was to determine how variations of cooking time of pasta could modify pasta digestion by simultaneously measuring parameters linked to either digestion in the small intestine (glycemic and insulinemic responses) or fermentation of indigested starch in the colon (hydrogen (H_2) breath excretion).

MATERIAL AND METHODS

Pasta (spaghetti) were cooked for 11 minutes (T1= standardized cooking time), 16.5 minutes (T2= T1 X 1.5) or 22 minutes (T3= T1 X 2).

Starch was characterized by X-ray diffraction, differential scanning calorimetry (DSC) and in vitro α-amylase susceptibility.

12 healthy subjects (6 males - 6 females; mean age: 22 years) were selected after a lactulose test (breath H_2 excretion with 10 g of ingested lactulose) and an oral glucose tolerance test (glycemic and insulinemic responses with 55.5 g of ingested glucose). They received in a randomly assigned order the 3 types of pasta (50 g of starch = 55.5 g of glucose) on 3 different days. Peripheric venous blood was sampled for

3 hours and analyzed for glucose and insulin. Expired
breath air was sampled for 9 hours and analyzed for H_2.

RESULTS AND DISCUSSION

X-ray diffraction and DSC showed that starch was
completely gelatinized whatever cooking time. Moreover,
in vitro α-amylase susceptibility was identical with the
3 times of cooking.
Glycemic (fig. 1) and insulinemic (fig. 2)
responses were identical whatever the cooking time as
already shown by WOLEVER et al. (1986)[3].

FIGURE 1
INFLUENCE OF PASTA COOKING TIME
ON POSTPRANDIAL PLASMA GLUCOSE CONCENTRATION

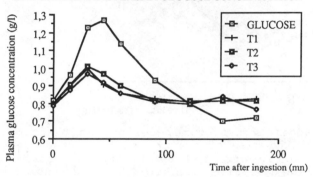

FIGURE 2
INFLUENCE OF PASTA COOKING TIME
ON POSTPRANDIAL PLASMA INSULIN CONCENTRATION

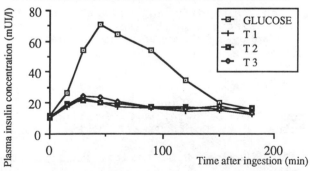

Glycemic indexes (59±15, 65±15, 46±10) and insulinic
indexes (26±4, 28±6, 26±6) for T1, T2 and T3
respectively were not significantly modified by cooking

time.
  Increased breath H_2 excretion with the 3 meals
(fig. 3) indicates that a fraction of pasta starch
escaped intestinal digestion: this result is in
agreement with the findings of ANDERSON et al.(1981)[2].
The absence of significative difference in H_2 excretion
shows that ileal starch digestibility was not affected
by cooking time.

FIGURE 3
INFLUENCE OF PASTA COOKING TIME
ON BREATH HYDROGEN CONCENTRATION (ppm)

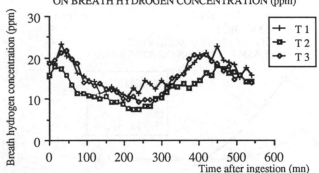

  Mean oro-caecal transit time, defined as the time
between ingestion and rise of breath H_2 above baseline,
was not significantly affected by length of cooking
(274±27, 238±33 and 278±18 min for T1, T2 and T3
respectively).

CONCLUSION

  Overcooking does not modify nutritional value of
pastas which remain caracterized by low glycemic and
insulinemic indexes and by small amounts of indigestible
starch.

REFERENCES

1. D.J.A. Jenkins, T.M.S. Wolever R.H. Taylor, H.
Barker, H. Fielden, J.M. Baldwin, A.C. Bowling, H.C.
Newman, A.L. Jenkins, D.V. Goff, Am. J. Clin. Nutr.,
1981, 34, 362.
2. I.H. Anderson, A.S. Levine, M.D. Levitt, N. Engl. J.
Med., 1981, 304, 891.
3. T.M.S. Wolever, D.J.A. Jenkins, J. Kalmuski, C.
Giordano, S. Guidici, A.L. Jenkins, L.U. Thompson, G.S.
Wong, R.G. Josse, Diabetes Care, 1986, 9, 401.

THE UTILISATION OF α-AMYLASE RESISTANT CORN AND PEA STARCHES IN
THE RAT

R.M. Faulks, S. Southon and G. Livesey

Institute of Food Research Norwich Laboratory
Colney Lane
Norwich NR4 7UA

1 INTRODUCTION

A proportion of the starch in cooked foods may become resistant to
α-amylase hydrolysis in vitro[1] due to retrogradation[2] and the
formation of starch complexes[3].
It is not known to what extent resistant starches (RS) escape
digestion and absorption in the small intestine, if they undergo
fermentation, whether there is an adaptation to long term feeding
or if they have any of those properties normally associated with
dietary fibre.
In this study the utilisation and physiological effects of in
vitro α-amylase resistant starches isolated from retrograded pea
and maize starch gels was investigated in the rat.

Experimental Design

Male Wistar rats (150) 100g. were randomly allocated to
one of 5 dietary treatments. All animals were given a fibre free
semi-synthetic control diet (SS) ad-lib for 13d. On day 14 rats
in each dietary treatment given one of the following diets: diet
1. fibre free (SS) diet (Control) diets 2-5, control (SS) diet
with the addition of 100g/kg of sucrose (Sucrose group), Solka-
floc (Cellulose group), resistant corn starch (RSC group) or
resistant pea starch (RPS group). In order to assess any
adaptation the animals were fed the experimental diet for up to
30d.
Each of the dietary groups consisted of 3 groups of 10 rats which
were killed after 8/9, 17/18 or 29/30 days respectively. From day
14 of the study food intake was limited to 12g/d for 20 days and
14g/d thereafter for rats fed diet 1, animals fed diets 2-5
received 10% more diet each day to allow for the addition of the
test material.

Faecal collections were made daily and body weights recorded
regularly.
Small intestinal (SI) length, ileal (distal 50% of SI) and caecal
tissue wet and dry weights were recorded. The ileal and caecal
contents were collected for wet and dry weights and the caecal pH
measured. The carbohydrate content of the dry digesta from the
ileum, caecum and faeces was measured as glucose after acid
hydrolysis.

Results and Discussion

        Only traces of carbohydrate were found in the ileal and
caecal digesta from the Control and Sucrose groups. Carbohydrate
found at these sites in other groups was attributable to
unabsorbed carbohydrate from cellulose or the resistant starches.
The dry ileal contents contained 50% carbohydrate in the Cellulose
and RPS groups but only 25% in the RCS group at both 8/9 and
17/18d. This indicated that RPS is as resistant to digestion as
cellulose in the SI and that RCS undergoes some limited digestion.
There was no indication of adaptation in the SI in any of the
groups over this period. The percentage carbohydrate in the dry
ileal and caecal contents was similar in the rats fed the
cellulose supplemented diet for 8/9 and 17/18d. However in the
RCS and RPS fed rats the percentage carbohydrate in the dry caecal
contents was much lower than that in the dry ileal contents
falling from 25% to 7% and 45% to 11% between the two sites at
8/9d and 28% to 0.6% and 50% to 18% by 17/18d for RCS and RPS
respectively.
After the first few days on the test diets the dry faeces from the
Cellulose group contained a relatively constant amount of
carbohydrate (65% w/w) but in the RPS and RCS groups the
percentage faecal carbohydrate declined with time from values of
40% and 20% respectively (Fig. 1) After 4d the carbohydrate
content of the dry faeces from the RCS group had fallen to 2% and
then remained constant but that from the RPS group fell gradually
to 10% over the 17/18d period. Faecal dry matter output was
relatively constant within groups throughout the study but
increased significantly between Sucrose, RCS, RPS and Cellulose
groups respectively; Control and Sucrose groups having similar
values at all times. The fall in carbohydrate content of the dry
caecal contents and faeces with time in the RCS and RPS groups
indicated that there is an adaptation to increased utilisation
through increased fermentation in the caecum. This is further
supported by the finding that caecal tissue dry weight for the two
RS fed groups was significantly greater than for the other 3
groups. Furthermore the pH of the caecal contents of the two RS
fed groups was significantly lower than the other 3 groups.
Increases in faecal dry matter output in those groups fed the

complex carbohydrates was only partially acounted for by the
presence of carbohydrate in the faeces.

Conclusion

<u>In vitro</u> isolated α-amylase resistant starches appear to vary in
their availability as carbohydrate and in the extent to which they
are fermented <u>in vivo</u>. Differences were also observed in the rate
and degree of adaptation to RS in the diet. The increase in
faecal dry matter in the RS fed rats was only partially accounted
for by the presence of carbohydrate. RS therefore appears to have
some of the properties associated with dietary fibre.

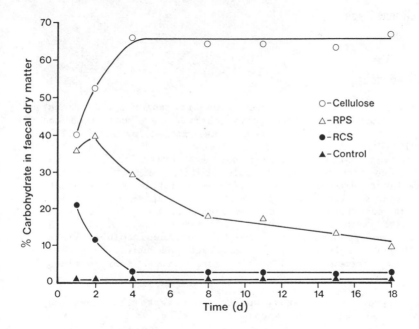

Figure 1 Changes in carbohydrate content of dry faeces with time

REFERENCES

1. R.W. Kerr, "Chemistry and Industry of Starch", Academic Press,
   New York, 1950, 166-167.
2. R. Collinson, "Starch and its Derivatives", Chapman and Hall,
   London, 1968, 194-201.
3. I. Bjorck, M. Nyman, B. Pedersen, M. Siljestrom, N-G. Asp and
   B.O. Eggum, <u>Journal of Cereal Science</u>, 1986, <u>4</u>, 1-11.

DIGESTION OF FIBRE CARBOHYDRATES OF PEA HULLS, CARROT AND CABBAGE
BY ADULT COCKERELS

M.A. Longstaff and J.M. McNab

AFRC Institute for Grassland and Animal Production
Poultry Department
Roslin
Midlothian EH25 9PS

1 INTRODUCTION

The increased use of methods whereby neutral sugar constituents
from the hydrolysis of fibre polysaccharides are converted to
alditol acetates and the acidic sugars measured colorimetrically[2]
has permitted a more informed discussion on the relationship
between polysaccharide structure and its digestion[3,4,5]. The
recent clinical interest on the role of fibre digestion in man
has stimulated numerous studies with monogastric animals that
have implicated fibre in a plethora of digestive and physiological gut functions. The few studies on fibre digestion in
chickens have given estimates of implied fermentation of about 15
to 33% of graminaceous fibre[5,6] and none of the insoluble fibre
from lupin seeds[4]. In contrast, pigs, rats and humans have been
reported[3,7] to ferment considerably more fibre from various
sources[3,7].

The purpose of this study was to investigate the digestion
of fibre in pea hulls (secondary cell walls) and carrot and
cabbage (primary cell walls) using an adult cockerel bioassay
which achieves total collection of excreta voided from a known
amount of foodstuff eaten.

Characterisation of Neutral and Acidic Polysaccharides of Total (Insoluble + Soluble) and Insoluble Fibre

Total fibre polysaccharides were measured as the sum of
neutral sugars and uronic acids after acid hydrolysis of the
insoluble precipitate remaining after 50 mg of de-starched
feedingstuff was washed three times with 30 mls 80% ethanol.
Insoluble fibre polysaccharides were measured after acid
hydrolysis of the precipitate remaining after 50 mg de-starched

322

feedingstuff was washed three times with 30 mls buffer, pH 7. The amount of soluble polysaccharides could be derived by difference. Carrot and cabbage were freeze dried to bring them to about the same moisture content as pea hulls. Table 1 shows that pea hulls contained the greatest amount of neutral polysaccharides and a slightly higher quantity of acidic polysaccharides than carrot and cabbage fibre. Almost equal amounts of neutral and acidic polysaccarides were found in carrot and cabbage. The neutral polysaccharides which were most soluble were those containing rhamnose, arabinose and galactose. The acidic polysaccharides of carrot and cabbage were the most soluble.

Table 1   Monosaccharide composition of fibre in pea hulls, carrot and cabbage

g/kg D.M. + S.D.

	Pea hulls	
	Insol.	Total
Rha	2.5+ 0.9	7.1+ 0.3
Fuc	1.7+ 0.4	2.8+ 0.3
Ara	12.0+ 4.2	32.2+ 3.8
Xyl	99.2+ 4.4	112.3+ 9.3
Man	1.8+ 0.1	2.4+ 0.2
Gal H+C	10.0+ 0.8	21.0+ 3.5
Gluc	350.0+60.7	430.0+39.7
Sum neutral sugars	436.2+51.8	607.9+49.2
Uronic acids	83.8+25.3	145.6+10.4

	Carrot		Cabbage	
	Insol.	Total	Insol.	Total
Rha	0.7+0.2	3.0+0.6	0.6+ 0.4	2.2+ 0.5
Fuc	0.2+0.1	0.4+0.1	0.9+ 0.3	1.3+ 0.8
Ara	4.2+0.6	12.7+1.0	9.4+ 1.8	19.3+ 3.1
Xyl	4.7+2.0	4.3+0.4	9.6+ 1.1	11.3+ 1.9
Man	4.4+0.4	4.7+0.3	4.0+ 0.9	4.8+ 0.7
Gal H+C	6.6+0.3	20.8+0.8	6.8+ 0.6	13.0+ 1.1
Gluc	68.3+0.5	73.0+4.1	59.8+16.1	74.7+ 9.0
Sum neutral sugars	88.5+1.8	118.9+1.2	91.4+18.8	128.2+15.9
Uronic acids	17.8+4.1	111.6+6.4	20.3+ 2.6	88.6+ 5.0

Digestion of Total (Insoluble + Soluble) Fibre

Table 2 shows that the overall digestibility of the neutral polysaccharides (sum of neutral sugars) was very low in all three feedingstuffs, mainly due to the large amount of indigestible cellulose present. Polysaccharides containing rhamnose, arabinose and galactose were preferentially better digested. The acidic polysaccharides of carrot and cabbage were digested best.

Table 2 Digestibility of total neutral and acidic
         fibre sugars

	Pea hulls	Carrot	Cabbage	SEM	P
Rha	0.24+0.10	0.04+0.07	0.18+0.02	0.05	.002
Fuc	0.01+0.09	-1.20+0.59	-0.58+0.56	0.19	.001
Ara	0.22+0.07	0.12+0.06	0.05+0.20	0.05	.01
Xyl	0.01+0.06	-0.22+0.52	-0.26+0.56	0.18	NS
Man	0.23+0.05	-0.09+0.08	0.03+0.02	0.05	.001
Gal $_{H+C}$	0.19+0.11	0.11+0.06	0.09+0.02	0.05	NS
Gluc	0.03+0.09	-0.01+0.07	-0.03+0.01	0.04	NS
Sum neutral sugars	0.04+0.08	0.01+0.06	-0.04+0.16	0.04	NS
Uronic acids	0.05+0.12	0.24+0.10	0.28+0.14	0.05	.001

The results suggest that the most soluble polysaccharides, belonging to the pectins were digested best. The lower digestion of the acidic polysaccharides in pea hulls was presumed to be because of the presence of acidic xylans, based on xylose and glucuronic acid, as well as pectin.

REFERENCES

1. A.B. Blakeney, P.J. Harris, R.J. Henry, and B.A. Stone, Carbohydr. Res., 1983, 113, 291.
2. N. Blumenkrantz and G. Asboe-Hansen, Analyt. Biochem., 1973, 54, 484.
3. H.Graham, P. Aman, R.K. Newman, and C.W. Newman, Br. J. Nutr., 1985, 54, 719.
4. B. Carre and B. Leclercq, Br. J. Nutr., 1985, 54, 669.
5. M. Longstaff and J.M. McNab, Br. Poult. Sci., 1986, 27, 435.
6. W. Bolton, World's Poultry Congress, 1954, 28, p. 94.
7. M. Nyman, N-G. Asp, J. Cummings, H. Wiggins, Br. J. Nutr., 1956, 55, 487.

A PROPOSED METHOD FOR DETERMINING THE UTILIZATION OF UNDIGESTIBLE SUGARS IN MAN

N. Hosoya and H. Hidaka*

Vice President
Kokusai Gakuin,
Saitama Junior College,
2-5, Yoshiki-cho,
Ohmiya-shi, 330 JAPAN

*) Bio Science Laboratories,
Meiji Seika Kaisha, Ltd.,
580 Horikawa-cho, Saiwai-ku,
Kawasaki-shi, 210 JAPAN

INTRODUCTION

Several kinds of undigestible sugars and sugar alcohols have recently been developed as low caloric sweeteners and bulking agents.[1,2] To estimate the available energy of undigestible sugars, a new method of radiorespiratory study combined with a feces incubation has been done using fructooligosaccharides.

Utilization of [U-^{14}C]-Fructooligosaccharides in Man

Fructooligosaccharides. 1^F-(β-fructofuranosyl)$_n$sucroses (n=1-3) are naturally occurring in plants, and a mixture of them are now commercially produced from sucrose by the action of fungal β-fructofuranosidase.[3] The saccharides are undigestible,[4] and they have useful physiological properties through selective utilization by bifidobacteria in human intestinal canal.[5]

Radiorespiratory Study in Man. Six healthy male volunteers participated in the study. After daily intake of unlabeled fructooligosaccharides for 7 days, 6.1 g of ^{14}C-fructooligosaccharides (66.4 μCi) was given and radioactivity of expired $^{14}CO_2$, flatus, urine and feces were determined during 48 hours. The respiratory pattern of $^{14}CO_2$ expiration is presented in Fig. 1. The total $^{14}CO_2$ production was 48.9 ± 1.3% for 24 hours and 55.2 ± 1.6% for 48 hours, and the maximum expiration rate was found at 8 hours, after which the rate decreased rapidly. The recovery in the feces was 10.1 ± 1.5% for 48 hours, and urinary radioactivity was 1.9 ± 0.2%. The amount of $^{14}CO_2$ of flatus was very low and this result strongly suggested that the $^{14}CO_2$ produced by fermentation in the colon must be absorbed from the colon and expired in the breath.

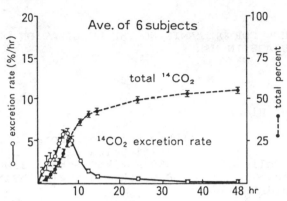

Figure 1 $^{14}CO_2$ Expiration after ingestion of
            ^{14}C-fructooligosaccharides in six subjects

Anaerobic Incubation of ^{14}C-Fructooligosaccharides
with Subjects' Feces. In parallel with radiorespiratory
study, the study was carried out in order to simulate the
degradation of the sugars in colon. After 8 hours incubation, direct $^{14}CO_2$ production was 9.6 ± 1.2% and more than
half (57.9 ± 2.7%) was volatile fatty acids (VFAs) including acetic acid (24.1 ± 1.8%).
    Determining the Utilization of Undigestible Sugars.
The individual end products derived from labeled undigestible sugar were measured in the radiorespiratory
study. Amount of radioactivity in feces and urine shows
that of loss by those routes, and the expired $^{14}CO_2$ indicated the sum of energy utilized directly to man as well
as indirectly after the fermentation by the intestinal
bacteria. Therefore, it is necessary to subtract the
fermentative $^{14}CO_2$ (9.6%) from the total respiratory $^{14}CO_2$
(49.8%), and the remainder (39.3%) resulted from the actual utilization in mammalia for 24 hours. Then the
caloric utilization of undigestible sugars will be estimated by the following equation.

$$\text{energy of undiges-} \atop \text{tible sugar (kcal/g)} = \sum \text{each amount of} \atop \text{absorbed VFA (g)} \times \text{energy of} \atop \text{VFA (kcal/g)}$$

REFERENCES

1. N.Hosoya, Nutr.Proc.Int.Congr., 9th, 1972, 1, 164.
2. S.K.Figdor and J.R.Bianchine, J.Agric.Food Chem., 1983, 31, 389.
3. H.Hidaka, M.Hirayama and N.Sumi, Agric.Biol.Chem., 1988, 52, 1181.
4. T.Oku, T.Tokumaga and N.Hosoya, J.Nutr., 1984, 114, 1574.
5. H.Hidaka, T.Eida, T.Takizawa, T.Tokunaga and Y.Tashiro, Bifidobacteria Microflora, 1986, 5, 37.

ENERGY AND MACRONUTRIENT BIOAVAILABILITY FROM RURAL AND URBAN MEXICAN DIETS.

Jorge L. Rosado, María Morales and Lindsay H. Allen.
Department of Nutritional Physiology, National Institute of Nutrition. Vasco de Quiroga No. 15, Tlalpan, México, D.F. 14000 and Department of Nutritional Sciences, University of Connecticut, Storrs CT 06268.

Compositional information on dietary constituents is at best only a rough estimate to the nutritional value of the human diet. A complete understanding of the nutritional value of the diet requires consideration of a number of dietary, physiological and possible genetic factors which affect nutrient utilization. Several studies indicate that components which are abundant in plant foods, such as dietary fiber, phytic acid and tannic acid may significantly reduce the absorption and consequently the utilization of several nutrients. Plant foods are staple for diets regularly consumed by a great majority of the population in Mexico and many other countries, specially in rural areas. The degree to which this inhibitory effects may be ocurring when mixed diets are consumed is at present unknown. In the present study we evaluated the effect of mixed diets, representing average consumption of the rural and urban population in Mexico, on the absorption and utilization of several nutrients.

Methods

Sixteen healthy Mexican adult females were studied during two metabolic periods lasting from 12 to 21 days each. Two diets, a typical Mexican diet of the rural areas (RMD) and an Urban Mexican diet (UMD) were given to each subject in a crossover design each one on a different metabolic period. Diets in both experiments represent average diets consumed by a majority of the population in rural communities (RMD) and the more "modernized" cities (UMD). The diets differed mainly in the source of nutrients. In general, they were from plant foods for the RMD while the UMD contained more animal sources of food.

327

With both diets there was an initial equilibration period for the elimination of pre-experimental diet residues from the intestinal tract. This period took from 4 to 12 days as indicated by the fecal excretion of polyethilene glycol 4000 (PEG). After equilibration was reached, 6-days metabolic balance of energy and nitrogen and digestility of dietary fiber and fat, were measured for the two metabolic periods. PEG was fed throughout the study and used as quantitative fecal marker.

Results

TABLE 1.   Stool output and characteristics of women consuming the rural and urban diets (g/d).

	R M D	U M D	P>|T|
Total weight	184.6 + 25	51.2 + 6	0.0001
Dry matter	36.6 + 4	13.3 + 1	0.0001
Water in feces (%)	78.2 + 1	72.1 + 1	0.0012
Laxation rate (defecations/d)	1.4 + 0.1	0.9 + 0.1	0.0002

TABLE 2.   Intake, excretion, apparent absorption and balance of energy and macronutrients of 16 women consuming the rural and urban diets.

	R M D	U M D	P >|T|
Nitrogen (g/d)			
Intake	7.6 + 0.6	10.5 + 0.4	0.001
Fecal	2.6 + 0.3	1.1 + 0.1	0.0001
Urine	4.7 + 0.5	6.8 + 0.4	0.0001
Apparent absorption (%)	64.8 + 3.4	89.8 + 0.4	0.0001
Crude balance	0.4 + 0.4	2.7 + 0.4	0.0005
Fat (g/d)			
Intake	34.4 + 2.5	55.2 + 3.2	0.0001
Feces	3.4 + 0.4	1.6 + 0.1	0.0001
Apparent absorption (%)	89.2 + 1.1	97.0 + 0.2	0.0001
Energy (kcal/d)			
Intake	1816 + 109	1983 + 101	0.036
Feces	199 + 19	101 + 4	0.0001
Apparent absorption (%)	89 + 0.9[1]	95 + 0.3	0.0001
ME Balance	1542 + 97[1]	1787 + 97	0.005
ME Atwater	1681 + 100[1]	1766 + 79	0.005

[1]p < 0.01 between balance and Atwater's

TABLE 3. Fiber intake, excretion and digestibility of 16 women consuming the rural and urban diets (g/d).

	R M D	U M D	P > |T|
Intake	39.9 + 2.6	9.2 + 0.8	0.0001
Fecal excretion	14.1 + 1.3	2.3 + 0.2	0.0001
Digestibility	25.7 + 2.4	7.1 + 0.8	0.0001

Conclusions

1.- Energy intake was spontaneously reduced by 166 kcal when subjects ingested the rural diet (RMD) based on plant foods compared to the urban (UMD) more refined mixed diet containing both animal and plant foods. The effect can be attributed to the high fiber content of the former and its effect on satiety.

2.- Fecal weight was increased 133 g/d by ingesting a plant-based rural Mexican diet compared to more refined urban Mexican diet. Both an increase in dry matter and an increase in water output were observed. The higher dry matter excretion was due to the presence of dietary fiber in feces as well as to increased malabsorption of nutrients.

3.- Nitrogen balance (crude) was significantly lower with rural diet compared with the urban diet. This observation was due to both lower intake and increased fecal excretion of nitrogen. Apparent absorption of nitrogen was 90% and 65% for the UMD and RMD respectively.

4.- Biological availability of energy was 1778 kcal/d with the urban diet and 1532 kcal/d with the rural diet. The difference was due to lower energy intake (ad libitum) combined with an increase in fecal energy of about 100 kcal per day with the rural diet. The application of the Atwater's factors accurately predicted metabolizable energy from the urban diet but overestimated energy bioavailability from the rural diet by about 10%. The factors of 0.975 suggested by FAO/WHO/UNU (1) to correct for energy availability in diets containing moderate amounts of dietary fiber is to high considering the 89% apparent absorption observed with the rural diet. The factor should be closer to 0.9 for the rural mexican diet.

5.- About 26 g/d of dietary fiber in the rural diet and 7 g/d in the urban diet were digested and thus contributed to energy bioavailability.

References

1.- FAO/WHO/UNU. Energy and protein requirements Technical Report Series # 724 World Health Organization Geneva, 1985

FACTORS INFLUENCING UPTAKE AND UTILISATION OF MACRONUTRIENTS.

Helmut, F. Erbersdobler

Institut für Humanernährung und Lebensmittelkunde der
Christian Albrechts Universität zu Kiel, Düsternbrooker
Weg 17, 2300 Kiel 1, FRG

1 INTRODUCTION AND DEFINITIONS

The nutrients measured by chemical analysis are not always
fully utilisable. Difficulties result e.g. from the unac-
cessibility of the nutrients because of undigestible cell
walls, a bulky or dense structure, a low solubility and
moreover from the presence of certain compounds inhibiting
the digestion. During food processing derivatisations of
nutrients occur as well as the formation of cross linkages
making the food inaccessible for digestion or/and metabolism. Parts of the nutrients are said to be unavailable.
In some cases, however, the utilisation is also improved
without being recognized.
　　　Strictly speaking the term bioavailability is defined
as the utilization of nutrient compounds after digestion
and absorption. In a wider sense, however, also the digestibility is included, namely if the course of digestion is
limited to the section between the mouth and the large intestine (the so called **ileal digestibility**). The latter
definition was mainly and widely used by many authors in
the last years. Another important point is the question of
"availability for what?" - availability for energy utilisation in general (e.g. in dietary fibers), for blood
glucose levels or for protein synthesis (amino acids)?

2 FACTORS AFFECTING NUTRIENT AVAILABILITY
Positive and negative effects

　　　The favourable influence of cooking on the digestibility of raw potato starch is as well known as the beneficial effect of toasting of soy beans on protein digestibility. But also other techniques of food processing and

preparation like extracting, milling and washing are able
to improve the utilisation of nutrients or to eliminate
adverse components like e.g. tannins. A positive effect of
a mild heat treatment of proteins on their utilisation is
well known (see also table 4). Similar results were obtained with starches of different origin where a wet heating
and gelatinisation improved the digestibility and the pro-
vision of blood glucose[1]. On the other hand a decrease in
starch utilisation by the formation of enzyme resistant
starch can occur. The details of these phenomenons will be
discussed in other papers of the congress.

The main factors influencing negatively the utilisation of macro nutrients are caused by reactions during
food processing and preparation. Table 1 gives a synopsis
of the different effects on nutrient availability.

Experiments with model compounds.
For a long time it was not possible to understand the
mechanisms making a nutrient unavailable. With our more
advanced knowledge of the main reactions occuring during
food processing and by using several substances suitable
as models, however, we are now able to understand the most
important effects. Some models used are given in figure 1.

Table 1 Influence of technological treatment on the utilisation and
nutritive value of the energy producing macronutrients

	main technical influences	main reactions and the nutritional consequences
1. PROTEINS	oxidation, heat treat- ment, chemi- cal deriva- tisation	Maillard- and other reactions, cross linking, racemisation, total destruc- tion - reduced availability of amino acids, reduced digestibility of the protein, adverse effects of several derivatives
2. CARBO- HYDRATES	heat treat- ment, arti- ficial crosslinking	gelatinisation, pyrolysis - partially improved, partially reduced digestibility, production of colour and flavour
3. FATS	hydrogenation oxidation	isomeric (e.g. trans-) fatty acids, products of the fat oxidation - reduced utilisation and metabolism, adverse effects on other metabolic reactions, in vivo oxidation of body fats and fat soluble vitamins

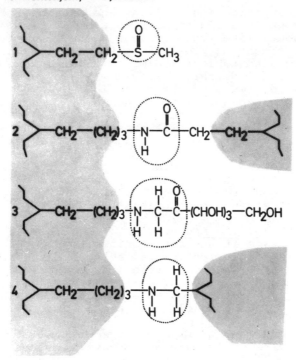

1 = Methioninesulphoxides; 2 = Glutamyllysine;

3 = Fructoselysine; 4 = Lysinoalanine

Figure 1 **Amino acid derivatives and cross linking products used as models**

Methioninesulphoxides (two diastereoisomers) are formed by the reaction of proteins with lipid peroxides or by peroxide treatment of foods. Because of being reduced to methionine during hydrolysis and chromatography they are not detected in routine amino acid analysis. Generally methionine sulphoxides are regarded to be highly digestible and available[2,3]. The availability as a total was estimated to be between 62% for chicken[4] and 85-90% for rats[5].

Fructoselysine (FL) is the most abundant amino acid derivative in human nutrition and is found after the reaction of lysine with glucose, lactose (forming lactuloselysine = galactose-FL) or maltose (maltuloselysine = glucose-FL) respectively. As table 2 shows the FL moiety (given as "glycosylated" lysine) represents in many dried foods the main lysine damage. FL is calculated from its analytical artefact and indicator furosine as is described elsewhere[6]. High lysinoalanine values in several products show that also cross linking reactions occured.

Table 2 Contents in lysine, glycosylated lysine (in g/16 g of N) and lysinoalanine (in mg/160 g of N) and the calculated lysine losses in several foods

	n	total analysed lysine*	glycosy-lated lysine**	lysino-alanine	% lysine losses	
					des-troyed#	inacti-vated#
Pasta and other items	20	2.6 +0.6	0.2 +0.1	nd***	0%	8%
Biscuits and similar items	8	1.3 +0.5	0.3 +0.1	180(0-710)	50%	10%
Zwieback	2	1.4 -1.5	0.7-0.8	80(40/120)	45%	35%
Breakfast cere-als processed	7	2.9 +1.3	0.5 +0.6	210(0-890)	9%	16%
UHT*** milks	27	8.7 +0.4	0.1 +0.1	50(0-110)	1%	1%
Condensed milks	11/8##	8,3 +0.3	1.2 +0.3	310 +50	6%	14%
Skim milks, spray dried	33	8.8 +0.5	0.6 +0.5	nd	0%	7%
Skim milks, roller dried	42	8.5 +0.5	0.9 +0.6	nd	5%	10%
Whey, spray dried	33	8.6 +0.4	0.6 +0.5	nd	2%	8%
Infant milk formula, dried	44	8.4 +0.6	0.7 +0.6	tr***	5%	7%
Infant milk formula, steril.	23/15##	8.0 +0.4	0.9 +0.3	420 +290	9%	11%
Formula diets for tube feeding, sterilized	19/33##	8.3 +1.1	0.2 +0.2	1150 +480	5%	3%

* total lysine = free lysine + inactivated lysine;
** calculated from the furosine values
*** UHT = Ultra Heat Treated; nd = not determined; tr = traces
# destroyed lysine = suggested lysine in the raw material - total analysed lysine; inactivated lysine = lysine bound as FL and LAL
number of samples determined for lysinoalanine

FL is poorly liberated by digestion and not actively transported out of the intestine but slowly absorbed by diffusion as shown in earlier experiments with laboratory animals using the ^{14}C-labeled compound[7].It is not metabolized by the organism and excreted <u>via</u> the kidneys in unchanged form within 24 hours[7,8]. Experiments with student volunteers, using the furosine determination in the urine as a measure, showed that only about 1.2-1.5% of the ingested FL were absorbed and excreted[8]. FL penetrates

slowly into the cells of kidney tubules, but only poorly
into the liver and muscle cells. This demonstrates a poor
availability for the transport systems at the cells[7,8,9].

Lysinoalanine (LAL). An example for crosslinking is
the formation of LAL which occurs mainly in proteins heated under alkaline conditions by the reaction of the ε-
amino group of lysine with dehydroalanine, which itself is
formed by ß-elimination of 0-substituted serine or of cystine. The metabolic transit of LAL is somewhat similar to
fructoselysine as is measured by several authors and summarized by Finot[12]. In contrast to FL[7], LAL is excreted in
the urine mainly in combined form and as catabolites.
About 11-25% of the ingested LAL appeared in the urine.
Undigested and excreted in the feces remained 33-65%[12].
This is similar to results with FL[9]. The results with
rats, however, are contradictory to the findings with student volunteers[8]. Results of Robbins et al.[13] indicated
that the lysine moiety of LAL is completely unavailable to
the rat but partially available (about 36%) to chicken.

Glutamyl- and aspartyllysine. These "isopeptides" are
formed by crosslinking between lysine on the one hand and
glutamine or asparagine on the other. They are partially
still available but reduce protein digestibility[14]. This
type of reaction is discussed more in detail below.

Other reactions like that with aldehydes or phenolic
compounds lead to derivatives of different availability
and/or to crosslinking as is demonstrated by Hurrell et
al. on the example of lysine with caffeic acid[15]. A type
of modification not mentioned until now is racemisation of
certain amino acids, namely serine, aspartic acid, phenylalanine, tyrosine, glutamic acid, alanine, lysine and leucine, in the protein molecule due to heat and/ or alkaline
treatment of the food[16]. The D- amino acids resulting from
these reactions are only partially metabolized to the biological active L- forms and in this way not fully available for protein synthesis. The practical relevance for
human nutrition is uncertain until now.

Proteins which are not digested and absorbed may lead
to a desamination and ammonia production in the hind gut
as was shown with fructoselysine and lysinoalanine elsewhere[10,11]. Also in carbohydrates these hind gut fermentations are of big biological importance. Generally by these
processes misleading results of digestibility experiments
can be obtained. In severely damaged proteins, however,
not all of the crosslinks can be split by the microorga-
nism (see below figure 2 and tables 4 and 6).

3 INFLUENCE ON BIOAVAILABILITY OF MICRONUTRIENTS

It is well known that many macronutrients have a positive influence on the absorption and utilisation of minerals and trace elements. Other structures, however, act as inhibitors like presumable casein in the absorption of zink. These effects will certainly be discussed in other papers. Finot and Furniss[17] examined the in vitro findings of Hayashi[18], in which LAL acted as a metal chelator, for Maillard products on rats. They found that the feeding of heated casein glucose mixtures was associated with increased kidney levels and urinary losses of zinc and copper. This confirms results with parenteral solutions of Steglink et al.[19] The relevance of these effects, however, for the practical nutrition remains doubtful. More work is necessary to examine whether the positive or negative effects of certain proteins, peptides and amino acids on micronutrient absorption are modified by e.g. food processing.

4 INFLUENCE OF AMINO ACID REACTIONS ON PROTEIN DIGESTIBILITY

The results with model compounds (e.g. with volunteers) indicate that in the amino acid derivatives, which result from food processing, the problems of digestion and absorption would be more important than utilisation after absorption[7,8]. This is also valid for exogenous factors influencing availability like tannins[20], protease inhibi-

Table 4 Correlation of lysine damage in heated soy proteins with the digestibility of the protein in rats[21]

Heat treatment*	Total lysine**	FDNB-reactive lysine	Portal-plasma lysine***	Digestibility of the protein
0	6.6=100	5.3=100	540µM=100	not determined
95°C	95	94	112	91% = 100
138°C	91	72	58	91
160°C	80	32	18	19

*   Heating a mixture of isolated soy protein with 10% tap
     water in the open air for 24 h
**   Amino acid analyser after hydrolysis with 6M HCl
*** Measured 60 min after the test meal (4 rats pooled)
     minus a residual level (200 µM = 2/3 of fasting level)

tors and others. Synthetical produced amino acid derivatives, however, like succinyllysine may behave differently. As can be seen from table 4 lysine reactions, namely at more severe heating, lead to a depression of protein digestibility, presumable by the formation of crosslinks.

The mechanism making the protein undigestible seems to be a more or less unspecific inhibition of the access of the digestive enzymes to the sites of cleavage. The simple derivatisation of lysine, e.g. by forming lysine sugar complexes, on the other hand appears not to be too unfavourable for digestion (see also table 6). A certain catalysing effect of glucose, however, enhancing the damage to the whole protein is most likely.

Table 5 shows results of De Groot and Slump[22], modified in order to compare the amount of LAL crosslinking with protein digestibility. As can be seen, a LAL crosslinking of about 1% was equivalent to a reduction of the digestibility of ten percent, in isolated soy protein as well as in casein. This suggests that besides LAL also other crosslinks existed like in the results from table 4, where probably glutamyl- and aspartyllysine were predominant.

The influence on digestibility appears to be highly dependent on the amount and distribution of the crosslinks over the whole protein molecule. If there is a nonuniform distribution, the part of the protein with lower amounts of crosslinks should be digestible. Figure 2 shows a model situation in which a schematic protein molecule (ribonuclease) was furnished with its lysyl and aspartinyl or glutaminyl groups, which then were assumed to have reacted

Table 5 Correlation of the lysinoalanine- (LAL-) content in an isolated soya protein and casein with the digestibility of the proteins for rats (from: De Groot and Slump[22])

ppm LAL in the proteins		Crosslinking in % of the proteins	Digestibility in %	
			absolute	relative
0	soya protein	0	95	100
1000	"	0.09	96	100
8300	"	0.70	86	91
0	casein	0	101	100
11500	"	0.97	90	89.

b = supposed reactions between Lys and Asn or Gln
additional reactions under more severe conditions
suggested formation of lysinoalanine
c = supposed undigested residues = 30-40%
d = supposed undigested residues = 20-25%

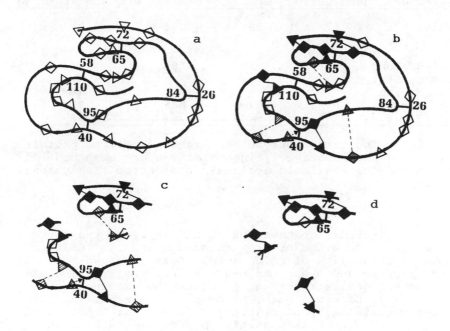

<u>Figure 2</u> **Suggested reactions of the lysyl- △ and asparti-
nyl + glutaminyl- ◇ residues in a model protein**

at the sites favourable for crosslinking. The model shows
a relatively unpolar distribution of the crosslinks, opening a chance for digestion of the undamaged parts. Two
conceptions of a moderate or more severe heat damage were
assumed representing digestibilities of 75-80% vs. 60-70%
respectively. This concept of a model corresponds well
with first digestibility studies using the **homoarginine
labeling** technique[23,24]. Homoarginine, obtained by derivatisation of lysine in the protein chain with methyliso-
urea[25] is not used for protein synthesis and does not
appear in the endogenous proteins. Its absorption represents in this way the true digestibility of the protein.
Table 6 shows that in spite of a severe lysine damage and
a reduction in protein digestibility, the parts with undamaged lysine (guanidation) remained highly digestible.

Table 6　Relationship of lysine availability and protein digestibility as measured with rats or by the "homoargini-ne method" with pigs (from data of Hagemeister et al.[24])

Casein, heated at	Degree of guanidation	True digestibility lysine	protein	Disappearance of homoarginine
Native	97	98	96	99
Heated alone (110°C, 24h)	80	91	96	97
Heated with 20% glucose (105°C, 24 h)	65	67	79	93

* High lysine damage but better digestion of the protein
** Most of the reactive lysine molecules are absorbed
***Some of the available lysine is undigested (inclusion?)

5 CONCLUSIONS

It may be stated that nowadays we have a clear knowledge about many mechanisms of protein damage and its influence on the availability of amino acids. Less is known for other factors and other macro-nutrients. Crosslinking ei-ther by endogenous reactions or caused by external com-pounds (e.g. tannins) seems to be the main negative factor on the digestibility of proteins (and also of other nutri-ents?). Although it is possible to predict the protein quality from the chemical determined amino acids together with indicators like furosine or lysinoalanine it is just now very difficult to predetermine the actual amino acid utilisation and to foresee all influences on the protein molecule, especially in more complex systems like plant foods. Unclear are also many reactions in complex carbohy-drates and in fats. Namely the influence of the hind gut fermentations on bioavailability of nutrients and energy are to be solved in the future.

6 REFERENCES

1. J. Holm, I. Lundquist, I. Björk, A.-C. Eliasson and N.-G. Asp, Am.J.Clin.Nutr., 1988, 47, 1010.
2. H.F. Erbersdobler, In: D.J.A. Cole, K.N. Boorman, P.J. Buttery, D. Lewis, R.J. Neale, and H. Swan, Eds., `Protein Metabolism and Nutrition´. Butterworths, London, Boston, 1976, p. 139.
3. A.U. Gjoen, and R.L. Njaa, Br.J.Nutr. 1977, 37, 93.

4. P. Slump, K.D. Bos and C. Verbeek, In: Proc. of the European Conference on Food Chemistry EURO Food Chem II, Rome, 323, 1983.
5. J.-L. Cuq, P. Besancon, L. Chartier and C. Cheftel, Fd.Chem., 1978, 3, 85.
6. H.F. Erbersdobler, In: M. Fujimaki, M. Namiki and H. Kato, Eds., `Amino-Carbonyl Reactions in Food and Biological Systems´. Elsevier, Amsterdam, Oxford, New York, Tokyo and Kodansha, LTD, Tokyo, 1986, Development in Food Science, Vol. 13, Chapter 49, p. 481.
7. H.F. Erbersdobler, A. Brandt, E. Scharrer and B. v. Wangenheim, Prog.Fd.Nutr.Sci., 1981, 5, 257.
8. H.F. Erbersdobler, A. Groß, U. Klusmann and K. Schlecht, In: M. Friedman, Ed. `Absorption and Utilization of Amino Acids´. CRC Press, INC, Boca Raton, in the press.
9. H.F. Erbersdobler, Kieler Milchwirtschaftliche Forschungsberichte, 1983, 35, 301.
10. H.F. Erbersdobler, I. Gunsser and G. Weber, Zentrbl.Vet.Med. A., 1970, 17, 573.
11. M. Sternberg, and C.Y. Kim, J.Agric.Food Chem., 1979, 27, 1130.
12. P.A. Finot, Nutrition Abstracts and Reviews in Clinical Nutrition - Series A, 1983, 53, 67.
13. K. R. Robbins, D.H. Baker and J.W. Finley, J.Nutr, 1980, 110, 907.
14. R.F. Hurrell and K.J. Carpenter, In: M. Friedman, Ed., `Protein Crosslinking. Nutritional and Medical Consequences. Advances in Experimental Medicine and Biology´, Plenum Press, New York, 1977, Vol 86 B, Chapter 16, p. 225.
15. R.F. Hurrell, P.A. Finot and J.L. Cuq, Br.J.Nutr., 1982, 47, 191
16. M. Friedman and P.M. Masters, J.Food Sci.,1982, 47, 760.
17. P.A. Finot and D.E. Furniss, In: M. Fujimaki, M. Namiki and H. Kato, Eds., `Amino-Carbonyl Reactions in Food and Biological Systems´. Elsevier, Amsterdam, Oxford, New York, Tokyo and Kodansha, LTD, Tokyo, 1986, Development in Food Science, Vol. 13, Chapter 50, p. 493.
18. R. Hayashi, J.Biol.Chem., 1982, 257, 13896.
19. L.D. Stegink, J.B. Freeman, P.D. Meyer, L.J. Filer Jr., L.K.Fry and L. Den Besten, Fed.Proc., 1975, 34, 931.
20. B.O. Eggum, B. Pedersen and I. Jacobsen, Br.J.Nutr., 1983, 50, 197.
21. H.F. Erbersdobler and T.R. Anderson, ACS Symposium Series, 1983, 215, 419.
22. A.P. De Groot and P. Slump, J.Nutr., 1969, 98, 45.
23. H. Hagemeister and H.F. Erbersdobler, Proc.Nutr.Soc., 1985, 44, 133A.
24. H. Hagemeister, M. Schmitz and H.F. Erbersdobler, In: Ch. Barth and E. Schlimme Eds., `Milk Proteins in Human Nutrition´ Steinkopff, Darmstadt, in the press
25. J. Mauron and E. Bujard, In: Proc. 6th Int. Nutr. Conf. Edinburgh, Livingstone, London, 1963, p. 343.

RELATIONSHIP BETWEEN IN VITRO AND IN VIVO PARAMETERS OF AMINO ACID BIOAVAILABILITY

I. Galibois, C. Simoes Nunes (x), A. Rérat (x) and L. Savoie

Centre de Recherche en Nutrition, FSAA,
Université Laval, Québec, G1K 7P4 Canada;
(x) Laboratoire de Physiologie de la Nutrition,
CRJ, INRA, 78350 Jouy-en-Josas, France.

1 INTRODUCTION

The bioavailability of amino acids (AA) is a primary determinant of protein nutritional quality, but few techniques allow its measurement. An interesting but quite elaborate procedure is the method of Rérat et al. in the pig (1), that enables to measure the pattern of appearance of dietary AA in the portal bloodstream. At that point, AA availability is the resultant of many phenomena of digestion, transport and metabolization in the intestinal wall. Of these, the sequence of hydrolysis during the luminal digestion process might be the most important factor. In that case, AA availability could be conveniently studied and partly predicted by an in vitro method reproducing in vivo proteolysis conditions, such as the one developed by Savoie and Gauthier (2). In this work, the degree of correspondence was determined between the pattern of in vitro hydrolysis and the pattern of in vivo absorption of essential AA (EAA) from two protein sources.

2 MATERIALS AND METHODS

Protein sources and amino acids. The sources of casein (Na caseinate, UCCP, France) and rapeseed proteins (concentrate 00 Tandem, CETIOM, France) were the same in the in vitro and in vivo studies. For calculation of correlation between in vitro and in vivo profiles, the following nine EAA were used: threonine, valine, methionine, leucine, isoleucine, phenylalanine, histidine, lysine and arginine.

In vitro data. After a 30-min pepsin predigestion, the protein sources (250 mg aliquots) were submitted in four replicates to a 24-h pancreatin hydrolysis in dialysis tubes, with the continuous removal of digestion products by circulation of a phosphate buffer. The EAA composition of digesta collected at 3-h intervals were determined by ion-exchange chromatography (Autoanalyser model 6300, Beckman, Palo Alto, CA).

Table 1. Correlation between in vitro and in vivo EAA profiles, casein.

in vitro / in vivo	0-3H	3-6H	6-9H	9-12H r^1	12-15H	15-18H	18-21H	21-24H
0-1H	0.83**	0.92***	0.94***	0.93***	0.77**	0.61	0.58	0.29
1-2H	0.93****	0.98***	0.95***	0.88****	0.65*	0.48	0.44	0.13
2-3H	0.91***	0.93***	0.90***	0.82**	0.56	0.34	0.33	0.04
3-4H	0.81**	0.86**	0.84**	0.81**	0.67*	0.50	0.43	0.33
4-5H	0.81**	0.76*	0.65*	0.54	0.36	0.20	0.18	0.23
5-6H	0.85**	0.83**	0.75*	0.68*	0.45	0.27	0.28	0.11
6-7H	0.74*	0.74*	0.67*	0.58	0.30	0.13	0.17	-0.05
7-8H	0.25	0.34	0.40	0.39	0.34	0.22	0.22	0.04

^{1} Coefficient of correlation, n=9. * $p<0.05$, ** $p<0.01$, *** $p<0.001$

Table 2. Correlation between in vitro and in vivo EAA profiles, rapeseed proteins.

in vitro / in vivo	0-3H	3-6H	6-9H	9-12H r	12-15H	15-18H	18-21H	21-24H
0-1H	0.81**	0.91***	0.95***	0.90***	0.91***	0.86**	0.85**	0.82**
1-2H	0.69*	0.86**	0.94***	0.91***	0.85**	0.76*	0.76*	0.73*
2-3H	0.56	0.72*	0.83**	0.87**	0.88**	0.81**	0.84**	0.82**
3-4H	0.55	0.71*	0.84**	0.90***	0.94***	0.88***	0.92***	0.84**
4-5H	0.56	0.69*	0.79**	0.82**	0.88***	0.81**	0.84**	0.81**
5-6H	0.53	0.71*	0.86**	0.91***	0.90***	0.83**	0.84**	0.76*
6-7H	0.42	0.57	0.73*	0.78**	0.86**	0.82**	0.82**	0.80**
7-8H	0.16	0.28	0.41	0.41	0.54	0.56	0.48	0.56

<u>In vivo data</u>. Six pigs, fitted with catheters in the portal vein and
in the carotid artery as well as with an electromagnetic flow probe
around the portal vein, received 800-g test meals containing either 12%
casein or 12% rapeseed proteins. Blood samples were collected and blood
flow rate recorded during a period of 8 hours. For each 1-h interval,
the profile of EAA absorbed was determined by coupling blood flow rate
with porto-arterial differences in plasma EAA concentrations.

<u>Statistics</u>. The degree of correspondence between <u>in vitro</u> and <u>in vivo</u>
EAA profiles was calculated with Pearson's test of correlation.

3 RESULTS AND DISCUSSION

Tables 1 and 2 indicate the coefficients of correlation obtained
when comparing the profiles of EAA released <u>in vitro</u> to the profiles of
EAA absorbed in the portal vein of pigs after the ingestion of the 12%
protein diets. With casein (table 1), the best correspondences were
found when comparing EAA patterns measured during the first half of
<u>in vitro</u> digestion and <u>in vivo</u> absorption periods. This is consequent
with the observation that the <u>in vitro</u> dialysis method allows to col-
lect during early proteolysis the AA that are preferentially attacked
by digestive enzymes (3), and that these AA have a high probability to
be those rapidly released in portal blood in an <u>in vivo</u> situation.

With rapeseed proteins, however, correspondences between <u>in vitro</u>
and <u>in vivo</u> data were distributed differently (table 2). The EAA profile of the first <u>in vitro</u> interval was poorly correlated to the <u>in vivo</u>
patterns. Contrarily to casein, all EAA profiles of the subsequent <u>in</u>
<u>vitro</u> digesta had significant coefficients of correlation with most <u>in</u>
<u>vivo</u> profiles. This suggests that enzymatic hydrolysis of rapeseed pro-
teins released EAA in such proportions they could avoid in part the
well-known competition for intestinal transport sites (4), and be
absorbed in portal vein within similar kinetics.

These original results show that luminal proteolysis, as reprodu-
ced by the <u>in vitro</u> technique, is a key determinant of absorption of AA
in portal bloodstream. The EAA patterns of <u>in vitro</u> digesta thus appear
to be good indicators of AA bioavailability, to a degree varying with
the nature of the protein source.

4 REFERENCES

1. A. Rérat, P. Vaissade and P. Vaugelade. <u>Ann. Biol. anim. Bioch.</u>
    <u>Biophys.</u>, 1979, <u>19</u>, 739.
2. L. Savoie and S.F. Gauthier. J.Food Sci., 1986, <u>51</u>, 494.
3. C. Vachon, S.F. Gauthier, J.D. Jones and L. Savoie. <u>Nutr.Rep.Int.</u>,
    1983, <u>27</u>, 1303.
4. B.G. Munck. 'Physiology of the Gastro-Intestinal Tract', Raven
    Press, New York, 1981, vol. 2, Chapter 44, p. 1097.

IN VITRO TECHNIQUE TO EVALUATE AMINO ACID AVAILABIL...

L. Savoie, G. Parent, R. Charbonneau and I. Galibois

Centre de recherche en nutrition
et Département de nutrition humaine et de consommation
Pav. Paul-Comtois, Université Laval, Québec
Canada G1K 7P4

1 INTRODUCTION

Several methods have been proposed to evaluate protein quality. However, it has become clear that neither amino acid profile or nitrogen digestibility can be considered as the sole determinant, and that individual amino acid digestibility must also be considered. Results obtained by fecal or ileal measurements are affected by the variable contributions of endogenous secretion of proteins and alterations in amino acids brought about by microorganisms in the gut, and cannot take into account the sequence and form of release of amino acids. The digestibility of a protein is a spatio-temporal event implying that the kinetics of release of a given amino acid will determine the intestinal site where it will become available for absorption.

Materials and Methods

The in vitro digestion of proteins (Na Caseinate, N x 6.25 = 86.8% and rapeseed concentrate, N x 6.25 = 52%) was carried out in a dialysis system involving a two-step hydrolysis at $37^{\circ}C$[1]. Forty (40) mg of proteic nitrogen were first digested in 0.1N HCl, at pH 1.9, with 1 mg of pepsin (hog stomach mucosa, 1:60 000). The peptic digestion was stopped by raising the pH to 7.5 with the addition of 1N NaOH. The suspension was then transferred to the dialysis bag with a molecular weight cutoff of 1000 Daltons of the digestion cell[2] and 10 mg of pancreatin (hog pancreas 5X) was added. The digestion products were collected by a circulating sodium phosphate buffer (10 mM, pH 7.5) every 3 hours for 24 hours.

The dialysate was chromatographied on a Copper Sephadex G-25 column[3] in free amino acid and oligopeptide fractions. Digestibilities were calculated as followed:

$$\text{Protein digestibility (\%)} = \frac{\text{N in dialysate (mg)}}{40 \text{ mg}} \times 100$$

$$\text{AA digestibility (\%)} = \frac{\text{AA in dialysate (mg \%)}}{\text{AA in protein (mg \%)}} \times 100$$

Results and discussion

Throughout the experimental period, casein had a higher cumulative digestibility than rapeseed. Amino acids followed various pattern of digestion. For casein, arginine, tyrosine, lysine, methionine, leucine and phenylalanine, were preferentially hydrolysed in the first period, while threonine, serine, glutamic acid and proline were released much more slowly. In rapeseed, amino acids were hydrolysed more gradually and only three amino acids followed the same kinetics than casein (tyrosine, methionine and serine). Marked differences involved arginine, cystine, lysine. For casein, isoleucine, valine and threonine were mostly found in peptide form while arginine and lysine were released as free amino acids. With rapeseed, leucine, phenylalanine and tyrosine appeared in the free form while histidine, threonine and valine were rather found in the peptide fractions.

As shown by Table 1, there was a significant negative correlation between the digestibility of individual amino acids (that is, their overall release) and their percentage of release in peptides with both proteins during the first 3 hours of digestion. The correspondence remained negative and significant with rapeseed protein as digestion proceeded, but disappeared rapidly with casein.

Table 1 Correlation Between the Digestibility of Amino Acids (%) and their Proportions as Peptides (%) in the Digestion Products.

Period of digestion	Casein	Rapeseed
	r values[†]	
0- 3 h	- 0.85 ***	- 0.72 **
3- 6 h	- 0.29	- 0.64 *
6- 9 h	- 0.21	- 0.51 *
9-12 h	0.03	0.10

[†] Coefficient of correlation, n=16; *$p<0.05$; **$p<0.01$; ***$p<0.001$.

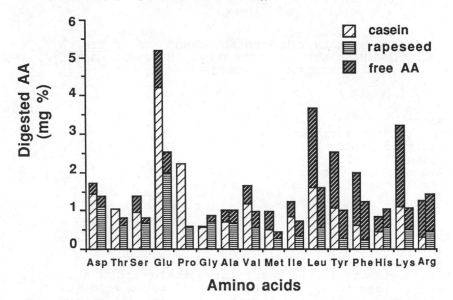

<u>Figure 1</u> Nature of digestion products in the first quarter of <u>in vitro</u> digestion of çasein and rapeseed. Adapted from Savoie <u>et al</u>., 1988[4].

The sequential release of amino acids can be attributed, in part, to the specificity of proteolytic enzymes for target amino acids. However, the protein nature has hindered protease specificity, due to the conjugated effect of primary, secondary and tertiary structures. As a result, the nature of the material offered (free amino acids and oligopeptides) to brush-border final digestion and absorption, varies according to the period of digestion and to the protein ingested. This is illustrated in Figure 1.

REFERENCES

1. S. Gauthier, C. Vachon and L. Savoie, <u>J. Food Sci.</u>, 1986, <u>51</u>, 960.
2. L. Savoie and S. Gauthier, <u>J. Food Sci.</u>, 1986, <u>51</u>, 494.
3. L. Savoie and G. Parent, <u>Nutr. Rep. Intern.</u>, 1987, <u>35</u>, 783.
4. L. Savoie, I. Galibois, G. Parent, R. Charbonneau, <u>Nutr. Res.</u>, 1988, <u>8</u>, in press.

A COMPARISON BETWEEN THE SIBBALD METHOD AND AD LIB. FEEDING ON TME$_n$ VALUES OF FEEDSTUFFS IN NORMAL AND CAECECTOMISED ROOSTERS

J.P. HAYES
Department of Poultry Science
University of Stellenbosch
Stellenbosch   7600
Republic of South Africa

1 INTRODUCTION

Microbial activity in the gastrointestinal tract of the chicken can lead to an overestimation of amino acid availability values[1,2] and it can affect the efficiency of utilization of metabolisable energy[3]. With regard to feedstuff evaluation it is important to know whether the nutrient content is not overestimated due to microbial breakdown to non-nutritive substances in the caecum. In previous experiments[2] lysine availability of heat-damaged fish meal was 56% in normal roosters but only 42% in caecectomised roosters. The aim in our experiments was to determine the effect of caecectomy on true metabolizable energy (TME$_n$) values of feedstuffs within two feeding regimes, viz. force-feeding by tube as opposed to ad lib intake. Lysine availability was also determined.

2 EXPERIMENTAL PROCEDURE

Intact and caecectomised[4] adult roosters were either precision-fed by the method of Sibbald[5] with 48hr excreta collection or were allowed free access to diets for four days with feed intake and excreta collection measured during the last three days of the period according to the so-called Dual Semi Quick (DSQ) method[6] which is generally practiced in our laboratory. Endogenous energy was deter- mined by feeding dextrose, 40g/bird, as a slurry 24 hours after feed removal. In the DSQ procedure products which are normally readily consumed, eg. grains, were supple- mented with 2 parts per 100 with a vitamin/mineral premix and fed as such. Unpalatable products, however, were mixed in equal proportions with a "basal" diet which consisted of 98 parts ground corn and 2 parts of the vitamin/mineral premix. Each feedstuff was fed to 7 intact or 7 caecectomised roosters and as excreta samples were not pooled, values obtained for the different roosters served as replicates to determine the effect of caecectomy.

3 RESULTS AND DISCUSSION

Caecectomy caused a general decrease in TME_n values for several feedstuffs if the Sibbald method of evaluation was employed (Table 1). Differences were significant for corn, lupins, sunflower oil cake (SOCM), groundnut oil cake (GNOCM) and fish meal (FM). The results of other workers are thus confirmed who found the same effect of caecectomy for distillers' dried grains[7]. For the DSQ method on the other hand which utilized a four day ad lib feeding period, TME_n values for most feedstuffs were practically unaffected by caecectomy (Table 2). An exception was SOCM where two samples were tested and only in one sample TME was significantly higher in intact roosters than in caecectomised roosters.

With regard to lysine availability caecectomy resulted in lower values only for the sorghum sample in the DSQ method. For the other feedstuffs no differences between intact and caecectomised roosters could be found. In the literature a number of workers have reported lower amino acid availability values due to caecectomy[7] in roosters while other workers[8] found that certain amino acids eg. lysine were not affected by the removal of the caecum. It was pointed out[9] that the endogenous excretion of amino acids, especially lysine, can be positively influenced by the caeca due to bacterial synthesis and that this will significantly affect amino acid digestibility values. In the present study it was found that the endogenous lysine excreted by intact roosters amounted to 16.85 mg/rooster/d and by caecectomised roosters to 31.1 mg/d.

It was concluded from the present experiments that more work is needed to establish with certainty whether caecectomised roosters have to be used for TME_n and amino acid availability determinations or not. There are indications that especially the so-called rapid methods might yield higher TME_n values for certain feedstuffs in intact roosters than in caecectomised roosters and that this could be due to a degradation of indigestible material in the intestinal tract and not to a higher bio-availability of energy.

Table 1   Effect of caecectomy on TME_n and lysine
           availability values (Sibbald method)

Feedstuff	TME_n MJ/kg		% Lys. avail.	
	Intact	Caecect	Intact	Caecect
Corn A	14.3*	13.6	92.8	87.8
Corn B	12.9	13.2	69.2	69.9
Lupins	11.7*	10.0	82.8	81.6
Fish Meal A	13.6*	12.7	96.4	96.1
Fish Meal B	12.9	12.5	--	--
Sunflower oc	9.0*	7.9	84.0	83.3
Groundnut oc	9.7	8.5	71.4	--

Table 2   Effect of caecectomy on TME_n and lysine
           availability values (DSQ method)

Feedstuff	TME_n MJ/kg		% Lys. avail.	
	Intact	Caecect	Intact	Caecect
Corn	14.0	13.8	92.3	--
Sorghum	13.4	13.6	69.7	83.5
Sunflower oc	9.0	8.6	88.6	79.4
Sunflower oc	8.0*	6.9	80.4	82.3
Fish meal	12.0	12.6	92.3	93.6

*   denotes significance at 5% level of probability

REFERENCES

1. Nesheim, M.C. and K.J. Carpenter, 1967. Brit. J. Nutr.
   21, 399-411.
2. Hayes, J.P., R.E. Austic and M.L. Scott, 1984. Proceedings and Abstracts of the XVII World's Poultry Congress and Exhibition. Aug. 8-12 p. 303-305.
3. Campbell, L.D., A. Chwalibog, R.B. Eggum and Grete
   Thorbek, 1979. 8th Symposium on Energy Metabolism,
   Cambridge, England. p. 1.
4. Payne, W.L., R.R. Kifer, D.G. Snyder and G.F. Combs,
   1971. Poultry Sci. 143-150.
5. Sibbald, I.R., 1976. Poultry Sci. 55, 303-308.
6. Du Preez, J.J., A. du P. Minnaar and J.S. Duckitt,
   1984. World's Poultry Sci. J. 40, 121-126.
7. Parsons, M.C., 1985. J. Agric. Sci., Camb. 104, 469-472.
8. Raharjo, Y. and D.J. Farrell, 1984. Aust. J. Agric.
   Anim. Husb. 24, 516-521.
9. Green, S., Solange, L., Bertrand, Madelein, J.C. Duron
   and Maillard, R., 1987. Brit. Poultry Sci. 28, 643-652.

Maintenance of Biochemical Parameters During Weight
Reduction Regimes Using Foods Made With Isolated Soy
Protein

M.N. Volgarev (1) and F.H. Steinke (2)

(1) Institute of Nutrition, Academy of Medical
    Sciences, Moscow, USSR.
(2) Protein Technologies International, St. Louis, MO.
    USA.

Five basic food products, oatmeal porridge, a
nutritional beverage, two low fat (15%) sausages and a
pasta were developed using Isolated Soy Protein. These
foods were incorporated into Soviet menus to provide
1300 and 1700 Kcal balanced meals with protein intakes
of 90g per day.

Seventeen obese, hospitalized, hypercholesterolemia
patients were given the 1300 Kcal diet for 30 days, and
fourteen moderately overweight outpatient volunteers
were given the 1700 Kcal diet for 28 days. Twenty
blood chemistry measurements remained normal or
unchanged based on initial and final blood samples.
Weight losses were 7.0 and 4.1kg for the 1300 and 1700
Kcal diets, respectively.

Evaluation of nitrogen balance demonstrated a slightly
positive balance for the subjects on the 1300 Kcal diet
with estimated true nitrogen digestibility of 97.7%.

Blood cholesterol values were markedly improved in both
the hyper-cholesterolemia obese and the outpatient
group. Blood cholesterol was reduced 41% in the obese
group and 16% in the outpatient volunteers while
consuming the low calorie menus with isolated soy
protein containing foods.

NUTRITIONAL AND SAFETY EVALUATION OF A RECENTLY PRODUCED ANIMAL BLOOD PROTEIN

M. Antal, K. Nagy, K. Tóth, E. Dworschák, Ö. Gaál, A. Pegöly-Mérei, J. Szépvölgyi, A. Pintér[x], P. Baráti, G. Bíró

National Institute of Food- Hygiene and Nutrition
[x]National Institute of Hygiene
Budapest

INTRODUCTION

Nowadays a lot of comprehensive studies are performed to discover new protein sources. In this respect, the animal blood plasma which is currently wasted is ponderable. The bioavailability of a novel protein from plasma produced in Hungary was investigated.

NUTRITIONAL VALUES

Growth rate, protein efficiency ratio (PER), biological value (BV), true digestibility (TD) and net protein utilization (NPU) using N-balance technique of plasma protein (PP) were determined[1]. Casein completed with methionine (C) served as reference protein. NPU, BV and TD values of plasma protein were similar to those of reference protein. PER value was rather low since rats rejected the diet and so the development of animals fell significantly behind that of the casein group. For increasing the nutritive value PP was mixed with egg white protein (EP) in a ratio of 4:1, 2:1 and 1:1. Already a 4:1 mixture had a favourable effect and PER value of a 1:1 mixture corresponded to that of C (Table 1).

SAFETY EVALUATION

Plasma protein (PP) or the mixture of plasma protein and egg white protein (PP/EP) in a ratio of 3:1 or casein completed with methionine (C) was added as a sole source of protein at 8, 18 and 38 % respectively (Table 2). Proteins were tested in a 3 months experiment.

RESULTS AND DISCUSSION

The weight gain of male and female rats consuming the 8 % PP and males fed 8 % PP/EP containing diets fell significantly behind that of the other groups. Increasing the PP concentration of the diet gain was accelerated.

Pathologic differences could not be observed in rats kept either on
8 % PP or PP/EP and 18 % PP or PP/EP and 38 % PP/EP containing
diets in the following cases: haematological values (Hb, Hc, RBC,
WBC, thrombocyte, smear); urine parameters (quantitative); biochemical measurements (ASST, ALT, acidic and alkaline phosphatases,
serum albumin, urea-N, serum and liver total protein, triglyceride,
cholesterol, liver total lipid); oral glucose tolerance test: relative masses and histology of organs but kidney of rats consuming
PP containing diets.

In rats consuming 38 % PP containing diet: serum urea-N level was
elevated and AST and ALT activities were in few cases (AST: 87, 91,
269 U/1 ALT: 83, 101, 225 U/1 pathologically high; the relative
kidney-mass of females and the relative liver-mass in both sexes
increased and significant accumulation could be observed in the
hepatic total lipid content of males and in the cholesterol content
of both sexes (Table 3).
Nephrocalcinosis was developed in all groups consuming PP most
pronouncedly in animals fed by 8 % PP.

Lysinoalanine (LAL) could influence the nutritional value and
produce nefrocalcinosis[2]. Plasma protein did not contain lysinoalanine, methionine-sulfone and hydroxy-methylfurfural. Moderate to
severe kidney calcification was noticed due to high P and low Mg,
Ca containing diet[3]. Ca, P and Mg content of the diet was in
accordance with NRC recommendation, Ca, P and Mg content of PP was
300, 130 and 1080 mg/100 g. So PP could not shift the ratio of
minerals toward low dietary Ca, Mg and high P. The abnormalities
observed could be explained by the low methionine and isoleucine
content of PP (2,34 and 0,35 g/100 g resp.)

   CONCLUSION
Nutritional value and safety of blood plasma protein from animal
source prove that it could be a suitable protein source if its
amino acid composition is balanced.

Table 1 Nutritional Value of Plasma Protein

	PER	TD	BV	NPU
C	3,1+0,31	95+2,2	90+1,4	89+2,8
PP	1,1+0,16	96+9,6	81+5,9	79+6,6
PP/EP (4:1)	2,3+0,27	95+5,4	86+7,1	82+9,8
PP/EP (2:1)	2,8+0,12	96+4,5	93+3,5	91+2,8
PP/EP (1:1)	3,2+0,14	92+2,8	95+3,0	91+3,0

Table 2 Composition of Diets (g/100 g)

Protein[x]	8	18	38
Sunflower oil	10	10	10
Potato starch	8	8	8
Vitamin mix	1	1	1
Mineral mix[xx]	1	1	1
Wheat starch up to 100		100	100

[x]Protein content of casein, plasma protein, the mixture of plasma protein-egg white protein (3:1) and that of diets was measured by Kjeldahl technique. Diets containing casein were completed with 0,1, 0,2 and 0,4 g of DL-methionine, respectively.
[xx]According to NRC recommendations-Ca:600 mg, P:500 mg, Mg 40 mg/100 g diet.

Table 3 Hepatic Cholesterol (mg/g)

	C			PP			PP/EP		
Protein %:	8	18	38	8	18	38	8	18	38
					male				
x	4,9	4,7	5,3[c]	4,5	6,1[b]	10,3[a]	4,0	4,6	4,1[d]
±SD	1,5	1,1	1,3	1,1	1,5	2,5	0,9	0,9	0,7
					female				
x	3,6	3,6	3,5[c]	4,0	4,2[b]	7,5[a]	3,0	3,3	2,5[d]
±SD	0,8	0,3	0,6	1,1	1,0	1,8	1,1	1,0	1,6

$$p < 0,01$$
$$a \longrightarrow b; c; d$$

REFERENCES
1. P. L. Pellett and V. R. Young eds. Nutrition evaluation of protein foods pp 104, 108 UNU 1980.
2. P. A. Finot, Nutr. Abstr. Rev in Clin. Nutr. - Series A, 1983, 53, 67.
3. R. M. Forbes, J. Nutr. 1963, 80, 321.

BIOAVAILABILITY OF AMINO ACIDS, MINERAL BALANCES AND
VITAMIN B₁ STATUS AMONG MALES CONSUMING FABA BEAN DIETS
WITH HIGH PROANTHOCYANIDINS.

Laila Hussein, Hesham Mottawei and Ronald Marquardt*

Department of Nutrition, National Research Center,
Giza, Dokki, Egypt.

* Department of Animal Nutrition - University of Manitoba,
  Winnipeg, Canada.

1 INTRODUCTION

Vegetable proteins have recently received increased attention as low cost replacement for animal protein. Although
the quality of soybean proteins had been extensively studied in man[1]; other plant proteins did not receive the same
interest. Faba beans (Vicia faba) are the staple food in
Egypt. The seeds of some faba bean varieties are rich in
proanthocyanidins (PA); and their inclusion in the diet
had been reported to depress the apparent digestibility of
proteins and some amino acids in experimental rats[2].

This report describes the availability to humans of
proteins, amino acids and minerals in diets, differing in
their PA content.

2 SUBJECTS AND METHODS

Seventeen healthy boys aged 12-14 y participated in the
study. Each subject consumed each of 4 diets for 10 days.
The proximate composition and chemical analysis of the
diets are presented in Table 1. Bioavailability was
assessed based on apparent absorption (feces and urine
collected quantitatively during the whole metabolic study).

Nitrogen content of daily urine specimens, fecal
composites and composites of the total daily diets were
analyzed by the micro-Kjeldahl method. PA was assayed by
Folin Denis reagent in the absence or presence of polyvinyl
pyrrolidone, and the intensity of the developed blue color
was measured spectrophotometrically[3]. The proanthocyanidin
(anthocyanidin formation assay) was also assayed in HCl-
butanol[4]. The enzymatic gravimetric method was used for

Table 1   Food Ingredients and Chemical Composition of the
           4 Experimental Diets

| Food Ingredients | D i e t | | | |
	A	B	C	D
	Mean Dry Matter Consumed/Subject/Day			
Faba beans,	50.1			
Giza 3, with hulls			33.2	
" ", without hulls		40.3		
Triple white with hulls				39.5
Starch	20.4	26.9	22.8	21.6
Oil, vegetable	22.5	31.5	31.8	27.6
Margarine	15.5	19.9	26.8	26.2
Protein intake g/KG/d	1.15	1.32	1.43	1.41
PA mg/d	563	493	792	467

Cellulose to keep fibre content constant.

determination of dietary fibre[5], whereas fibre in stool
was determined without enzymatic pre-treatment. The amino
acid contents of the food and stool samples were determined after hydrolysis in 6N hydrochloric acid using a
LKB Biochron 4151 Alpha plus Amino Acid Analyzer. Mineral
analyses were carried out after digestion using a combination of wet and dry ashing[6] using atomic absorption
spectrometry (Beltsville Human Nutrition Research Center,
U.S.A).

3   RESULTS AND DISCUSSION

Table 2 presents the% apparent digestibilities of crude
protein, fat and fibre among subjects consuming diets
with increasing levels of PA. Significant lower mean
protein digestibilities were obtained after consuming
diets containing 160 or 126 mg% PA ($P < 0.05$) compared to
corresponding mean levels obtained after consuming diets
containing 90 or 78 mg% PA. The % digestibility (disappearance) of fibre was similarly affected. The % bioavailability of Met was very low in diet C containing
126 mg% PA, compared to corresponding mean level of 47%
in diet D, with 76 mg% PA. The AA scores (absorbed AA
in mg/g N/FAO scoring) improved significantly upon
supplementation of Diet D with Met.

Table 2   Digestibilities of Protein, Fat and Fibre

	D I E T			
NUTRIENT	A	B	C	D
PA(mg %)*	160	90	126	78

	Apparent Digestibilities (%)							
	$\bar{X}$	SE	$\bar{X}$	SE	$\bar{X}$	SE	$\bar{X}$	SE
Crude Protein	69	0.3^a	77	0.8^b	69	0.3^a	79	0.3^b
Ether Extract	85	1.0	85	1.3	89	1.1	91	0.7
Crude Fiber	67	1.8^a	76	0.5^b	68	0.3^a	76	1.1^b

* PA Proanthocyanidin level in the diets.

Mean values not sharing a superscript differed significantly ($P < 0.05$).

The absorption of Ca, P and Mg was improved significantly ($P < 0.05$) in diets containing dehulled faba beans and PA = 88mg %. The absorption of Zn was highest among subjects consuming diets containing faba beans, var. Triple white with PA = 78mg %. No uniform trend was found for the absorption of Fe from the different diets. This in agreement with the fact that non haem iron is affected by different factors during absorption. The subjects were negative Zn balance with mean levels of 2.4 and 0.5 mg/day for subjects consuming diets C,D, respectively.

REFERENCES
1. Miles, CW., Ziyad, J., Bodwell, CE., Steele, PD. J.Food Sci. (1984), 49, 1167.
2. Eggum, BO., Christensen, KD in:"Breeding for seed protein improvement using nuclear techniques". Intern. Atomic Energy Agency, Vienna (1975),pp.135–143.
3. Sjodin, J., Matersson, P., Magyaresi, T. Pflanzenzuchtung (1981) 86,231.
4. Butler, L.G. in "Proc.Intern. Symp. on Sorghum Grain Quality" Intern. Crop Res. Institute Semi-arid Tropics (ECRISAT)(1982), pp.294–311.
5. Asp,N., Johansson, GG., Hallmer, H., Siljestrom, M. J. Agr. Food Chem. (1983), 31, 476.
6. Hill, AD., Patterson, KY., Veillon, C., Morris, ER. Anal. Chem. (1986), 58, 2340.

FOLATE BIOAVAILABILITY

G. Farrar and J. A. Blair

Department of Pharmaceutical Sciences
Aston University
Aston Triangle
Birmingham B4 7ET

Folic acid (pteroyl glutamic acid, figure 1) is the
parent molecule for a large number of derivatives
collectively known as folates. These compounds are
required by mammals for 1-carbon transfer reactions
(synthesis of purines, deoxythymidylic acid, glycine and
methionine)[1]. Since these folate co-enzymes are not
synthesised in-situ, they are required by mammals as
vitamins. Although the minimum requirement in man is
50 µg/day, an intake of 200 µg/day is recommended[2].

Folic acid (FA) is not present in food or mammalian
tissues except when added as a dietary supplement. It
has no metabolic role, but it can enter folate metabolism
by reduction of the pterin ring to 7,8-dihydrofolate (DHF).
Major folate metabolites are 5,6,7,8-tetrahydrofolate
(THF) and the substituted tetrahydro forms 5-methyltetra-
hydrofolate (5MeTHF) and 10-formyltetrahydrofolate
(10CHOTHF) (figure 1). They are transported in urine,
plasma and CSF as monoglutamates with 5MeTHF as the major
species. In tissues where they function as coenzymes,
the major species are polyglutamates (figure 1) formed by
the further addition of glutamate residues; monoglutamates
are present only in trace amounts[1].

The interconversions of the various species, together
with some key enzymes are shown in figure 2.

Folate bioavailability is best described as the
proportion of dietary folate incorporated into liver as
it is the largest polyglutamate pool[1]. Other tissues
(eg. brain or kidney) may have different changes in
incorporations.

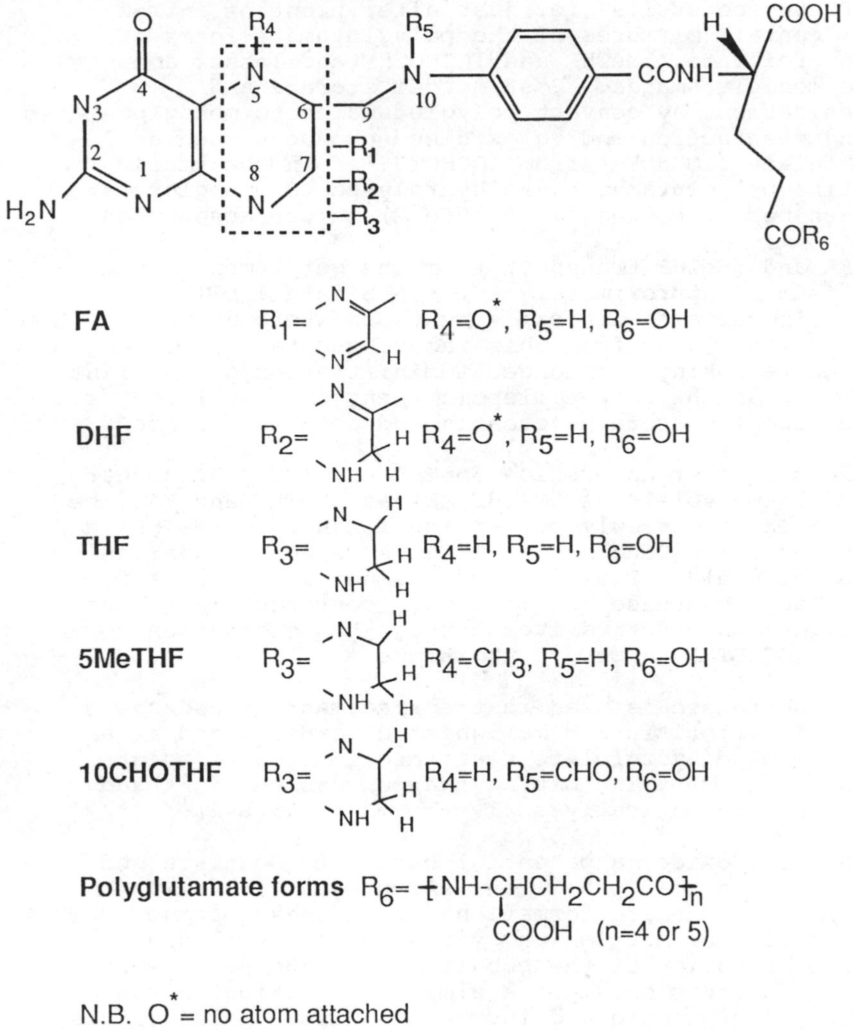

FIGURE 1. FOLIC ACID AND DERIVATIVES.

Fresh foodstuffs (ie. just after plant or animal death) contain mixtures of the polyglutamate forms of tetrahydrofolate, 5MeTHF and 1OCHOTHF and lesser amounts of the monoglutamates. Post mortem storage and homogenisation may convert polyglutamates to monoglutamates by conjugase action and to oxidised products such as 10-formylfolate (1OCHOFA) from 1OCHOTHF[1]. In the small intestine polyglutamates are hydrolysed to monoglutamates by brush border conjugase (figure 2) before absorption.

FA and 5MeTHF transport from the gut lumen have a pH optimum of approximately 6[3]. FA bioavailability is reduced in certain clinical situations where jejunal lumen pH moves away from this value, such as in sodium bicarbonate dosing, prolonged administration of alkaline drugs such as the anti-epileptic phenytoin, achlorohydria in the elderly, acute pancreatis and coeliac disease[3].

In man after absorption 5MeTHF and 1OCHOTHF appear in the plasma solely as 5MeTHF, FA as 5MeTHF and FA (the latter then only slowly converting further to 5MeTHF) and 1OCHOFA as only 1OCHOFA (ie. 1OCHOFA is not an available folate for man)[4]. Plasma 5MeTHF is not a substrate for polyglutamyl synthase but is slowly converted in tissues to polyglutamate derivatives through transformation to THF and 1OCHOTHF which are substrates[1].

Methotrexate is used in the treatment of psoriasis, rheumatoid arthritis and malignant disorders, and as an inhibitor of dihydrofolate reductase it reduces folate bioavailability by inhibiting the conversion of FA and DHF to the enzymatically active forms (figure 2)[1].

Nitrous oxide, a potential hazard to dentists and also used as a food propellant and present in saliva(?), reduces polyglutamate formation and increases urine 5MeTHF by inhibition of methionine synthase[1]. This is due to specific oxidation of the cobalt ion of the B_{12} coenzyme required for this enzyme. A similar situation in man of lowered polyglutamate and increased plasma 5MeTHF occurs with reduced uptake of dietary B_{12} (pernicious anaemia, achlorohydria, vegans)[1].

Methionine synthase is also probably inhibited by the oxidising action of peroxides in polyunsaturated oils[5], with a consequent decrease of liver polyglutamates and increased output of urinary 5MeTHF. The rise of MeTHF in the urine of alcoholics suggests reduction of methionine synthase activity[6].

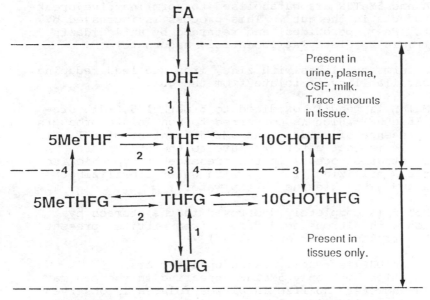

LEGEND.

1). DHFR (dihydrofolate reductase)
2). Methionine synthase (Vitamin B_{12} dependent)

3). Polyglutamate synthase
4). Conjugase.
FA - folic acid
DHF - dihydrofolate
THF - tetrahydrofolate
5MeTHF - 5-methyltetrahydrofolate
10CHOTHF - 10-formyltetrahydrofolate
THFG - tetrahydrofolate polyglutamate
DHFG - dihydrofolate polyglutamate
5MeTHFG - 5-methyltetrahydrofolate polyglutamate
10CHOTHFG - 10-formyltetrahydrofolate polyglutamate

N.B. Enzymes 1-4 are the major participating enzymes,
they are not however, the sole enzymes responsible for the
conversions.

FIGURE 2. FOLATE METABOLISM AND ENZYMES.

FA and 5MeTHF are catabolised to form inactive break-down products in the gut[7]. This process is increased by oxidants (Fe^{3+}, peroxides) and retarded by antioxidants (eg. vitamin E, diethylstilboestrol, ascorbate)[5,8].

FA forms complexes with zinc, iron and lead reducing the bioavailability of folate from the gut.

5MeTHF is readily oxidised to 5-methyl 5,6-dihydro-folate (5MeDHF) which is converted to non folate products in the presence of acid[8]. The 5MeTHF content of UHT milk for example is lost after exposure to the atmosphere. A similar situation occurs in the presence of hypochlorite (Milton's sterilizing fluids), with water sterilizing tablets and with chlorine in tap water[9].

5MeTHF is completely destroyed in the stomach by oxidation with nitrous acid formed from nitrite (present in food, drinking water and saliva)[9,10].

In man DHF is readily taken up after oral administration with only 5MeTHF appearing in the plasma[8]. After THF however, no rise in plasma folates is observed due to very rapid oxidation to non folate compounds.

10CHOTHF is very rapidly oxidised in neutral or alkaline solutions to form 10-formyl folic acid. This species however does not enter the folate metabolic cycle in man[8], but does so in rats probably due to gut bacterial action[11]. Therefore care must be taken when considering animal models to study folate metabolism.

SUMMARY

1. Folate bioavailability is complex.

2. Bioavailability in animal models can be estimated by liver polyglutamate formation.

3. In man bioavailability is estimated by the oral administration of FA and the 24 hour collection and analysis of urine, faeces and serum for folate content.

4. Available food folate is best measured as 5MeTHF and 5MeTHFG.

5. Analysis of samples from 2-4 can be performed using high performance liquid chromatography.

6.   Exposure to oxidising species (O_2, $OH^{\bullet}$, Fe^{3+}, peroxides, nitrite, hypochlorite, water sterilising agents, chlorine in tap water, nitrous oxide) should be avoided.

7.   Adequate intake of antioxidant (vitamin C, vitamin E) and vitamin B_{12}, is required for maximum bioavailability.

REFERENCES

1.   P.B. Rowe, 'The metabolic basis of inherited disease', Ed J.B. Stanbury et al, (1983), 5th Edition McGraw-Hill (New York) p498.

2.   J. Lindenbaum, Current Concepts Nutr (1980), 9, 105.

3.   A. Benn, C.H.J. Swan, W.T. Cooke, J.A. Blair, A.J. Matty, M.E. Smith, Brit. J. Med, (1971), 1, 148.

4.   K. Ratanasthien, J.A. Blair, R.J. Leeming, W.T. Cooke, V. Melikian, J. Clin. Path, (1974), 27, 875.

5.   M.J. Stankiewicz, Ph.D thesis, (1988), Aston University.

6.   D.A.R. Al-Haddad, Ph.D thesis, (1984), Aston University.

7.   A.E. Pheasant, M.J. Connor, J.A. Blair, Biochem. Med, (1981), 26, 435.

8.   K. Ratanasthien, J.A. Blair, R.J. Leeming, W.T. Cooke, V. Melikian, J. Clin. Path, (1977), 30, 438.

9.   C.G.B. Hamon, J.A. Blair, (manuscript in preparation).

10.   S.J.R. Heales, J.A. Blair, A.E. Guest, A.E. Pheasant, 'Biochemical and Clinical Aspects of Pteridines, Vol 4, Ed H. Wachter et al, (1985), Walter de Gruyter, (Berlin and New York) p17.

11.   M.J. Connor, J.A. Blair, 'Chemistry and Biology of Pteridines', Eds Kisliuk/Brown, (1979), Elsevier North Holland, Inc. p531.

USE OF THE RAT FOR MEASURING THE BIOLOGICAL
AVAILABILITY OF FOLATES IN FOODS

J.M. Gee, A. Bhabuta and I.T. Johnson

Department of Nutrition & Food Quality
AFRC Institute of Food Research - Norwich Laboratory
Colney Lane, Norwich NR4 7UA

1   INTRODUCTION

Folates exist in foods in a variety of substituted and
conjugated forms[1]. Their bioavailability depends both
upon their efficiency of absorption and their capacity
to interact with the appropriate metabolic pathways.
This report describes a method for the assessment of
folate availability from human foods by measuring the
response to diet of selected tissue stores in the
folate-depleted rat.

2   METHOD

Male Wistar rats(ca.200g) were fed for at least 28 days
on a semi-synthetic diet supplemented with all
necessary vitamins other than pteroylglutamic acid
(PGA). Depleted animals were subsequently transferred
to a test diet containing a source of folate, or
maintained as controls on the depletion diet. The
experimental diets were supplemented with PGA, freeze-
dried cooked liver, or freeze-dried raw cabbage. At
the end of a defined period of repletion all the
animals were killed and samples of liver, serum and
small intestinal mucosa were recovered for folate
analysis by radio-immunoassay (RIA). The folate
contents of the diets were determined by
microbiological assay with <u>Lactibacillus. casei</u>[2].

Table 1   Tissue folate levels in folate depleted and
PGA-supplemented rats

Group	Liver	Mucosa	Serum
Depleted	2.7	0.2	15.2
Supplemented	11.4	1.7	305.0

Results are means of pairs

3   RESULTS

During this depletion period the animals continued to
gain weight and remain healthy; however radio-
immunoassay showed a significant reduction in folate
levels in liver, serum and intestinal mucosa (Table 1)
compared to those of rats fed a PGA-supplemented diet
(50mg/Kg).

After a 7 day repletion period there was a significant
recovery of serum folate stores in animals fed PGA-
supplemented diets.   The extent of recovery was closely
related to the dietary folate content, with evidence of
saturation at a level of 50mg/Kg diet (Figure 1).   The
total folate intake and serum-folate response to a diet
supplemented with freeze-dried liver (125g/Kg diet) is
shown in Figure 2.

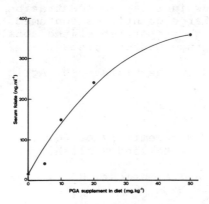

Figure 1 Serum folate response to PGA repletion

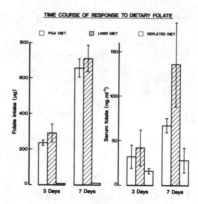

<u>Figure 2</u> Serum folate response to liver supplement diet

4 CONCLUSION

The use of RIA to measure the serum folate response to supplemented diets in the folate-depleted rat provides a relatively fast and inexpensive approach to the measurement of folate availability in human foods. The sensitivity of the serum folate response as a biological end-point should enable the method to be applied to foods such as potatoes and cereal products which are relatively low in folate concentration but which, because of the large quantities consumed, provide a relatively high proportion of the total folates consumed in average western diets[3].

This work was supported by the Ministry of Agriculture, Fisheries and Food.

REFERENCES

1.   R.L. Blakley, 'The Biochemistry of Folic Acid and Related Pterdines',   North Holland Publishing Co. 1969.

2.   D.R. Phillips and A.J.A. Wright, <u>Brit. J. Nutr.</u>, 1983, <u>47</u> 183.

3.   J.E. Spring, J. Robertson, and D.H. Buss, <u>Brit. J. Nutr.</u>, 1979, <u>41</u> 487.

Increase In The Bioavailability of Vitamin A In The Rat By Dietary Lignin.

G. L. Catignani and K. H. Myers

Department of Food Science, Box 7624
North Carolina State University
Raleigh, North Carolina 27695   USA

Within the past several years, considerable effort has been directed toward the study of the physiological and pharmacological effects of various types of purified fiber or fractionated natural material enriched in fiber. Certain of these have been shown to lower serum cholesterol in man and experimental animals. One of the effects of dietary fiber on lipid metabolism centers around its interactions with bile acids, resulting in an increased loss of bile acids by fecal excretion and thus a decreased absorption of fats and fat soluble substances.

In vitro studies have confirmed the ability of certain dietary fibers to absorb bile acids(1). These studies prompted an investigation into determining whether this property of fiber was sufficient to affect the uptake of vitamin A, the absorption of which is influenced by the presence of bile.   Lignin and cellulose were chosen as test materials.   Both were readily available and represent the strongest and weakest affinity respectively for a variety of bile acids in vitro(1). In addition, cholestyramine was included as a positive control, known to lower vitamin A absorption via a bile sequestration mechanism.

Male weanling Sprague Dawley rats were used. Food and water were supplied ad libitum. Rats were maintained on AIN-76A semi-purified diet(2) for two weeks prior to each study. In initial experiments, rats were fed diets containing 10% cellulose, 10% lignin, 4% cholestyramine or a fiber-free diet. All test materials were of an equal particle range of 200-400 mesh. At the end of a four-week period of dietary modification, plasma and liver retinol concentration were determined(3). For absorption experiments, animals were fasted for 12 hr. Each group was then given 5 gm of their respective diets free of vitamin A. Within 1 hr the animals had consumed the diet. Each was then intubated intragastrically (i.g.) and administered 0.1 ml of corn oil containing 7 microgram of 14C retinyl acetate. Animals from each group were sacrificed at times 0,1,2,4,6,9,13 and 18 hr. Following saponification, retinol was determined as described above(3) with peak fractions being collected to measure radioactivity.

Weight gain, liver weight and food consumption did not differ significantly among the experimental treatments. Plasma and liver retinol values are shown in Table 1. Cholestyramine lowered the concentration of liver retinol as previously reported. The 10% lignin diet doubled the liver concentrations of retinol compared to the fiber-free or the 10% cellulose groups.

An increase in the efficiency of absorption could result in such findings. Therefore, the effect of dietary lignin on the absorption of vitamin A was determined.

The rate of absorption of total radioactivity and the specific activity of retinol were estimated by area under the curve calculation following an i.g. administered dose of 14C retinyl acetate. Total radioactivity per 18 hr (absorption 95% completed) was not significantly different nor were plasma retinol values (microgram/dL).

TABLE 1

Dietary Treatment	Retinol	
	Plasma microgram/dL	Liver microgram/g
Fiber Free	52.3±4.1	7.3±1.1
10% Lignin	46.1±2.2	14.8±1.4*
10% Cellulose	45.7±4.6	7.7±0.5
4% Cholestyramine	42.1±8.3	4.7±0.6*

*Significantly different from fiber free and 10% cellulose (P<0.01).

TABLE 2

Dietary Treatment	dpm/microgram retinol/18 hrs
Fiber free	11803 $\pm$ 2180
10% Lignin	19932 $\pm$ 2270*
10% Cellulose	13368 $\pm$ 2660

*Significantly different from the fiber free and 10% cellulose (P<0.05).

The specific activity of retinol (disintegration per minute per 18 hr) was calculated and the results are shown in Table 2.

These data demonstrate that the amount of radioactivity absorbed as unchanged (intact) retinol was approximately 50% to 70% greater in the lignin fed animals as compared to the other dietary treatments. Since the total absorbed radioactivity was not different among treatments, a larger proportion of the radioactivity must exist in compounds other than retinol in the fiber free and 10% cellulose fed rats. As previously reported, these data support the action of lignin as an antioxidant protecting the retinol from oxidative destruction during digestion and absorption (4). The results of this study demonstrate that the consumption of dietary lignin increased the efficiency of absorption of a single dose of vitamin A in the rat. Such nutrient-dietary component interactions are important, particularly when the dietary requirement for animals or humans is determined. This study suggests that the amount of dietary vitamin A might be reduced by as much as 50% of the amount currently considered adequate and still meet the needs of the organism when sufficient dietary lignin is included in the diet.

REFERENCES:

1. Story J.A. and D. Kritchevsky. 1976. J. Nutr. 106, 1292.
2. AIN Ad Hoc Committee on Standards for Nutritional Studies. 1977. J. Nutr. 107, 1340.
3. Catignani G.L. et al. 1983. Clin. Chem. 29, 708.
4. Catignani G.L. & M. E. Carter. 1982. J. Food Sci. 47, 1745.

The Workshop Reports

SPECIATION WORKSHOP: REPORT

Chairpersons: Dr. D. J. McWeeny; Dr. G. R. Moore

In the context of bioavailability, the speciation of an
element is the chemical form(s) in which it exists in the
lumen of the small intestine in the presence of the
products of digestion of food together with any substances
naturally present there, eg. gastric secretions.

The workshop addressed four questions:

1/   How are the levels of particular species, both
     in vivo and in vitro, best determined?

2/   What are the kinetic and thermodynamic stabilities
     of these species?

3/   Can physiological uptake and distribution patterns
     be predicted, given these levels and stabilities?

4/   What elements should first be addressed?

Advances in instrumentation over the last 5-10 years have
opened up possibilities for separating chemical species
at concentrations typical of those existing in food after
digestion.   A range of techniques now exist - including
a number of chromatographic separative techniques (GC,
HPLC, FPLC, SEC, ion-exchange) coupled to sensitive
detectors (AAS, ICP-MS).   By contrast, measurement of
certain species can be achieved by DPASV without prior
separation.   This latter electrochemical technique gives
a 'snapshot' estimate of its situation;   by contrast the
chromatographic procedures may allow extensive changes
to occur as the abundances of any species in equilibrium
with each other change in response to the separative
process.   Care must be taken to ensure that changes

during analytical procedures do not result in the formation
of artefacts or irrelevant species.

A major difference was noted in the views of the participants over the merit of in vitro analysis of foods. Some
felt that since the food would spend 2-3 hours in the
stomach at pH2-3 before passing into the gastrointestinal
tract, many of the chemicals would be degraded and the
metal-ligand adducts broken up. Thereafter, on passage
into the intestine at pH7-8, metal-ligand complexation
would take place with the resulting complexes bearing
little resemblance to those present in the food. Whilst
this general scheme was accepted by all participants some
felt that it was not necessarily true that most metal-
ligand adducts would be broken up by a relatively short
exposure to acid, haem being cited as an example. Also,
in vitro methods were defended on the grounds that supple-
menting foods with materials that made trace elements more
bioavailable required the chemical composition of the food
to be defined. Another point in their favour is the
relative ease of measurement compared to in vivo methods.
It was finally concluded that both approaches were needed.

The prediction of physiological uptake and distribution
patterns from analytical thermodynamic and kinetic data
was described by participants as "impossible" and "far
in the future". Even its strongest advocate declared
that once active uptake mechanisms and surface (eg.membranes)
phenomena were considered it was "a fantasy" to believe
modelling would provide good predictions in food systems -
although considerable success had been achieved in some
simpler environmental studies. Many people felt the work
should be encouraged, particularly in respect to toxic
elements.

Defining the priority areas was acknowledged by most to
be difficult, there being political and social considerations as well as nutritional ones. For example, priority
topics in Western Europe may be very different from those
in Africa. However, with regard to dietary composition
in Western Europe it was felt that zinc, iron, selenium
and possible iodine were the most important nutrient
elements; of the toxic elements cadmium, arsenic and
aluminium require attention.

ISOTOPE WORKSHOP: REPORT

Chairpersons: Dr. B. Sandstrom;   Dr. M. J. Jackson.

The aim of this workshop was to put into perspective
the current and future roles of isotopes in the study
of bioavailability.   Two major themes were discussed;
recent developments in experimental and analytical
techniques and the limitations and roles of isotopes.
Dr. Fairweather-Tait lead a discussion on the use of
dual isotopes in the study of mineral absorption.
Emphasis was placed in this discussion on the need to
undertake preliminary work to examine the plasma kinetics
of the isotope of choice and the need to carefully define
the quantity of isotope given intravenously so as not to
disturb normal physiological mechanisms.   Professor
Lonnerdal presented data on the relevance of extrinsic
isotopic labelling of foodstuffs, especially milk.
Recent data suggests that iron isotopes added to milk
may not exchange completely with the native iron and
therefore may not be a good technique for the study of
iron absorption from milk.   However, these problems do
not appear to occur with calcium, copper, zinc or
manganese.

The recent controversy in the U.S.A. concerning the
necessary time for which faecal sampling should be
continued following an oral isotopic zinc load was
discussed by Professor Hambidge.   He presented data
demonstrating that at more than 5-7 days post oral load
the majority of the isotope found in the faeces was
derived from re-excreted isotope rather than residual
non-absorbed material.   Dr. Mellon showed data comparing
the isotopic ratio values obtained by fast atom bombardment mass spectrometry (FAB), thermal ionisation mass
spectrometry (TIMS) and inductively-coupled plasma mass
spectrometry (ICPMS).   These were found to be in generally

good agreement although the FAB system gave results
about 2% different to TIMS.   Good precisions were
obtained by all systems (relative standard deviations:
FAB 0.5%, TIMS 0.5%, ICP with continuous nebulisation 0.3%
and with flow injection 4.8%).

In the second part of the workshop Professor Greger
pointed out the potential problems with isotopic techniques
(particularly stable isotopes).   She stressed that in
many isotopic studies the cost/benefit ratio was too high,
that the added sensitivity obtained from use of the isotope
was of questionable value in the light of normal biological
variation and that in many studies the sensitivity gained
by the use of isotopes is lost during sample collection
and preparation.   Dr. Sandstrom compared the relative
benefits of radioactive and stable isotopes with particular reference to the magnitude of the dose received by
subjects during studies involving radioactive isotopes.
It was shown that providing a sensitive whole-body counter
is used the dose involved in a single meal absorption
study was roughly equivalent to that received during a
trans-Atlantic flight or a normal dental X-ray.

Many members of the audience contributed to the discussion
at this workshop and it was generally felt to have been
a worthwhile forum for exchange of ideas and experiences.

REFERENCE MATERIALS WORKSHOP: REPORT

Chairpersons: Dr. G. V. Iyengar;   Dr. P. J. Wagstaffe

Dr. Iyengar introduced the workshop and proposed that
six participants give a ten minute overview of their
particular expertise relative to RM. Their reports are
summarised as follows:

Dr. Iyengar discussed the concept of multi-purpose
biological and dietary RMs, giving particular attention
to the development of a total human mixed diet.   This
would be characterised for a range of commonly determined
inorganics, proximates and organic constituents (mainly
nutrients); of special interest were vitamins and
cholesterol. A brief report was given on an ongoing and,
so far successful, study of the stability of vitamins in
both fresh and freeze dried material.

Dr. Wagstaffe gave an overview of BCR RM activities for
nutritional analyses. Ten CRMs were available covering
22 elements and 140 reference values for inorganics.
In addition three edible oil/fat RMs were available for
fatty acids, sterols and other relevant properties.
Five simple food RMs (rye and plain flour, haricot beans,
milk powder and pork muscle) will be characterised with
respect to proximates, amino-acids, vitamins, fatty acids
and, if possible, fibre. Dr. Wagstaffe took the occasion
to invite proposals to the Community Bureau of Reference
for further projects.

Dr. Parr summarised the biological RMs available from the
IAEA mentioning especially H9, a mixed diet material, all
these being characterised for inorganics only. He reported
on the preparation of a document designed to give guidance
on the proper use of CRMs and drew attention to an International Atomic Energy Agency report which listed all

available biological RMs characterised for inorganics
from the main products.

Mr. R. Alvarez supplemented his earlier lecture with a
number of remarks.   Of particular interest were the total
mixed diet for inorganics, proximates and organics;
cholesterol in egg-powder;   renewal of the oyster-tissue
material;   cod liver oil for α-tocopherol (determined by
normal and reversed-phase HPLC) PCVs, PHHs and bovine-
serum for 12 elements.   In addition several agricultural
materials were being prepared in a joint project between
Agriculture Canada and the National Bureau of Standards.

Professor Southgate focussed on the importance of RMs
in validating nutrient data used for food composition
tables and added that CRMs could be very helpful to third
world countries.   Citing the very poor results obtained
for ash in collaborative studies, he stressed the needs
for quality assurance (QA) even for apparently simple
properties such as total fat, protein etc. Detailed
information on carbohydrate (individual sugars, starch
components etc.) were very important.   There were
particular needs for labelling (eg fatty acids) and he
considered that data to be published should show evidence
of validation with RMs.

Professor Ashmead expressed the needs of a researcher in
the field of bioavailability.   He doubted the usefulness
of RDA values without an insight into the chemical form
of the element.   For example, the RDA for iron could
appear to be met by a food which in fact had very low
bioavailability.   He noted that because of food processing
the RDAs for several nutrients, notably copper, zinc,
calcium and some vitamins were not met for some population
groups in the USA.

The meeting was then opened to general discussion, the
conclusions of which are briefly summarised as follows:

1/   It is more important to characterise factors which
inhibit or enhance bioavailability (amino acid, phytate,
ascorbic acid, fibre etc.) in a RM than the actual chemical
species of that element;   that is, in general the element
will be transformed in the intestine regardless of its
original form.   Important exceptions include haeme/
non-haeme iron, methylmercury and arsenobetaine.

2/   In general researchers in this area seem to be
largely unaware of the availability and importance of
RMs in the validation of their measurement.   In extreme

cases this can totally invalidate their work.

3/ Steps should be taken to ensure that researchers are aware of the availability of RMs.

4/ Researchers should let RM producers know of the shortcomings of available RMs and of their particular needs.

5/ RMs should always be incorporated in the experimental design. The preparation of "in house" RMs characterised by means of certified RMs should be encouraged.

IRON METHODOLOGY WORKSHOP: REPORT

Chairperson: Dr. C. Mills

The significance of iron-related disorders in man was
considered briefly in relation to other nutritional
problems.   Suggestions are that iron deficiency diseases
rank closely after protein/energy malnutrition and iodine
deficiency disorders in order of importance.   However
the proportion of the former that is related to dietary
practices involving consumption of poorly available
sources of iron is not clearly defined.   Despite this,
a recent World Health Organisation Experts Group on vitamin and mineral requirements identified as important
research priorities the need to assess dietary iron
availability and its variability in individual subjects.

The workshop recognised the need for improved precision
and accuracy in the conduct of bioavailability studies
with human subjects.   Assessments of bioavailability are
essential in attempts to define iron economy during
studies of iron requirements.   For such purposes there
is a particular need to standardise conditions of measurement and to identify those features in the dietary sources
of iron which govern iron availability and those physiological variables which influence responses during such
studies.   The importance of defining the existing iron
status of subjects used in such studies was universally
agreed.   However, there was debate about the relevance
of currently-used indices for the depletion or saturation
of specific pools and whether, for example, the inverse
relationship frequently claimed between plasma ferritin
and the fractional efficiency of iron absorption was
continuous (linear) or discontinuous.

Other evidence suggested that further validation of
criteria of iron status in infants was needed to

facilitate additional iron availability studies with such
subjects. Discussion of the origins of variability in
isotopic measurements of iron absorption within single
subjects over short intervals of time suggested that
'memory' effects reflection iron absorption from immediately previous meals were a significant cause of such variability. The practice of starving subjects for 24 hours
before such tests was recommended by one participant but
the merits and limitations of this were not discussed.

After reaching general agreement on the importance of
greater standardisation of the conditions for in vivo
testing, the merits and limitations of in vitro and
in vivo testing were considered. In vitro methods have
the advantage of rapidity but the disadvantages introduced
by arbitrary decisions such as:

> (i)   the selection of complexing agents of
>   appropriate affinity for iron in methods
>   for the determination of 'ionic' iron;
>
> (ii) the composition of the medium used in enzymic
>   methods simulating gastric and duodenal
>   digestion, and
>
> (iii) the cut off (eg. 6-8k Dalton) in membranes
>   employed for 'dialysable' iron studies.

Typical of the general conclusions derived from a
comparison of data derived from in vitro and in vivo
availability studies was evidence that the stability of
the iron complex rather than complex size per se was an
important determinant of stability.

A fact strongly emphasised by several contributors was
that, despite their limitations, many in vivo techniques
produced useful information on the likely physico-chemical
characteristics of iron sources differing in bioavailability. During a discussion of 'valency shifts'
influencing iron absorption disquiet was expressed that
the influence of variation of gut redox potential on iron
availability was not more extensively studied in view of
the effects of ascorbate on this variable.

In vitro techniques may well have particular value for the
rapid screening of foods with extremes of iron availability.
In general insufficient attention was given to the importance of conducting concurrent studies with human subjects.

Although rankings of iron availability for a series of
foods derived from rat studies may well be broadly similar
to those derived from human studies, the efficiencies of

of absorption tended to be markedly higher in rats.   The
origins of this phenomenon were not known, nor were they
currently being studied.   Other differences included the
apparently greater susceptibility of man to inhibition of
iron absorption by phytate.   Again there were apparently
no investigations planned to elucidate this difference.

Emphasis was given to the fact that while the value of
iron for fortification could be reasonably assessed by
haemoglobin repletion, extrinsic isotopic tagging was
inappropriate for such purposes.

There was no evidence to suggest that more effective
potentiators of iron absorption than ascorbate remained
to be discovered.   The suggested role of peptidyl
cysteine in the 'meat enhancement' of iron absorption
was considered to require confirmation.

The influence of supranormal calcium intakes of the
postmenopausal woman on vegan diets may merit greater
emphasis in future studies of iron availability.
Insufficient attention has been given to the action of
iron absorption when dietary iron intake is high.

FIBRE AND PHYTATE, EFFECT ON MINERAL BIOAVAILABILITY
WORKSHOP: REPORT

Chairpersons: Dr. A.E.Harmuth-Hoene;   Dr. N. G. Asp

During the last 15-20 years phytic acid (PA), and possibly
also dietary fibre (DF) itself have been shown to reduce
the bioavailability (BA) of minerals and trace elements.
In foods containing both PA and DF, it is well documented
that PA is the main factor responsible for inhibition,
due to the formation of insoluble mineral complexes.
In vitro binding studies, as well as animal experiments
and some human studies on ileostomy subjects, indicate
that DF polysaccharides with a high content of uronic
acid residues - especially pectin - have the capacity
of binding cations.   It was agreed, however, that there
is no data indicating that DF in mixed diets may lead to
mineral deficiencies.   It was also stressed that an
increased intake of foods rich in DF usually implies a
simultaneously increased mineral intake. DF supplements,
on the other hand, are usually depleted of minerals.

Major progress is being made in the understanding of how
variously degraded PA, i.e. penta- to triphosphates of
inositol, will affect mineral availability.   New
analytical methods have been developed to differentiate
between these compounds.   Such methods should be used
whenever possible instead of the less specific iron
precipitation or phosphate determination methods,
especially when studying the influence of food processing
aiming at reducing PA.

Many factors in foods modify the inhibitory effect of PA
and possible DF.   These include amino acids and peptides
(ligands), ascorbic acid (antioxidant), other minerals -
particularly calcium (increased stability of phytate/
mineral complexes) and other inhibitory compounds such
as polyphenols.   Other discussions centred on whether

381

minerals liberated from ligands in the colon could be absorbed.   The importance of such a mechanism is not well documented in man.

The following points were considered especially important in future studies of bioavailability:

1)   To standardize and define as far as possible both methods of PA and DF analysis, as well as the experimental model.

2)   Dietary composition in relation to levels of the mineral under study.

3)   Length of the study in relation to adaptive mechanisms.

4)   The assessment of the mineral status of the experimental subjects or animals.

It was suggested that the problems in defining DF would be best solved by abandoning this term.

INTERACTIONS WORKSHOP: REPORT

Chairperson: Dr. D. T. Gordon.

The bioavailability of any nutrient is affected by both
intrinsic and extrinsic factors.   Intrinsic factors are
those internal to the animal or human and include sex,
age, nutritional and health status.   Components of the
diet are thus classified as extrinsic factors.   The action
of these extrinsic factors on nutrient bioavailability
can also be envisaged as interactions among dietary
components and nutrients.

Interactions among nutrients which affect bioavailability
may be classified as competitive, non-competitive or
multi-nutrient.   Competitive interactions, or one-way
interactions, are negative, mutual and are a consequence
of the similarity in chemical and physical nature of the
nutrient.   The interaction between Zn and Cu exemplifies
competitive interaction.   Low dietary copper concentration
will impair iron nutriture and represents a one-way positive, non-competitive interaction.   Multinutrient interactions have only recently begun to be addressed and
comprise a complex set of variables represented as a set
or chain of reactions being the result of alterations in
the dietary concentrations of more than 2 nutrients.

To adequately understand and determine the bioavailability
of a nutrient, an investigator must appreciate the importance of interactions among and between intrinsic and
extrinsic factors.   The first step that such an investigator must take after deciding upon an interaction study
is to seek the advice of a statistician in developing a
proper experimental design.   Prior to administering the
test materials, the nutritional status of the animal model
or human subjects should be known.   In addition to knowing the accurate nutritional status of the host and the

nutrient concentration in the diet, it is important to
know the ratio of nutrients that are varied. This is
especially important if more than 2 concentrations of a
nutrient are to be evaluated.

The method by which the nutrients are to be administered
to the test animal or human subject, must be considered.
Results may vary, depending upon how the nutrients are
provided, for example ad libitum in the diet, in a simple
meal or by gavage in solution.

Appropriate consideration must also be given to the animal
model used so that results are obtained which can ultimately be related to the human.   For this reason the use of
the rat model in interaction studies may not always be
appropriate;   rather the use of food production animals
such as the pig is recommended.   There is a wealth of
nutritional information available on this animal model.

In the area of mineral interactions, it is important to
consider the total levels of dietary cations and anions.
As the concentration of various minerals used specifically
as their salts, may be increased to achieve the desired
concentration of one or more specific cations, an investigator has the option of providing anions as the chloride,
sulphate, phosphate, oxide or carbonate.   The two anions,
oxide or carbonate, will not affect the net urinary
excretion of anions as compared to chloride, phosphate or
sulphate.

The fortification of foods and the supplementation of
diets with added nutrients offer the most important
justification for continued studies on interactions and
investigations into the way in which these interactions
among nutrients affect their bioavailability.

ENERGY AND COMPLEX CARBOHYDRATES WORKSHOP: REPORT

Chairperson: Dr. G. Livesey

The workshop examined the difficulties of assessing both
the availability of carbohydrates in vivo and the energy
value of the unavailable carbohydrates, and sought
suggestions for improved methodology and scientific
understanding.   The term unavailable carbohydrate (UC)
was used;   dietary fibre was omitted from the vocabulary
of the workshop because of debate about whether resistant
starch should be classified as fibre – a problem of
policy not of science.

Two approaches to the assessment of energy value were
recognised.   Chemical balance experiments gave apparent,
and energy balance experiments gave partial digestible
and metabolizable energy values.   The partial values
were recommended for use when calculating the energy value
of whole diets because it accounts for interactions
between UC and other energy sources.

Losses of protein and fat to faeces with increased UC
intake explained the difference between partial and
apparent energy values.   Available data showed that for
mixed meals the sum of these additional losses was higher
for UC which showed least fermentation!   Hence these
losses did not seem to be explained by additional loss of
bacterial protein and fat which would be expected with the
fermentation of UC.   The observation for mixed meals
seemed not to apply to isolates.   The insoluble, least
fermentable UC gave least additional losses of energy in
protein and fat when compared with soluble viscous
polymers.   Soluble polymers (e.g. polydextrose) and
sugar alcohols (e.g. palatinit) gave rise to little additional loss of fat but did increase nitrogen losses.
Hence it seemed that these fermentations gave faecal

bacteria without much additional fat.   This was further
evidence that the losses of fat due to UC in mixed meals
was not bacterial lipid.

With palatinit, only 3.5% of the energy utilized could be
recovered as H_2 and CH_4.   A similar observation was made
for UC in mixed meals.   This was much less than the 22%
expected in ruminants.   Some in vitro data was consistent
with lactic acid production, otherwise anaerobic conditions required that reducing equivalents be produced in
the large bowel.   It was recommended that studies be
undertaken to assess the pathways of hydrogen utilization
in the human colon.   The implication of the observation,
that gaseous energy was not a large loss in man, was
advantageous.

Fermentation is associated with increased bacterial
biomass in the faeces.   It was recommended that the cost
of their synthesis be accounted for when calculating
physiological fuel values.   The exact cost remained to
be debated.

Losses of energy to faeces were related to the fermentability of the UC.   Cross linkages in non-starch polysaccharides (NSP) and gelatinization and retrogradation
of starches were major factors affecting their degrada-
bility.   Processing affected both carbohydrates, and
caused some depolymerization of the starch.   Appropriate
methods needed development for characterising the NSP
and starches in foods as eaten, for use in the experimental
feeding studies.   It was suggested that knowledge of the
food source and treatment, sugar composition of the NSP
and lignin content would help prediction of fermentability.
Fluorescence microscopy for examination of phenolics may
be possible.   When lignin content was low a sequential
extraction (hot water, oxalate, 1M KOH, 4M KOH) with
sugar analysis may be useful in determining the strength
of binding of the pectins and hemicelluloses.   Alternatively fermentability might be examined directly with
bacteria in vitro.

A problem arose when analysing resistant starches in
uncooked foods since the procedure may involve effectively
cooking the starch to solubilize it prior to analysis.
Cooking of meat may also give rise to products which
analyse as AOAC total dietary fibre.   Resistant starch
produced by heat treatment had a high energy value
relative to the value for UC.   The AOAC method of total
fibre determination was therefore not recommended as
appropriate for assessing food energy values and gives

rise to an underestimate of total dietary energy value.

The use of breath hydrogen tests to assess carbohydrate availability was recommended as useful for subject groups needing about 10 subjects, but H_2 responses were too variable to make it applicable to individuals. Suggestions for improvement included use of hydrogen-labelled carbohydrates as an internal marker of individual variation, use of whole-body H_2 collection (not just breath), and use of 24h collections to decrease the variance.

Many participants felt that more time for discussion would be valuable and perhaps the subject deserved a separate symposium.

PROTEIN AND AMINO ACID WORKSHOP: REPORT

Chairpersons: Dr. L. Savoie;   Dr. A. Kerat

The existence of a close relationship between the
biological value of proteins and the pattern of their
constituent amino acids has been mainly derived from
knowledge of the limiting factors.   However, physio-
chemical characteristics of the food proteins vary
considerably due to their different origins, mode of
preparation and the presence of other food constituents.
This affects their behaviour during the complex physiological process of digestion and absorption.   Their
further utilization, mainly but not exclusively for
protein synthesis, will then depend upon the synchronous
supply to specialized tissues.

It should therefore be most proper to define amino acid
availability as "the proportion of amino acids in a food
or a diet that is digested and absorbed in a form and at
a time suitable for various biological uses".

It is necessary to "sharpen" the tools used to estimate
properly the amount, nature and chronology of amino acids
absorbed.   The effects of time on the utilization of
nutrients by the tissues could then be derived according
to the various targets.   This will vary between animal
species, as gut length affects the duration of transit
and absorption, and the feeding habits (meal eater or
nibbler) affect the time interval between meals.

An in vivo technique capable of measuring qualitatively
and quantitatively the kinetics and pattern of appearance
of amino acids in the portal venous blood should serve
as a reference method.   Patterns of blood amino acids
considered optimal for various and specific physiological
needs should then be defined.

<u>In vitro</u> methods are needed to mimic the various steps of protein digestion and absorption and to measure the hydrolysis rates and the nature of hydrolysis products. Correlation studies with the reference method will then point out the exact <u>in vitro</u> technique needed for a practical day to day analysis, more rapid and less expensive, adapted to a specific purpose of protein utilisation.

VITAMINS WORKSHOP: REPORT

Chairperson: Dr. C. Bates

The following practical questions were raised concerning
the importance of bioavailability measurements on
vitamins in human diets:

   a) do the food composition tables require
      adjustment (e.g. revision, new format)?;

   b) how should diet and survey data be interpreted,
      in the light of bioavailability information?;

   c) how should food labelling be tackled, to take
      account of limited bioavailability?;

   d) what are the implications for the Recommended
      Dietary Amounts (RDAs) of vitamins?

The limitations of food table data were briefly discussed:
it is clearly mistaken to consider that the tables contain
'definitive' values, because of imperfect assay methods
and the wide variations between samples, e.g. of variety,
season, processing, storage, cooking-damage, etc. The
poor correlation observed between estimated individual
intakes of nutrients, and the biochemical or clinical
indices of status was discussed. Clearly the food table
approach has considerable value if cautiously applied,
but improvements are needed, and these ought to be defined.

The issue of recommended dietary amounts was raised: one
illustration of an approach from Germany was the definition
of an "RDI" (recommended dietary intake of total vitamin)
together with an "RBA" (recommended bioavailability factor,
ranging from 0 to 1) which, when multiplied together give
the "RDA" for the absorbed vitamin. Clearly, in practice
the RDA's do take bioavailability into account, and they
generally refer to the requirement for vitamins present

in real foods and diets, even though some of the
available evidence about minimum requirements is based
on data from forms of vitamins which do occur in food
(e.g. pteroylmonoglutamate), or which are not given with
food (tablet supplements).

The problem of active <u>versus</u> less-active forms, and
precursors, of vitamins was illustrated by the problem
of β-carotene isomers. Processing methods can produce
considerable isomerisation to 9-<u>cis</u> and 13-<u>cis</u> isomers
having only 40-50% of vitamin A precursor activity of
native β-carotene. Vitamin A itself can undergo similar
isomerisation. In view of the potential importance of
carotenoids, not only as precursors of vitamin A, but
also as free radical quenchers, there clearly is a need
to develop new techniques, both of measuring the
carotenoid isomers (including development of suitable
bioassays) and of interpreting the nutritional significance of changes which can occur during food processing,
or in the development of new foods. The need for non-
biological analytical techniques for vitamin bioavailability, where possible, was discussed as a general
concept.

Another topic of practical importance is the development
of vitamin derivatives with altered physical properties:
e.g. lipid solubility for water-soluble vitamins, which
may assist absorption. This was illustrated for thiamine,
for which Japanese manufacturers have produced several
derivatives, including thiamine propyldisulphide, which
are very effective in the treatment of thiamine deficiency,
for example, as caused by alcoholism. Derivatives of
vitamin B_{12}, absorbable by sufferers from pernicious
anaemia (P.A.) would likewise be welcomed, and the danger
of late recognition of P.A., when neuropathy is not
accompanied by megaloblastosis, was stressed.

Vitamin toxicity is a growing problem, and now includes
vitamin B_6 as well as vitamins A and D. Here, too,
bioavailability is important: the limited conversion
of carotenoids to vitamin A apparently prevents toxicity,
and likewise the limited conversion of cholesterol to
vitamin D by sunlight on the skin avoids the problem of
dietary vitamin D toxicity.

Clearly the original questions raised were only partly
answered and the discussions centred on some others which
relate to bioavailability of vitamins. New investigative
techniques, based on interdisciplinary research efforts,
may assist future progress.

WORKSHOP CONVENOR'S FINAL REMARKS

Convenor: Dr. A. E. Harmuth-Hoene

During the workshop sessions some questions and ideas of
a more general nature have emerged:

1)   How can we apply present and future knowledge of
      nutrient bioavailability to current food
      compositions tables?

This should be the final goal of current efforts to get
a better understanding of nutrient bioavailability. The
idea is to indicate those food items which will inhibit
or enhance the availability of certain nutrients. It
will be a slow, step-wise process with the aim to make
the consumer aware of the importance of bioavailability of
nutrients. There is much need to co-operate with food
producers and technologists, calling their attention to
possible changes in nutrient bioavailability during food
processing, especially when new methods or novel foods
are introduced.

2)   What is the relevance of decreased nutrient
      bioavailability to various population groups?

There is no general answer to this fundamental question.
One has to differentiate not only with respect to each
nutrient but also to the various population groups and
even sub-groups. In the case of carbohydrates and fats
we aim at reducing bioavailability by substituting
dietary fibre and non-absorbable fats. The consequences
of reduced bioavailability of vitamins and minerals
depend on dietary habits, nutritional status and nutrient
requirements of the individual. Thus the inhibitory
action of phytate and possibly dietary fibre on essential
minerals and trace elements will have no adverse effect
on people on a well balanced diet containing animal and

392

plant food with an ample supply of all essential nutrients. In the case of infants, pregnant or lactating women, or adolescents, or people on a strictly vegan diet (no eggs or milk) reduced bioavailability may lead to deficiency.

3)   One question that has been asked frequently concerns the ability of the living organism to protect itself - within certain limits - by adaptation against an insufficient supply of nutrients.

We know very little about adaptive mechanisms. More investigations should aim at elucidating homeostatic control instead of merely describing it.

4)   Have the workshop sessions been helpful to get a better understanding of the various aspects of bioavailability?

It was felt that there was not enough time to cover the various topics, because participation of the audience was quite active. Unfortunately there was too much over-lapping of the various workshop sessions. Three or four parallel sessions would have been optimal.

There was some disagreement as to whether the scope of a workshop should be to increase knowledge or to exchange experiences and opinions among equals. It was agreed that the organizers of the Conference had given the chairpersons very valuable and constructive support.

5)   What should we aim at in future work?

There is much need for standardization of analytical methods, which are basic for the assessment of bioavail-ability. More use of standard reference material from the European Community Bureau of Reference or the U.S. National Bureau of Standards should be made for cali-bration of methods. The need for standardization applies also to methods for bioassays which should enable us to obtain more meaningful and comparable data. The develop-ment of in vitro methods simulating in vivo conditions, which can be used as screening tests, is another promising step forward.

Bringing together chemists, food chemists, and nutrition-ists at this Conference was appreciated as very helpful and should be continued at future Conferences. Contacts to relevant international societies should be activated for more co-operation between various disciplines involved in problems of bioavailability.

Subject Index